D1703608

Text Atlas of Lymphomas

Text Atlas of Lymphomas

James O Armitage, MD
Professor and Chairman
Department of Internal Medicine
University of Nebraska Medical Center
Omaha, NE, USA

Franco Cavalli, MD, FRCP
Professor and Director
Department of Oncology
Ospedale San Giovanni
Bellinzona, Switzerland

Dan L Longo, MD, FACP
Scientific Director
National Institute on Aging
National Institutes of Health
Baltimore, MD, USA

Illustrations provided by

Judith A Ferry, MD
Associate Professor of Pathology
Massachusetts General Hospital
Boston, MA, USA

MARTIN DUNITZ

© Martin Dunitz Ltd 1999

First published in the United Kingdom in 1999 by
Martin Dunitz Ltd
The Livery House
7–9 Pratt Street
London NW1 0AE

All rights reserved. No part of this publication may be reproduced, stored in a retrieval system, or transmitted in any form or by any means, electronic, mechanical, photocopying, recording or otherwise, without the prior permission of the publisher or in accordance with the provisions of the Copyright Act 1988, or under the terms of any licence permitting limited copying issued by the Copyright Licensing Agency, 90 Tottenham Court Road, London, W1P 9HE.

A CIP catalogue record for this book is available from the British Library

ISBN 1-85317-705-9

Distributed in the United States by:
Blackwell Science Inc.
Commerce Place, 350 Main Street
Malden, MA 02148, USA
Tel: 1–800–215–1000

Distributed in Canada by:
Login Brothers Book Company
324 Salteaux Crescent
Winnipeg, Manitoba, R3J 3T2
Canada
Tel: 204–224–4068

Distributed in Brazil by:
Ernesto Reichmann Distribuidora de Livros, Ltda
Rua Coronel Marques 335, Tatuape 03440–000
Sao Paulo
Brazil

A 35 mm colour slide collection, based on 200 images from this Atlas, is also available.
ISBN 1-85317-838-1

Also available from Martin Dunitz Publishers
Textbook of Malignant Haematology; ed Degos, Linch, Löwenberg. ISBN 1-85317-322-3.
CD-ROM Atlas of Haematology; Cohen, Cycowitz, Djaldetti, Polliack. ISBN 1-85317-660-5.
An Atlas of Malignant Haematology; Mufti, Flandrin, Sandberg, Schaefer, Kanfer. ISBN 1-85317-054-2.

Composition by Scribe Design, Gillingham, Kent
Manufactured in Singapore by Imago

Contents

	Preface	vii
1.	Introduction and background	1
2.	Diffuse large B-cell lymphoma	5
3.	Follicular lymphoma	13
4.	Peripheral T-cell lymphomas	29
5.	Small lymphocytic lymphoma/Chronic lymphocytic leukemia	45
6.	Mantle-cell lymphoma	61
7.	MALT lymphoma (extranodal marginal-zone B-cell lymphoma)	69
8.	Burkitt's lymphoma/leukemia	83
9.	Anaplastic large T/null cell lymphoma	91
10.	Primary mediastinal large B-cell lymphoma	99
11.	Lymphoblastic leukemia/lymphoma	105
12.	Lymphoplasmacytic lymphoma	117
13.	Nodal and splenic marginal-zone B-cell lymphomas	123
14.	Lymphomas involving extranodal sites	133
15.	Hodgkin's disease	153
16.	Rare subtypes	177
17.	Summary	197
	Index	201

Preface

Our understanding of the 'solid' tumors of the immune system, namely, Hodgkin's disease and the non-Hodgkin's lymphomas, continues to evolve. These tumors have provided insights into tumor biology and therapy that have been widely applied in other malignancies. However, there is still considerable room for improvement in our ability to help patients afflicted by the lymphomas.

Over the past decade, a number of investigations into the immunology, genetics and etiology of non-Hodgkin's lymphoma have resulted in the identification of new subtypes. These entities, including mantle-cell lymphoma, anaplastic large-cell lymphoma, and MALT lymphoma, are clinically as well as histopathologically distinct. Their recognition provided the stimulus for a new classification of non-Hodgkin's lymphoma. This classification, termed the Revised European American Lymphoma (REAL) classification, divided non-Hodgkin's lymphomas into clinical/pathological entities (i.e. real diseases!), rather than simply morphological groupings. A recent test of the clinical applicability of the REAL classification showed it to be highly reproducible and clinically relevant.

This volume is meant to provide a guide to understanding the REAL classification. It provides the clinical characteristics, survival data and histological appearance of the major lymphoma subtypes. The ability to use this lymphoma classification will be key to providing optimal patient care for the foreseeable future.

The editors wish to acknowledge the major contribution of Dr Emanuele Zucca, Bellinzona, in the preparation of the book; and sincere thanks are also due to Alison Campbell and Martin Dunitz of the publishers.

JOA, FC, DLL

1 Introduction and background

The history of lymphoma classification

The distinction between Hodgkin's disease and non-Hodgkin's lymphoma became practical with the description of the Reed–Sternberg cell early in the 20th century. Since that time, the terminology to describe the non-Hodgkin's lymphomas has changed frequently and has often been confusing. The terms 'lymphosarcoma' and 'reticulum cell sarcoma' were developed to describe different types of non-Hodgkin's lymphoma. The description of follicular lymphoma by Brill et al and by Symmers set the stage for the first 'modern' lymphoma classification. This was proposed by Gall and Mallory, and divided non-Hodgkin's lymphomas into lymphosarcoma, reticulum cell sarcoma and giant follicular lymphoma.

In the 1950s, Henry Rappaport first proposed the lymphoma classification for which he remains well known. This classification divided lymphomas based on the pattern of cell growth and the size and shape of the tumor cells. It was shown to predict treatment outcome in a way that made it clinically useful. Unfortunately, the terminology in the Rappaport classification quickly became outdated when it became apparent that all non-Hodgkin's lymphomas were tumors of lymphocytes and that lymphocytes could be divided into those of T-cell origin and those of B-cell origin. The common large cell lymphoma with a diffuse growth pattern was termed 'diffuse histiocytic lymphoma' in the Rappaport classification.

Application of new understanding of the biology of the immune system led to new classifications. In the USA, Lukes and Collins proposed such a classification, and a similar system (the Kiel classification) was proposed by Lennert and colleagues in Europe. The Kiel classification became widely used and has remained popular up to the present time. For the first time, it defined lymphomas as being of low grade or high grade.

The use of widely different lymphoma classifications in different parts of the world hindered clinical research and clinical care. Because of this, an attempt was made by physicians from the US National Cancer Institute to reach a consensus system. This led to the development of the Working Formulation, which was not meant to be a classification per se but rather a means of translation between existing classifications. However, the Working Formulation became the most widely used system for classifying lymphomas in North America, while the Kiel classification remained popular in Europe. Since the development of the Working Formulation in the 1970s, new insights into the biology of the immune system have continued to be obtained. In particular, these include the identification of specific antigens associated with certain subsets of lymphocytes and their corresponding lymphomas, and the recognition of specific genetic abnormalities in certain subtypes of lymphoma. In several circumstances, these observations made it possible to recognize new subtypes of lymphoma that had not been widely accepted on purely morphological grounds. For example, the recognition of the t(11;14) and the resultant overexpression of the *BCL1* oncogene confirmed the existence of mantle-cell lymphoma. The discovery of the Ki-1 or CD30 antigen and the subsequent discovery of the t(2;5) cytogenetic abnormality that leads to overproduction of the ALK protein led to wide acceptance of anaplastic large T/null cell lymphoma as a specific entity.

In the 1990s, a group of hematopathologists from around the world proposed a new system of lymphoma classification that included the newly recognized entities. These pathologists, who referred to themselves as the International Lymphoma Study Group, proposed that specific lymphoma entities should be recognized on the basis of a combination of morphological and clinical characteristics. This is a major change from the purely morphological classifications of the past. For example, recognition of the entity of mediastinal diffuse large B-cell lymphoma requires knowledge of the existence of a large mediastinal mass. That tumor, morphologically, represents an otherwise typical diffuse large B-cell lymphoma. When this entity is recognized separately, the patients are found to be younger than those with other aggressive non-Hodgkin's lymphomas and have an unusual female predominance.

This new classification has been termed the Revised European American Lymphoma (REAL) classification (Table 1.1), and will form the basis of a new World Health Organization classification for lymphomas.

Clinical applications

Non-Hodgkin's lymphomas were almost uniformly fatal diseases early in the 20th century. The use of radiotherapy produced long survival on some rare occasions. However, the use of combination chemotherapy regimens in the early 1970s led to the recognition that some patients with diffuse large cell lymphoma could be cured, even when widespread disease was present. The development of an increasing number of chemotherapeutic agents and biologic therapies such as interferon and antibodies (with or without radiolabels) increases the importance of accurate lymphoma diagnosis. All the subgroups of non-Hodgkin's lymphoma do not respond equally to the same therapy.

Even in any particular, distinctive subgroup, all patients do not respond equally to a particular

---

Table 1.1
The REAL classification of non-Hodgkin's lymphomas[a]

B-cell lymphomas

Precursor B-cell lymphomas:
- B-lymphoblastic

Mature B-cell lymphomas:
- B-cell CLL/small lymphocytic
- Follicular
- Marginal-zone–nodal
- Extranodal marginal-zone (MALT)
- Splenic marginal-zone
- Lymphoplasmacytic
- Mantle-cell
- Diffuse large B-cell
- Primary mediastinal large B-cell
- Burkitt-like
- Burkitt's

T-cell lymphomas

Precursor T-cell lymphomas:
- T-lymphoblastic

Mature T-cell lymphomas:
- Mycosis fungoides/Sézary syndrome
- Peripheral T-cell (many subtypes)
- Anaplastic large T/null cell
- Adult T-cell leukemia/lymphoma

[a]Harris NL, Jaffe ES, Stein H et al, A revised European–American classification of lymphoid neoplasms: a proposal from the International Lymphoma Study Group. *Blood* 1994; **84**: 1361–92.

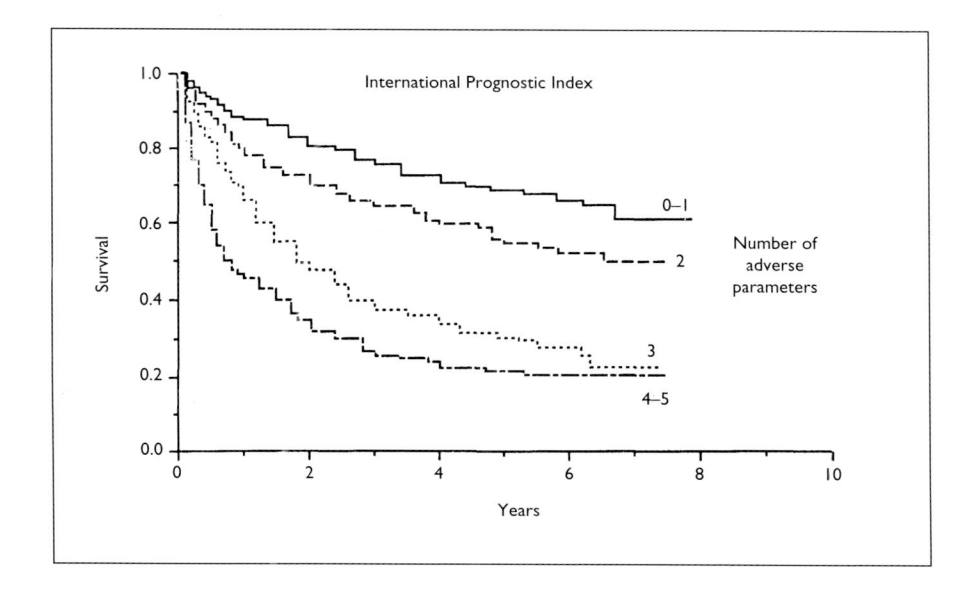

Figure 1.1
Overall survival with all types of non-Hodgkin's lymphoma grouped together by International Prognostic Index Score: 1254 lymphoma patients included in the ILSG Trial.

Table 1.2
The International Prognostic Index[a]

Factor	Adverse prognosis
Age	≥60 years
Ann Arbor stage	III or IV
Serum LDH	Above normal
Number of extranodal sites of involvement	≥2
Performance status	≥ECOG 2 or equivalent

[a]International Non-Hodgkin's Lymphoma Prognostic Factors Project, A predictive model for aggressive non-Hodgkin's lymphoma. *N Engl J Med* 1993; **329**: 987–94.

therapy. The best way to predict treatment outcome in a uniform group of patients is using the International Prognostic Index (Table 1.2). By simply summing the number of adverse characteristics, it is possible to divide patients into clinically relevant subgroups. As shown in Figure 1.1, this information divides non-Hodgkin's lymphomas of all subgroups into clinically relevant groups. However, the best distinction is when a particular subtype of non-Hodgkin's lymphoma as recognized in the REAL classification is subdivided based on the prognostic characteristics of the patients. Therapeutic decisions should currently be based on these two factors.

The following chapters illustrate the important characteristics of the major subtypes of non-Hodgkin's lymphoma recognized in the REAL classification. The order of the chapters is not entirely arbitrary. The non-Hodgkin's lymphomas (and lymphoid leukemias) are discussed in roughly their order of frequency. In addition, chapters are included on extranodal lymphomas, Hodgkin's disease and rare entities, some of which are not specifically included in the new classification schemes, but may nevertheless occasionally be diagnosed. We do not discuss plasma-cell disorders. The relevant histological, biological and clinical characteristics are presented, along with characteristic photomicrographs. This information should be used routinely by clinicians in the care of patients with non-Hodgkin's lymphoma.

Bibliography

Athan E, Foitl D, Knowles D, Bcl-1 rearrangement: frequency and clinical significance among B cell chronic lymphocytic leukemias and non-Hodgkin's lymphomas. *Am J Pathol* 1991; **138**: 591–9.

Brill NE, Baehr G et al, Generalized giant follicle hyperplasia of lymph nodes and spleen: a hitherto undiagnosed type. *J Am Med Assoc* 1925; **84**: 668–71.

DeVita VT Jr, Canellos GP, Chabner B et al, Advanced diffuse histiocytic lymphoma, a potentially curable disease. *Lancet* 1975; **i:** 248–50.

Ewing J, Reticulum cell sarcoma. *J Med Res* 1913; **32:** 1.

Gall EA, Mallory TB, Malignant lymphoma: a clinicopathological survey of 63 cases. *Am J Pathol* 1942; **18:** 381–432.

Harris NL, Jaffe ES, Stein H et al, A revised European–American classification of lymphoid neoplasms: a proposal from the International Lymphoma Study Group. *Blood* 1994; **84:** 1361–92.

International Non-Hodgkin's Lymphoma Prognostic Factors Project, A predictive model for aggressive non-Hodgkin's lymphoma. *N Engl J Med* 1993; **329:** 987–94.

Lennert K, Mohri N, Stein H, Kaiserling E, The histopathology of malignant lymphoma. *Br J Haematol* 1975; **31**(Suppl): 193–203.

Levitt M, Marsh JC, DeConti R et al, Combination sequential chemotherapy in advanced reticulum cell sarcoma. *Cancer* 1972; **29:** 630–6.

Lukes RJ, Collins RD, Immunologic characterization of human malignant lymphomas. *Cancer* 1974; **34:** 1488–503.

Mason D, Bastard C, Rimokh R et al, CD30-positive large cell lymphomas ('Ki-1 lymphoma') are associated with a chromosomal translocation involving 5q35. *Br J Haematol* 1990; **74:** 161–8.

Non-Hodgkin's Lymphoma Pathologic Classification Project, National Cancer Institute sponsored study of classifications of non-Hodgkin's lymphomas: summary and description of a working formulation for clinical usage. *Cancer* 1982; **49:** 2112–35.

Oberling C, Les reticulo-sarcoma et les reticulo-endothelio-sarcoma de la moelle ossense (sarcoma d'Ewing). *Bull Assoc France Etude Cancer* 1928; **17:** 259.

Rappaport H, Malignant lymphomas. In: *Tumors of the Hematopoietic System*. Publication 91, Armed Forces Institute of Pathology: Washington, DC, 1966.

Rappaport HW, Winter J, Hicks E, Follicular lymphoma: a re-evaluation of its place in the scheme of malignant lymphoma based on a survey of 253 cases. *Cancer* 1956; **9:** 792–821.

Reed DM, On the pathological changes in Hodgkin's disease, with especial reference to its relation to tuberculosis. *Johns Hopkins Hosp Rev* 1902; **10:** 133–96.

Stein H, Mason D, Gerdes J et al, The expression of the Hodgkin's disease associated antigen Ki-1 in reactive and neoplastic lymphoid tissue: evidence that Reed–Sternberg cells and histiocytic malignancies are derived from activated lymphoid cells. *Blood* 1985; **66:** 848–58.

Sternberg C, Uber eine eigenartige unter dem Bilde der Pseudoleukamie verlaufende Tuberculose des lymphatichon Apparates. *Ztschr Heilk* 1898; **19:** 21.

Symmers D, Follicular lymphadenopathy with splenomegaly: a newly recognized disease of the lymphatic system. *Arch Pathol* 1927; **3:** 816–20.

Vandenberghe E, De Wolf-Peeters C, Van den Oord J et al, Translocation (11;14): a cytogenetic anomaly associated with B-cell lymphomas of non-follicle centre cell lineage. *J Pathol* 1991; **163:** 13–18.

Virchow R, *Die Krankenhaften Geschwülste*. Herschwald: Berlin, 1864.

2 Diffuse large B-cell lymphoma

Definition and classification

Diffuse large B-cell lymphoma is an aggressive neoplasm with a short survival in the absence of effective therapy. However, it has been known for 25 years that this lymphoma can sometimes be cured with combination chemotherapy. Early reports of cure used older nomenclature, including the terminology 'diffuse histiocytic lymphoma', 'diffuse large cell lymphoma', 'large transformed cell lymphoma', 'centroblastic lymphoma' and 'immunoblastic lymphoma'.

The most common non-Hodgkin's lymphoma is diffuse large B-cell lymphoma. This lymphoma often presents de novo, but can also be seen as a result of histologic transformation of most low-grade B-cell lymphomas. Transformation to diffuse large B-cell lymphoma is a common occurrence in follicular lymphoma, and is also seen in small lymphocytic lymphoma and the marginal-zone lymphomas, including MALT lymphoma.

Diffuse large B-cell lymphoma can arise in essentially any site in the body. The most common site is in lymphatic tissue, but any organ system can be involved. With some sites of involvement, unique clinical problems or unusual clinical courses are often observed. Primary central nervous system diffuse large B-cell lymphoma is an increasingly important clinical problem. While seen often in patients with human immunodeficiency virus (HIV) infection, diffuse large B-cell lymphoma involving the central nervous system is being seen increasingly frequently in patients with normal immune function. Central nervous system presentation is associated with an aggressive clinical course. In contrast, diffuse large B-cell lymphomas confined to the skin sometimes pursue an indolent clinical course. Diffuse large B-cell lymphomas involving the sinuses, epidural tissue and, probably, testes have an unusual predilection to spread to the central nervous system. The unique characteristics of specific sites of involvement need to be taken into account in planning the management of any particular patient.

Frequency

Diffuse large B-cell lymphoma makes up approximately 40% of all non-Hodgkin's lymphomas; the frequency varies little geographically. It is the predominant non-Hodgkin's lymphoma in all parts of the world.

Diffuse large B-cell lymphoma is increasing in frequency. This is the major explanation for the dramatic increase in the incidence of non-Hodgkin's lymphoma that has occurred over the last several decades. In the USA, the increase in incidence has been 4% per year since 1950. The cause of this 'epidemic' remains a mystery. The frequency of diffuse large B-cell lymphoma is higher in patients with defective immune function. It is a frequent tumor in patients with HIV infection, but it also is seen with increased frequency in patients with other immune disorders such as rheumatoid arthritis. Diffuse large B-cell lymphoma occurs more frequently in individuals exposed to a variety of chemicals, including many used in agriculture. Despite this knowledge of predisposing factors, the reason for the development of the disorder in most patients is not known.

Pathology

Histology (Table 2.1)

Diffuse large B-cell lymphoma can be recognized accurately by pathologists. In the International Lymphoma Classification Study, diffuse large B-cell lymphoma could be diagnosed accurately 87% of the time when both histologic features and immunophenotype were taken into account.

Diffuse large B-cell lymphoma is a neoplasm of large cells growing in a diffuse (i.e. non-follicular) pattern. The nuclei of the tumor cells are usually at least twice as large as the nucleus of a small lymphocyte. The tumor cells have nuclei that are vasicular and often contain prominent nucleoli, and have basophilic cytoplasm. They usually represent a mixture of centroblasts and immunoblasts. Occasionally, the tumor cells can have an 'anaplastic' appearance similar to that seen in anaplastic large T/NK-cell lymphoma. In this situation, the tumors display B-cell antigens. There is usually a moderate to high growth fraction in diffuse large B-cell lymphoma.

Occasionally, diagnosis can be complicated by a predominance of infiltrating T lymphocytes. This can lead to confusion in immunophenotyping, if it is not recognized that the tumor cells mark as B cells. This entity, often called T-cell-rich B-cell lymphoma, follows the same clinical course as other diffuse large B-cell lymphomas.

Immunophenotype (Table 2.2)

The only characteristic immunophenotypic finding in diffuse large B-cell lymphoma is that the tumors mark as B cells and thus display the CD20 antigen. They stain negatively with T-cell markers such as CD3. As noted above, care must be taken to be certain that it is the immunophenotype of the tumor cells that is being observed and not that of infiltrating normal cells. Knowing the immunophenotype increases the accuracy of diagnosis by 10%.

Table 2.1
Histological features of diffuse large B-cell lymphoma

- Large cells (i.e. nuclei ≥ twice the size of a small lymphocyte) and diffuse growth pattern
- Vesicular nuclei, prominent nucleoli, basophilic cytoplasm
- Moderate to high growth fraction
- Usually a mixture of centroblasts and immunoblasts
- Can occasionally have an 'anaplastic' appearance
- Occasional predominance of infiltrating T cells can lead to confusion with peripheral T-cell lymphoma (i.e. T-cell-rich B-cell lymphoma)

Table 2.2
Typical immunophenotype and genetics of diffuse large B-cell lymphoma

Characteristic	Result
Immunophenotype	CD20$^+$
	CD3$^-$
Cytogenetics	t(14;18)(q32;q21)
	t(3;14)(q27;q32)
	t(8;14)(q24;q32)
Oncogenes	BCL2
	BCL6
	c-MYC

Genetics (Table 2.2)

Diffuse large B-cell lymphoma probably represents several subtypes of aggressive non-Hodgkin's lymphoma that have not yet been clearly delineated. This view is supported by the wide variety of cytogenetic abnormalities and oncogene abnormalities that are seen in this disorder. The most common cytogenetic abnormalities include the t(14;18)(q32;q21) that is characteristic of follicular lymphoma. This cytogenetic abnormality is seen in up to 30% of diffuse large B-cell lymphomas in various series. This cytogenetic abnormality is associated with overexpression of the *BCL2* oncogene. The protein overexpression rather than the translocation seems to have clinical significance.

Another common cytogenetic abnormality seen in diffuse large B-cell lymphoma is the t(3;14)(q27;q32). This cytogenetic abnormality is associated with overexpression of the *BCL6* oncogene. In some series, but not all, this has been reported to be associated with a good prognosis. A much less frequently seen cytogenetic abnormality in diffuse large B-cell lymphoma is the t(8;14)(q24;q32) that is associated with overexpression of the c-*MYC* oncogene. This cytogenetic abnormality is characteristic of Burkitt's lymphoma, but is also occasionally seen in patients with large B-cell lymphoma. A myriad other cytogenetic abnormalities have been reported in diffuse large B-cell lymphoma.

Clinical characteristics (Table 2.3)

Diffuse large B-cell lymphoma usually presents with lymphadenopathy, but extranodal presentations give a clinical picture that might be confused with carcinoma of the site of involvement. This lymphoma is more likely to be localized than other non-Hodgkin's lymphomas. While it can be seen in patients in any age, the median age is in the 60s. In the International Lymphoma Classification Study, the actual median age was 64 years, as seen in Table 2.3. This lymphoma is seen more frequently in males: 55% in the aforementioned study.

Approximately 50% patients with diffuse large B-cell lymphoma will have disease that is localized to one site (i.e. stage I) or confined to one side of the diaphragm (stage II). Approximately 50% of patients with localized lymphoma will have predominant extranodal involvement. The other 50% of patients with diffuse large B-cell lymphoma have more widespread disease. Approximately 60% of patients who present with stage III or stage IV disease will have extranodal involvement. Approximately 30% of patients will present with fevers, sweats or weight loss.

An elevation of the serum level of lactate dehydrogenase (LDH) is seen in approximately 50% of patients. While most patients will be fully active, approximately 25% of the patients have reduced performance status at the time of diagnosis. Thirty percent of patients will have a tumor mass of at least 10 cm diameter. The comparatively high frequency of elevated LDH, low performance status or large tumor mass account in part for the poorer prognosis associated with this lymphoma.

About 70% of patients with diffuse large B-cell lymphoma will have involvement of at least one extranodal site. Approximately 30% of patients will

Table 2.3
Clinical characteristics of diffuse large B-cell lymphoma

Characteristic	Result
Median age	64 years
Percent male	55%
Stage I	12%
Stage IE	13%
Stage II	13%
Stage IIE	16%
Stage III	13%
Stage IV	33%
B symptom	33%
Elevated LDH	53%
Karnofsky score ≤ 70	24%
Tumor mass ≥ 10 cm	30%
Any extranodal site	71%
Bone marrow positive	16%
GI track positive	18%
IPI score: 0/1	35%
2/3	46%
4/5	19%

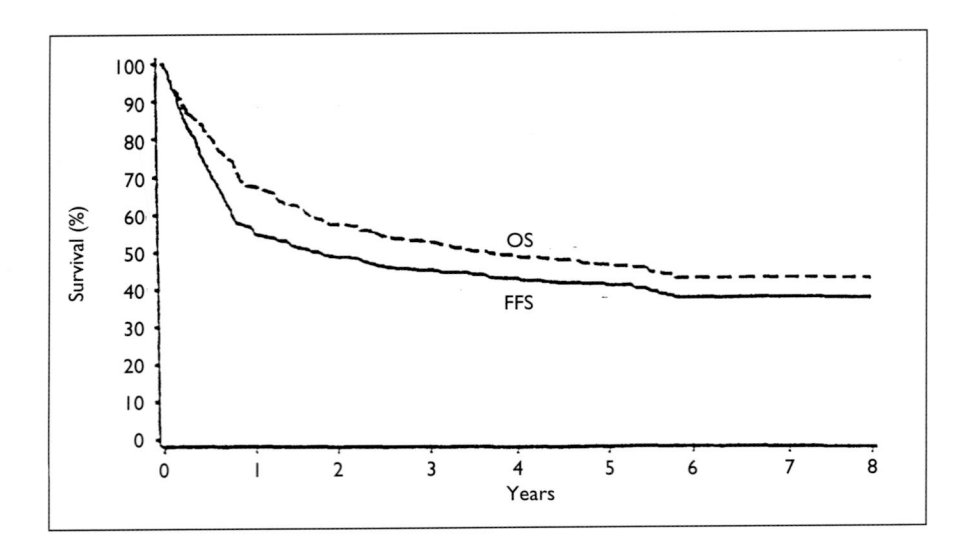

Figure 2.1
Overall survival (OS) and failure-free survival (FFS) for patients with diffuse large B-cell lymphoma.

have more than one extranodal site involved, and essentially any extranodal site can be involved. When the bone marrow biopsy is positive in these patients, the majority of patients will have small lymphocytes involving the marrow rather than large cells. The presence of small lymphocytes in the bone marrow in a patient with diffuse large B-cell lymphoma does not alter the overall prognosis. In contrast, the presence of large cells infiltrating the marrow has an adverse prognosis.

Approximately 30% of patients with diffuse large B-cell lymphoma will have none or only one adverse risk factor in the International Prognostic Index. About 50% of patients will have two or three adverse risk factors, and about 20% of patients will have four or five adverse risk factors.

Treatment and outcome

The treatment of patients with diffuse large B-cell lymphoma should emphasize the use of combination chemotherapy. The most popular regimen currently in use is the CHOP (cyclophosphamide, doxorubicin, vincristine and prednisone) (Table 2.4), although a variety of other regimens have at least equal activity. Even in patients with localized disease, the initial treatment should be combination chemotherapy. However, in patients with stage I, the total number of chemotherapy cycles can be reduced and involved-field radiotherapy substituted.

It has been known for at least 25 years that diffuse large B-cell lymphoma can be cured with combination chemotherapy – even in some patients with widespread disease. Unfortunately, experimentation with a wide variety of chemotherapeutic agents in varying combinations over the last two decades has not led to a definite improvement in treatment outcome. The consequence is

Table 2.4
The CHOP regimen: usually administered at 3-weekly intervals

Regimen	Drug	Dose (mg/m^2)	Day of cycle
CHOP	Cyclophosphamide	750	1
	Doxorubicin (Adriamycin)	50	1
	Vincristine	1.4 (maximum 2 mg)	1
	Prednisone	100 mg total dose (not per m^2)	1–5

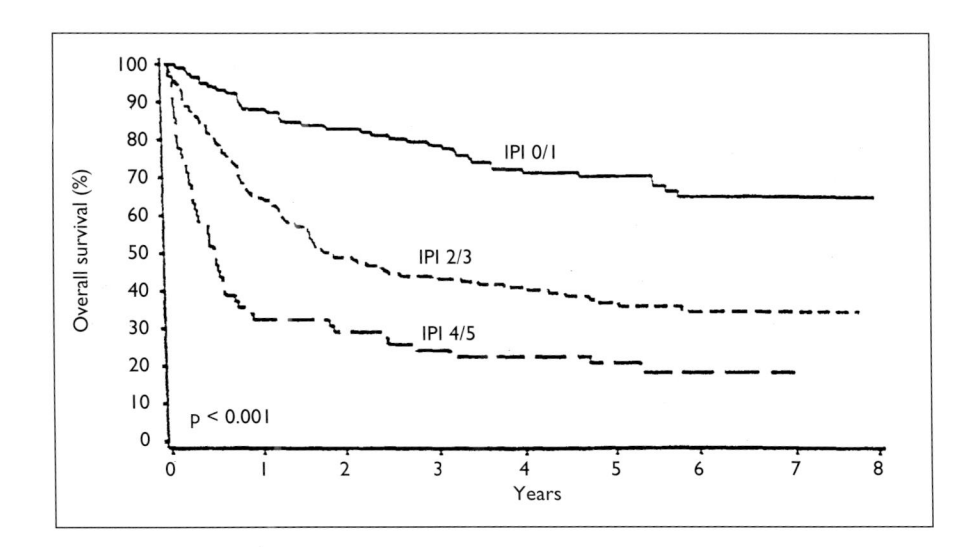

Figure 2.2
Overall survival according to International Prognostic Index (IPI) for patients with diffuse large B-cell lymphoma.

the failure-free and overall survival curves illustrated in Figure 2.1. Approximately 40% of all patients with diffuse large B-cell lymphoma can currently be cured. However, the chance for cure depends upon the risk factors in an individual patient. As illustrated in Figure 2.2, the International Prognostic Index can identify a subset of patients in which the five-year survival (i.e. usually very close to the five-year failure-free survival) is approximately 70%, and another subgroup of patients in which survival at five years is only approximately 20%.

Salvage therapy in patients with diffuse large B-cell lymphoma can occasionally be curative. It has recently been demonstrated that high-dose therapy and autologous hematopoietic stem cell transplantation can cure a significant proportion of patients with disease that remains chemotherapy-sensitive after relapse. In a randomized trial, this approach has been shown to be superior to standard-dose therapy. Studies are currently under way to see if earlier use of autotransplantation will improve results.

Involvement of specific sites in patients with diffuse large B-cell lymphoma can provide unique clinical problems. For example, patients with sinus involvement, epidural involvement or testicular involvement need to have prophylactic therapy to the central nervous system incorporated into their initial treatment, otherwise they have a high risk for a meningeal relapse. Patients who present with primary diffuse large B-cell lymphoma in the brain provide a particularly difficult clinical problem. However, intensive chemotherapy regimens including the use of high-dose methotrexate and early irradiation of the brain seem to improve treatment results. Finally, patients who present with diffuse large B-cell lymphoma confined to the skin sometimes pursue an indolent clinical course. Some investigators would suggest that these patients be treated very conservatively, with only excision or involved field radiotherapy.

Bibliography

Conlan MG, Bast M, Armitage JO, Weisenburger DD, Bone marrow involvement by non-Hodgkin's lymphoma: the clinical significance of morphologic discordance between the lymph node and bone marrow: Nebraska Lymphoma Study Group. *J Clin Oncol* 1990; **8:** 1163–72.

Devesa SS, Fears T, Non-Hodgkin's lymphoma time trends: United States and international data. *Cancer Res* 1992; **52:** 5432s–40s.

DeVita VT Jr, Canellos GP, Chabner B et al, Advanced diffuse histiocytic lymphoma, a potentially curable disease. *Lancet* 1975; **i:** 248–50.

Eby NL, Grufferman S, Flanelly CM et al, Increasing incidence of primary brain lymphoma in the US. *Cancer* 1988; **62:** 2461–5.

Filipovich AH, Mathur A, Kamat D, Primary immunodeficiencies: genetic risk factors for lymphoma. *Cancer Res* 1992; **52:** 5465s–7s.

Fisher RI, Gaynor ER, Dahlberg S et al, Comparison of CHOP vs m-BACOD vs ProMACE-CytaBOM vs MACOP-B in patients with intermediate or high-grade non-Hodgkin's lymphoma. *N Engl J Med* 1993; **328:** 1002–6.

Harris NL, Jaffe ES, Stein H et al, A revised European–American classification of lymphoid neoplasms: a proposal from the International Lymphoma Study Group. *Blood* 1994; **84:** 1361–92.

Hill ME, MacLennan KA, Cunningham DC et al, Prognostic significance of BCL-2 expression and *bcl-2* major breakpoint region rearrangement in diffuse large cell non-Hodgkin's lymphoma: a British National Lymphoma Investigation study. *Blood* 1996; **88:** 1046–51.

International Non-Hodgkin's Lymphoma Prognostic Factors Project, A predictive model for aggressive non-Hodgkin's lymphoma. *N Engl J Med* 1993; **329:** 987–94.

Jones SE, Miller TM, Connors JM, Long-term follow-up and analysis for prognostic factors for patients with limited-stage diffuse large-cell lymphoma treated with initial chemotherapy with or without adjuvant radiotherapy. *J Clin Oncol* 1989; **7:** 1186–91.

Kinlen LJ, Incidence of cancer in rheumatoid arthritis and other disorders after immunosuppressive treatment. *Am J Med* 1985; **78**(Suppl 1A): 44–9.

Levine AM, Lymphoma in acquired immunodeficiency syndrome. *Semin Oncol* 1990; **17:** 104–12.

Levine AM, Shibata D, Sullivan-Halley J, Epidemiological and biological study of acquired immunodeficiency syndrome-related lymphoma in the county of Los Angeles: preliminary results. *Cancer Res* 1992; **52:** 5482s–4s.

Levitt M, Marsh JC, DeConti R et al, Combination sequential chemotherapy in advanced reticulum cell sarcoma. *Cancer* 1972; **29:** 630–6.

Longo DL, Glatstein E, Duffey PI et al, Treatment of localized aggressive lymphomas with combination chemotherapy followed by involved-field radiation therapy. *J Clin Oncol* 1989; **7:** 1186–91.

Non-Hodgkin's Lymphoma Classification Project, A clinical evaluation of the International Lymphoma Study Group classification of non-Hodgkin's lymphoma. *Blood* 1997; **89:** 3909–18.

Offit K, LoCoco F, Diane C, Rearrangement of the *bcl* gene as a prognostic marker in diffuse large cell lymphoma. *N Engl J Med* 1994; **14:** 74–80.

Pearce N, Bethwaite P, Increasing incidence of non-Hodgkin's lymphoma: occupational and environmental factors. *Cancer Res* 1992; **52:** 5496s–500s.

Philip T, Armitage JO, Spitzer G et al, High-dose therapy and autologous bone marrow transplantation after failure of conventional chemotherapy in adults with intermediate-grade or high-grade non-Hodgkin's lymphoma. *N Engl J Med* 1987; **316:** 1493–8.

Philip T, Guglielmi C, Hagenbeek A et al, Autologous bone marrow transplantation as compared with salvage chemotherapy in relapses of chemotherapy-sensitive non-Hodgkin's lymphoma. *N Engl J Med* 1995; **333:** 1540–5.

Ramsay A, Smith W, Isaacson P, T-cell rich B-cell lymphoma. *Am J Surg Pathol* 1988; **12:** 433–43.

Snider WD, Simpson DM, Nielson S et al, Neurological complications of acquired immune deficiency syndrome: analysis of 50 patients. *Ann Neurol* 1983; **14:** 403–18.

Willemze R, Meister CJLM, Sentis HJ et al, Primary cutaneous cell lymphomas of follicular center-cell origin. *J Am Acad Dermatol* 1987; **16:** 518–26.

Yves Blay J, Conroy T, Chevreau C et al, High-dose methotrexate for the treatment of primary cerebral lymphomas: analysis of survival and late neurologic toxicity in a retrospective series. *J Clin Oncol* 1998; **16:** 864–71.

Zahm SH, Blair A, Pesticides and non-Hodgkin's lymphoma. *Cancer Res* 1992; **52:** 5485s–8s.

Diffuse large B-cell lymphoma

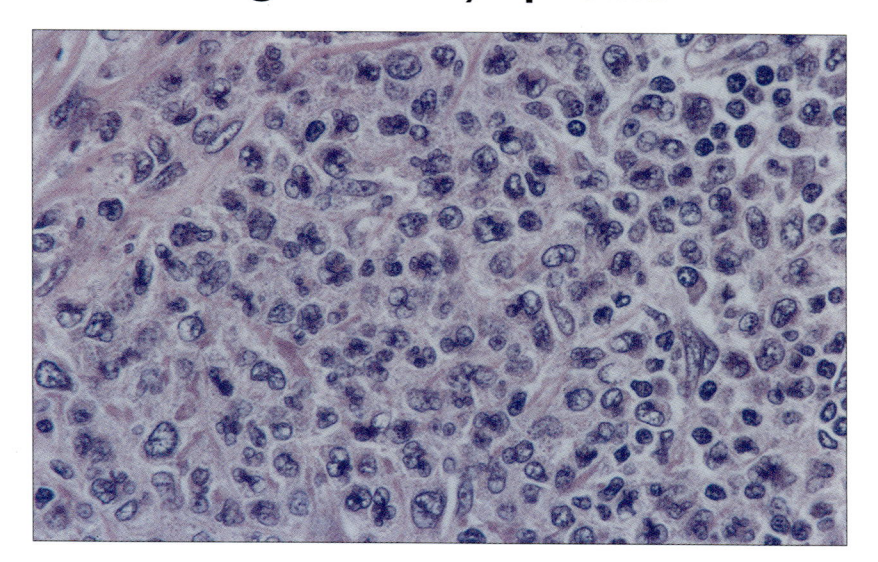

Figure 2.3

Diffuse large B-cell lymphoma – Lymph node:

This large B-cell lymphoma is composed predominantly of multilobated cells and large cleaved cells. (H&E stain)

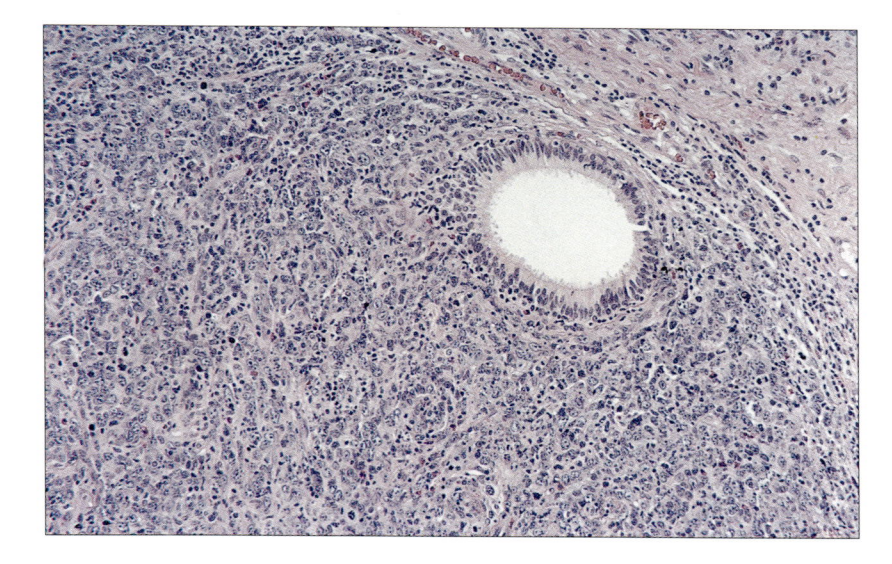

Figure 2.4

Diffuse large B-cell lymphoma – Epididymis:

(a) There is a diffuse infiltrate of large atypical lymphoid cells surrounding a residual tubule. (H&E stain)

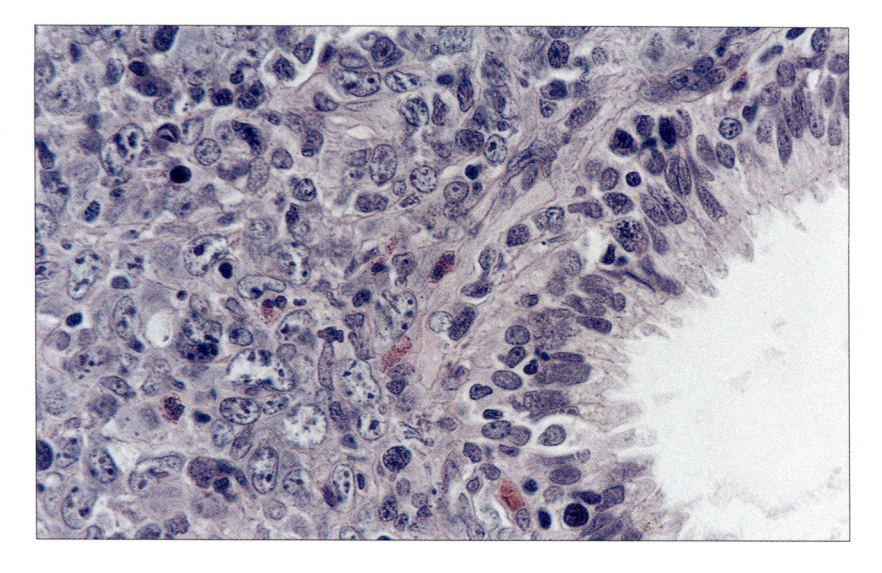

(b) The lymphoma is composed predominantly of centroblasts (large non-cleaved cells). (H&E stain)

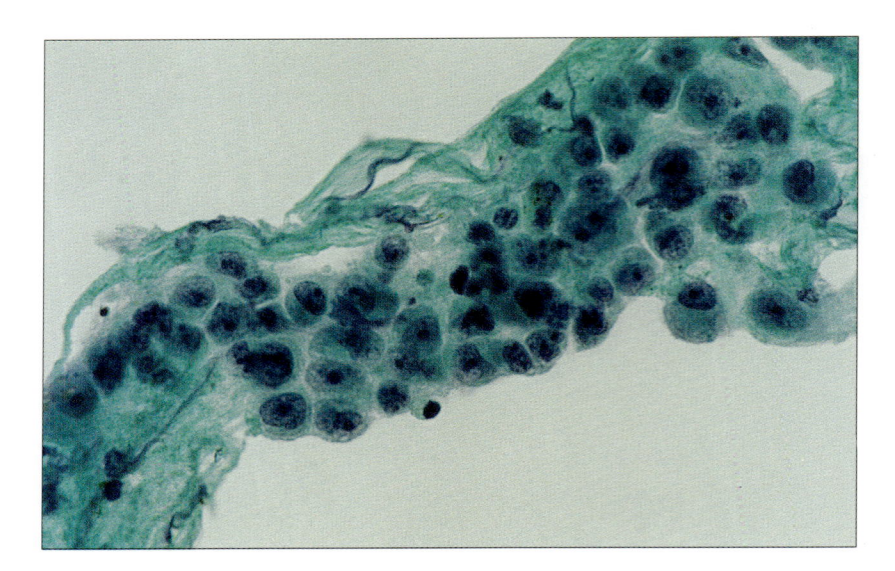

Figure 2.5

Diffuse large B-cell lymphoma – Eye:

This vitreous aspirate shows a lymphoma composed predominantly of immunoblasts. (Papanicolaou stain)

3 Follicular lymphoma

Definition and classification

Follicular lymphoma is a clonal malignancy of mature peripheral B cells derived from the follicular center of lymph nodes; the distinctive pathologic feature of this lymphoma is that it grows in a follicular or nodular pattern. The lymph node follicle is a site where antibodies of increasingly higher affinity for a particular antigen are generated through an antigen-driven process of selection. The B cells of the follicular center undergo regular genetic alterations in the form of somatic mutations and occasionally gene rearrangements in order to generate antibodies of increasing affinity (so-called 'affinity maturation'). When follicular center B cells become neoplastic, they retain the genetic instability. As a consequence, follicular lymphoma cells tend to change over time; in addition to spontaneous alterations in their surface immunoglobulin molecule related to ongoing mutations in the immunoglobulin genes, additional genetic lesions accumulate in these cells, and ultimately influence the rate of growth, natural history and response to treatment.

Frequency

Follicular lymphoma is the second most common form of lymphoma worldwide, behind diffuse large B-cell lymphoma. It accounts for 30–40% of all lymphoid tumors in adults in Western countries, occurring in a frequency of about 4 per 100 000 people annually. The disease is rare in the Orient. All lymphomas are increasing in frequency; however, follicular lymphoma is not increasing as rapidly as diffuse lymphoma.

Pathology

Histology

Follicular lymphoma has a nodular or follicular growth pattern; areas of diffuse growth may also be noted. Expanding tumor follicles efface the nodal architecture. The follicles are usually somewhat larger than normal follicles, and do not maintain the zones of lymphocyte maturation seen in normal follicles (Figure 3.1). The cytologic composition of the tumor includes normal and reactive T cells, follicular dendritic cells, and two predominant neoplastic cell types – a small cell with a cleaved nucleus (small cleaved cell or centrocyte), and a larger cell with a large nucleus with vesicular chromatin, prominent nucleoli and basophilic cytoplasm (large cell or centroblast). These two morphologic forms of the same malignant cell are present in varying proportions in different patients and even in different sites of the same patient and in different portions of the same tumor mass. They form a continuous spectrum of diseases that were

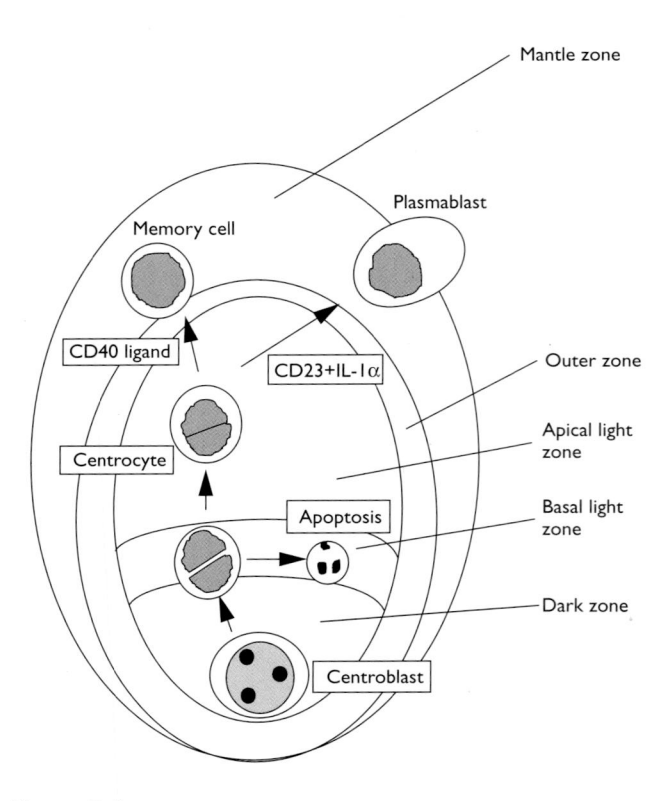

Figure 3.1

Normal lymphoid follicle structure and function. In a normal germinal center, dendritic cells carrying antigen stimulate the proliferation of B cells in the dark zone capable of recognizing the antigen. These cells take on the morphologic characteristics of centroblasts. As the cells mature into centrocytes, those with low-affinity antigen binding of the surface immunoglobulin die by apoptosis. Those with surface immunoglobulin molecules that have the appropriate antigen affinity mature into either memory B cells under the influence of T cells bearing CD40 ligand or into plasma cells by stimulation with CD23 and interleukin-1α (IL-1α). The dendritic cells in the basal light zone do not express CD23; those in the apical light zone do. Neoplastic follicles contain only a single clone of B cells that appear predominantly as centrocytes. A subpopulation of centroblasts is present, and its size determines the lymphoma grade. Other cell types present in normal follicles, such as dendritic cells and T cells, may also be present in neoplastic follicles, but these follicles do not have clear dark and light zones, and mantle zones are absent. (Reproduced from Magrath IT (ed) *The Non-Hodgkin's Lymphomas*, 2nd Ed, 1997, with permission from Edward Arnold.)

formerly divided into three entities empirically based upon the number of large cells present: follicular small cleaved cell lymphoma (<5 large cells per high-power field (hpf) in a tumor nodule), follicular mixed lymphoma (5–15 large cells/hpf) and follicular large cell lymphoma (>15 cells/hpf). Experience has demonstrated that the separation of follicular lymphoma into these three entities is difficult to do reproducibly.

In more recent histologic classifications (REAL, WHO), the spectrum of follicular lymphomas has been represented not by distinctly named entities but by histologic grades, with the presence of increasing numbers of large cells leading to the designation of a higher grade. In the new WHO classification, it was decided to consider the former follicular small cleaved as grade I, and follicular mixed as grade II. A tumor that was formerly called 'follicular large cell lymphoma' will be designated 'follicular lymphoma, grade III' in the WHO classification. Because of the difficulty in dividing the entities, discrete clinical differences to justify the effort have been hard to establish. Institutions where pathologists have developed skill and reproducibility find differences between patients with follicular small cleaved cell and follicular mixed lymphoma. Institutions where the pathologists have trouble with the distinction have not. Thus the arguments over whether to keep the entities separate or merge them together become contentious precisely because dividing them irreproducibly blurs the distinctions.

In the WHO classification, about 90% of patients with follicular lymphoma will have grades I or II disease and 10% will have grade III disease. Those with grades I and II disease will most likely follow the natural history outlined below that is typical of follicular lymphoma; those with grade III disease are considered to have a lymphoma with a more aggressive natural history that is more like diffuse large cell lymphoma.

Immunophenotype/immunohistology

Like other lymphomas, the cell surface phenotype of follicular lymphomas tends to reflect the phenotype of the normal lymphoid counterpart from which it is derived. Thus follicular lymphomas are surface immunoglobulin-positive (usually IgM only, but occasionally another isotype is also present), and CD19$^+$, CD20$^+$, CD22$^+$ and CD79a$^+$. Most tumors express CD10. They do not express CD5. The differential diagnosis is usually not difficult. Occasional patients with what was formerly called follicular mixed lymphoma were misdiagnosed with follicular hyperplasia. However, the neoplastic nature of the cells can be confirmed in several ways: the presence of a single light-chain isotype on the cells (polyclonal hyperplasia should contain both λ- and κ-expressing cells); the expression of BCL2 on immunohistology (normal follicular center cells do not express BCL2); or genetic analysis that shows clonal immunoglobulin gene rearrangement on Southern blotting or the presence of the t(14;18) translocation (absent in normal cells – see below). The proliferative fraction of follicular lymphomas (revealed by Ki-67 staining) is generally low (about 3%), but most of the proliferative activity is in the large cells, and as the number of large cells increases, so too does the proliferative fraction.

Genetics

The hallmark of follicular lymphoma is a gene translocation that brings the *BCL2* gene from chromosome 18 next to the immunoglobulin heavy-chain gene on chromosome 14. The t(14;18)(q32;q21) is present in about 85% of follicular lymphomas. Its role in the pathogenesis of follicular lymphoma is controversial. The molecular anatomy of the translocation suggests that it occurs early in the cell's development at a time when its immunoglobulin genes are rearranging. However, the maturation of the cell bearing the translocation is apparently not affected – it simply rearranges its other chromosome 14 to produce an immunoglobulin molecule and goes on to become a normally appearing mature peripheral B cell. The detection of cells bearing the t(14;18) translocation in otherwise completely normal individuals who never develop cancer, the finding that some follicular lymphomas bearing the translocation fail to express the BCL2 protein or even mRNA from the translocation, and the nearly universal presence of other genetic lesions in follicular lymphomas all suggest that *BCL2* translocation is neither necessary nor sufficient to transform a follicular center B cell into a malignant lymphoma or maintain the transformed state. However, the overexpression of BCL2 is capable of preventing the negative selection and apoptosis that normally occurs in the germinal center, and could keep alive a cell that was destined to die. The lengthened lifespan of a genetically unstable cell could then lead to the accumulation of other genetic lesions that produce the tumor.

The nature of the genetic lesions that contribute to follicular lymphomagenesis are not defined; however, the coexpression of certain cytogenetic abnormalities with t(14;18) in follicular lymphomas suggests that heterogeneous pathways may be involved. Trisomies involving X, 3, 5, 7, 8, 9, 12, 17, 18, 20 and 21, deletions involving 6q23 and 6q25–27, and abnormalities at Xp22, 1p21–22, 1p36, 3q21–27, 7q32 and 10q23–25 are among the many additional cytogenetic lesions that may be seen in follicular lymphoma.

Most follicular lymphomas progress to diffuse large cell lymphoma near the end of their course. This change in growth pattern is associated with an acceleration of the natural history and additional genetic lesions, including mutations in *p53* or *c-MYC* and others. Mutations involving *p53* are common in this setting; however, *p53* and *c-MYC* changes are apparently independent pathways for progression, since no cases with mutations in both genes have been noted.

Clinical characteristics/natural history

The majority of patients present with painless swelling in one or more lymph nodes. The neck is the most frequent site, followed by the groin and axilla. Patients often provide a history of having had lymph node swelling in the past that spontaneously regressed. The median age is 55 years; the disease is rare before age 30, and women and men are roughly equally affected. Splenomegaly is present in some patients, and may be a source of symptoms. More uncommonly, patients present with B symptoms (10–15%) or some manifestation of mass effects of enlarged lymph nodes, such as back pain, abdominal pain or bladder pressure. Despite the nodal presentation, the majority of patients have extranodal sites of disease – predominantly the bone marrow, where clusters of malignant cells are found next to trabeculae. The liver is involved in about 10% of patients, and 5–10% of patients have circulating malignant cells detectable on differential cell count of peripheral blood. More sophisticated molecular testing can identify circulating malignant cells in the vast majority of patients, because this disease spreads hematogenously early in its course.

Once a diagnosis has been made based upon an excisional lymph node biopsy, the assessment of the patient's prognosis requires additional testing (Table 3.1). On systematically performing anatomic staging based upon the Ann Arbor staging classification developed for Hodgkin's disease, it is found that 60–75% of patients have stage IV disease and 10–15% have stage I disease, with the rest equally divided between stages II and III. In some centers, patients of different disease stages had different survival probabilities. However, the most practical reason for performing anatomic staging is that the small percentage of patients with localized disease are potentially curable with radiation therapy (see below). For the 85% of patients who do not have localized disease, other features influence prognosis. Although no consensus has been reached on a standard method of assessing prognosis, the International Prognostic Index that was developed based upon treatment outcome for diffuse large cell lymphoma also divides patients with follicular lymphoma into distinct prognostic groups. This system uses age, stage, lactate dehydrogenase (LDH) level and performance status. Other systems use hemoglobin level instead of LDH, or a combination of LDH level and β_2-microglobulin level to determine prognosis. Most of the individual factors assessed are surrogate markers for two important determinants of survival: tumor bulk and the physiologic reserve of the patient.

The vast majority of patients respond to treatment (see below), but the duration of response is usually only a few years. Patients usually relapse in previously involved nodal sites of disease if the treatment was chemotherapy-based; they relapse in previously uninvolved non-irradiated nodes if treatment included radiation therapy to involved nodes. The response rate to a second intervention is generally about 15–25% lower than that to the first treatment, and the duration of the second remission is shorter than the first. Similarly, patients may continue responding to third, fourth, fifth, sixth or even later treatments – almost always with shorter remissions each time. The pace of disease progression becomes a little faster, much like the chronic phase of chronic myeloid leukemia. Then an acute acceleration of tumor growth becomes apparent, and rebiopsy of a rapidly growing lesion generally shows histologic progression to diffuse large cell or another aggressive-histology lymphoma. Transformed follicular

---

Table 3.1
Required and suggested staging procedures for follicular lymphoma

Required in all patients
- Excisional biopsy of an enlarged node: specimen processed for light microscopy, immunophenotyping and molecular studies
- Thorough history with attention to B symptoms
- Thorough physical examination; measure and record abnormalities
- Blood work:
    Complete blood count
    Serum lactate dehydrogenase
    Serum β_2-microglobulin
    Renal function tests
    Liver function tests
- Radiologic studies:
    PA and lateral chest radiograph
    Abdominal–pelvic CT scan
    Bilateral lymphogram
    Chest CT scan (unless chest radiograph is normal)
- Bilateral bone marrow biopsies and aspirates

Required under certain circumstances
- Percutaneous liver biopsy if bone marrow is negative and patient has early-stage disease
- Other tests to investigate specific symptoms:
    Gastrointestinal ultrasound or contrast radiographs
    Bone radiographs or scintigraphy
    Renal ultrasound or intravenous pyelography if paraaortic nodes are involved
- Serum calcium and uric acid

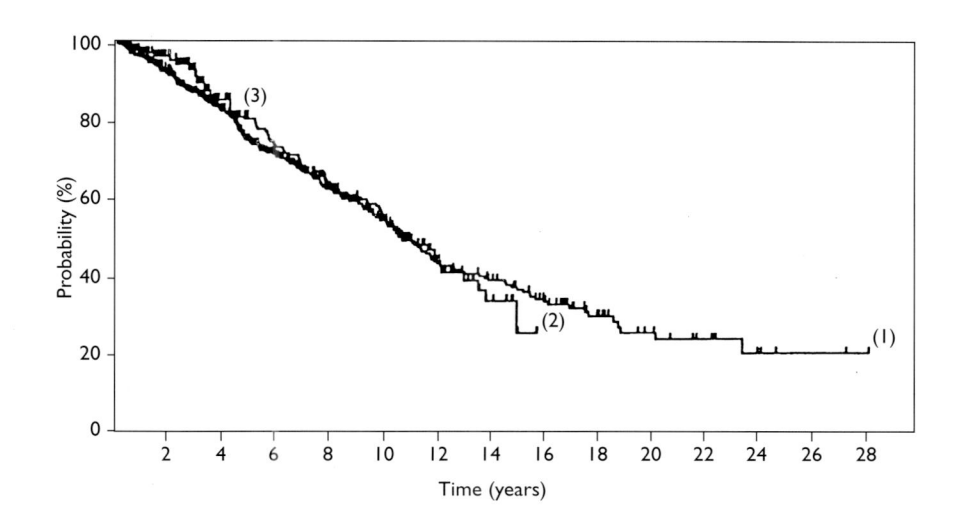

Figure 3.2
Survival curves of patients with follicular lymphoma treated at Stanford in different eras: (1) 1960–75; (2) 1976–86; (3) 1987–92. This is a Kaplan–Meier plot of survival of patients treated with diverse approaches at Stanford since 1960. Survival curves from diverse treatment centers all over the world look remarkably similar. (From Horning SJ, *Semin Oncol* 1993; **20**(Suppl 5): 75–88; with permission from WB Saunders.)

lymphoma has a poor prognosis, with a median survival of about six months. Only about 10–15% of these patients survive histologic transformation as a consequence of responding to aggressive treatment, and a portion of those who do survive relapse again with follicular lymphoma. According to autopsy series, 10% or fewer of patients with follicular lymphoma die with follicular lymphoma; in over 90%, the histology at death is diffuse aggressive lymphoma. About 6–8% of patients with follicular lymphoma will develop histologic transformation each year.

The average patient diagnosed with follicular lymphoma will follow a chronic remitting and relapsing course, and will die of aggressive-histology lymphoma about 10–12 years after diagnosis.

Treatment

Follicular lymphoma presents a paradox unlike any other in oncology. In most cancers, the difficulty in treatment lies in finding an intervention that causes tumor regression. In follicular lymphoma, nearly every kind of treatment produces tumor regression. However, it remains unclear whether treatment influences the natural history of the disease. A case can be made that the disease follows its own independent course that is predetermined by its genetic instability and the particular lesions in its genome, regardless of inter-vention. Survival curves from Stanford University reflect this possibility (Figure 3.2). Nevertheless, many recent developments promise to alter this picture. As several ongoing studies acquire longer periods of patient follow-up, it appears that treatment is associated with longer remissions, a reduced rate of histologic progression, and improved survival. Furthermore, the introduction of newer agents has led to a shift away from the nihilism that has pervaded the field for most of the last two decades.

Follicular small cleaved cell and follicular mixed lymphoma (follicular lymphoma, grades I and II)

The 15% of patients with follicular lymphoma, grades I and II who have clinical stage I or II disease appear to have a 50–60% chance of being cured by extended-field radiation therapy. In the Stanford experience, 80% of patients younger than age 40 were in their initial complete remission at 15 years after treatment with involved-field, extended-field or total nodal radiation therapy. Patients staged at laparotomy have similar outcome regardless of the extent of radiation; clinically staged patients do better with more extensive radiation. Some patients who receive curative radiation therapy succumb to radiation-induced second malignancy in the second and third decades after treatment. However, long-term survival is noted in over half of the treated patients. Adding combination chemotherapy to radiation therapy generally does not improve survival, though disease-free survival (remission duration) has occasionally been prolonged.

Radiation therapy is a curative modality in follicular lymphoma. The difficulty is that the disease often spreads to sites that cannot safely receive a curative dose of radiation therapy, especially the bone marrow. Even stage III patients (that is, patients with disease restricted to nodes, without marrow involvement) may have long-term disease-free survival similar to early-stage patients after treatment with total nodal radiation therapy. Long-term disease-free survival of 40–66% has been reported in stage III patients treated with total nodal radiation therapy. In the Stanford series, stage III patients without B symptoms and fewer than five sites of disease had an 88% relapse-free survival at 15 years. The addition of combination chemotherapy to radiation therapy does not appear to improve survival for patients with stage III disease.

Even though radiation therapy is curative for patients with follicular lymphoma, grades I and II, restricted to nodes, many patients with localized disease do not receive this therapy. Localized disease is rare; the average oncologist may see such a patient once every four or five years. Most physicians assume that a patient with follicular lymphoma has disseminated disease, and most often they are correct. However, the rare patient with localized disease is not well served by being carefully observed and followed monthly while the tumor becomes systemic, and no longer curable with radiation therapy.

Patients with stage III or IV follicular lymphoma are usually considered incurable with standard treatment approaches. Radiation therapy, single-agent chemotherapy, combination chemotherapy and combined-modality treatment approaches are all capable of inducing complete responses in the majority of patients. However, until recently, the median remission duration has been about two years, and it is not clear that patients being treated with curative intent have better survival than patients selected for no initial therapy or only palliative therapy.

Long-term follow-up of several studies and the introduction of new active chemotherapy and biologic agents is beginning to change this situation. Interferon has been demonstrated in several studies to prolong remission duration but not overall survival. However, in one study, overall survival has been significantly improved. The Groupe d'Etude des Lymphomes Folliculaires (GELF) compared six monthly cycles of CHVP (cyclophosphamide, doxorubicin, teniposide, prednisone), a CHOP-like regimen, with the same regimen plus interferon-α2b given three times a week for 18 months. Both disease-free and overall survival were significantly prolonged on the interferon arm. Although chronic interferon administration can produce significant fatigue, patients on interferon reported more time without symptoms of disease progression or toxicity in a quality-adjusted time without symptoms and toxicity (Q-TWiST) study.

Evidence is also emerging from studies using more aggressive treatment approaches that prolonged disease-free survival may be obtained in patients with advanced-stage follicular lymphoma. High-dose chemotherapy or high-dose radio-immunoconjugate therapy with autologous hematopoietic stem cell support appears to be capable of inducing median remission durations in excess of eight years, even in multiply relapsed patients. Critics argue that prolonged remission does not necessarily translate into prolonged survival; however, it is difficult to prolong survival without first augmenting remission duration. Furthermore, for the first time, salvage therapy in relapsed patients is inducing remissions that last longer than the initial remissions. Given that patients with follicular lymphoma usually have progressively shorter remissions with each treatment, this development looks like progress.

In the National Cancer Institute (NCI) randomized study comparing aggressive combined modality therapy using ProMACE–MOPP flexitherapy followed by low-dose total lymphoid radiation therapy with no initial therapy, significant differences have emerged between the two approaches. When patients who were randomly assigned to receive no initial therapy required systemic treatment, they received the same therapy as those randomly assigned to aggressive primary treatment.

Patients randomly assigned to aggressive treatment were significantly more likely to achieve a complete response than those in whom treatment was delayed (75% versus 43%). Thus the watch-and-wait approach resulted in patients coming to treatment with a greater tumor burden and being less responsive to therapy. The rate of histologic progression was significantly lower in the group of patients randomly assigned to aggressive therapy. Finally, remission durations with the combined-modality treatment approach were greater than nine years. With a median follow-up of 13 years, 55% of patients with follicular lymphoma treated with combination chemotherapy plus radiation therapy on the NCI study are in their first remission. It is not yet clear whether patients randomly assigned to aggressive treatment will have longer overall survival than those randomly assigned to watch and wait. The trend in favor of aggressive primary therapy is of borderline significance ($p = 0.06$). However, 75% of the surviving patients on the aggressive-treatment arm are in their initial complete remission and have been continuously free of disease, compared with 25% of the surviving patients on the watch-and-wait arm. In addition, those on the watch-and-wait arm more frequently reported feeling sad, concerned about their health, and fatigued than did those who underwent initial aggressive therapy.

Are these patients in long-term remission cured? It is not possible to say. No relapses have been seen after remissions longer than six years; however, the median follow-up time is just now approximately equal to the median survival. Additional follow-up is required to determine whether anyone is cured. Currently the data are consistent with either 40% or 0% of patients being cured.

New effective agents in follicular lymphoma may improve overall survival. Nucleosides such as fludarabine and cladribine are among the most active single agents in follicular lymphoma. They are being incorporated into combination regimens (for example FND: fludarabine, mitoxantrone (Novantrone), dexamethasone) with very high complete response rates, including molecular complete responses. In addition, a humanized anti-CD20 monoclonal antibody (Rituximab) has been developed that appears to induce complete responses in about 50% of treated patients, even in a salvage setting. This antibody works by a different mechanism than radiation therapy and chemotherapy, and is a prime candidate to be incorporated into primary treatment approaches, especially in the setting of low tumor burden.

Experimental agents are also promising. An ^{131}I-labelled anti-CD20 antibody (anti-B1) has been used in about 24 patients with follicular lymphoma who have not been previously treated; the response rate was 100%, with 75% complete responses including the clearance of t(14;18)-bearing cells from the bone marrow and peripheral blood. Other strategies using agents designed to interfere with signal transduction in tumor cells, such as the protein kinase C inhibitor bryostatin, or with programmed cell death, such as antisense oligonucleotides to BCL2, are in early phases of development. A variety of vaccine approaches also have enormous potential.

No consensus has been reached on the best approach to the management of advanced-stage follicular lymphoma, grades I and II (follicular small cleaved cell and follicular mixed lymphoma). An individualized approach to the patient may be optimal. For the 75-year-old woman who is asymptomatic from lymphoma, a conservative approach may be the most prudent one. For the 45-year-old executive whose life is likely to be foreshortened by the disease, a different set of considerations apply. Some people can adjust to the notion that they have an indolent lymphoma without undue concern, but are terrified of treatment. For others, the disease is a sword of Damocles over their heads that adversely affects the quality of their daily lives. The physician must strive to determine what approach is most likely to give an individual patient the most benefit, taking into account the nature of the disease, the side-effects of the interventions, and the patient's concerns.

Follicular large cell lymphoma (follicular lymphoma, grade III)

Follicular large cell lymphoma accounts for about 10–15% of all follicular lymphomas. It is reasonable to approach follicular large cell lymphoma in the same fashion as diffuse large cell lymphoma. All stages of follicular large cell lymphoma are curable with doxorubicin-based combination chemotherapy.

The treatment of choice for patients with stage I or II (non-bulky) follicular large cell lymphoma is four cycles of CHOP or CHOP-like chemotherapy plus involved field radiation therapy. Long-term survival has been reported in 84–90% of patients treated with this approach. The use of brief chemotherapy plus involved-field radiation therapy appears superior to chemotherapy alone.

Patients with bulky stage II disease (any mass larger than 10 cm) or with stage III or IV follicular large cell lymphoma, like patients with advanced diffuse large cell lymphoma, are treated with a doxorubicin-containing multiagent chemotherapy program. Although there is controversy about whether any regimen is better than CHOP in this setting, the GELA study using LNH87 demonstrated five-year overall survival of 58% in patients with follicular large cell lymphoma. This was not different from their results in diffuse large cell lymphoma using LNH87, and seems substantially higher than results reported with CHOP. Thus, physicians should consider using one of the more aggressive treatment programs such as LNH87, ProMACE–CytaBOM, MACOP-B, VACOP-B, F-MACHOP or COP–BLAM III. About 55–60% of patients with advanced-stage disease are curable with these regimens.

Patients with follicular lymphoma who relapse may have a variable course. Patients with follicular lymphoma, grades I and II who relapse with the same histology may respond to a second course of the primary therapy, but the second and subsequent remissions are usually shorter than the first. The success of salvage treatments diminishes with each relapse. Multiple relapses are common, and survival for several years with palliative treatment approaches is possible. If histologic progression occurs, the natural history of the disease accelerates, and the patient is either cured by salvage therapy (this occurs in a minority of patients: overall around 20%) or dies within a few months. Patients with follicular lymphoma, grade III who relapse may be cured with high-dose therapy and autologous stem cell transplantation in up to 40% of the cases.

Bibliography

Anderson T, DeVita VT Jr, Simon RM et al, Malignant lymphoma II. Prognostic factors and response to treatment of 473 patients at the National Cancer Institute. *Cancer* 1982; **50:** 2708–21.

Armitage JO, Sanger WG, Weisenburger DD et al, Correlation of secondary cytogenetic abnormalities with histologic appearance in non-Hodgkin's lymphoma bearing t(14;18)(q32;p21). *J Natl Cancer Inst* 1988; **80:** 576–80.

Bastion Y, Sebban C, Berger F et al, Incidence, predictive factors, and outcome of lymphoma transformation in follicular lymphoma patients. *J Clin Oncol* 1997; **15:** 1587–94.

Bierman PJ, Vose JM, Anderson JR et al, High-dose therapy with autologous hematopoietic rescue for follicular low-grade non-Hodgkin's lymphoma. *J Clin Oncol* 1997; **15:** 445–50.

Cole BF, Solal-Celigny P, Gelber RD et al, Quality-of-life-adjusted survival analysis of interferon alfa-2b treatment for advanced follicular lymphoma: an aid to clinical decision making. *J Clin Oncol* 1998; **16:** 2339–44.

Gallagher CJ, Gregory WM, Jones AE et al, Follicular lymphoma: prognostic factors for response and survival. *J Clin Oncol* 1986; **2:** 269–306.

Garvin AJ, Simon RM, Osborne CK et al, An autopsy study of histologic progression in non-Hodgkin's lymphomas. 192 cases from the National Cancer Institute. *Cancer* 1983; **52:** 393–8.

Ghia P, Boussiotis VA, Schultze JL et al, Unbalanced expression of bcl-2 family proteins in follicular lymphoma: contribution of CD40 signaling in promoting survival. *Blood* 1998; **91:** 244–51.

Gribben JG, Freedman AS, Neuberg D et al, Immunologic purging of marrow assessed by PCR before autologous bone marrow transplantation for B-cell lymphoma. *N Engl J Med* 1991; **325:** 1525–33.

Horning SJ, Rosenberg SA, The natural history of initially untreated low-grade non-Hodgkin's lymphoma. *N Engl J Med* 1984; **311:** 1471–5.

Hubbard SM, Chabner BA, DeVita VT Jr et al, Histologic progression in non-Hodgkin's lymphoma. *Blood* 1982; **59:** 258–64.

Korsmeyer SJ, Bcl-2 initiates a new category of oncogenes: regulators of cell death. *Blood* 1992; **80:** 879–86.

Litam P, Swan F, Cabanillas F et al, Prognostic value of serum β2-microglobulin in low-grade lymphoma. *Ann Intern Med* 1991; **114:** 855–60.

Lopez-Guillermo A, Cabanillas F, McLaughlin P et al, The clinical significance of molecular response in indolent follicular lymphomas. *Blood* 1998; **91:** 1955–60.

Lopez-Guillermo A, Montserrat E, Bosch F et al, Applicability of the international index for aggressive lymphomas to patients with low-grade lymphoma. *J Clin Oncol* 1994; **12:** 1343–8.

McLaughlin P, Fuller L, Redman J et al, Stage I–II low grade lymphomas: a prospective trial of combination chemotherapy and radiotherapy. *Ann Oncol* 1991; **2**(Suppl 2): 137–40.

McLaughlin P, Hagemeister FB, Swan F et al, Intensive conventional-dose chemotherapy for stage IV low-grade lymphoma: high remission rates and reversion to negative of peripheral blood bcl-2 rearrangement. *Ann Oncol* 1994; **5**(Suppl 2): 73–7.

Meerwaldt JH, Carde P, Somers R et al, Persistent improved results after adding vincristine and bleomycin to a cyclophosphamide/hydoxorubicin/Vm-26/prednisone combination (CHVmP) in stage III–IV intermediate- and high-grade non-Hodgkin's lymphoma. The EORTC Lymphoma Cooperative Group. *Ann Oncol* 1997; **8**(Suppl 1): 67–70.

Miller TP, Dahlberg S, Cassady JR et al, Chemotherapy alone compared with chemotherapy plus radiotherapy for localized intermediate- and high-grade non-Hodgkin's lymphoma. *N Engl J Med* 1998; **339:** 21–6.

Non-Hodgkin's Lymphoma Classification Project, A clinical evaluation of the International Lymphoma Study Group classification of non-Hodgkin's lymphoma. *Blood* 1997; **89:** 3909–18.

Paryani SB, Hoppe RT, Cox RS et al, Analysis of non-Hodgkin's lymphoma with nodular and favorable histologies, stages I and II. *Cancer* 1983; **52:** 2300–7.

Paryani SB, Hoppe RT, Cox RS et al, The role of radiation therapy in the management of stage III follicular lymphomas. *J Clin Oncol* 1984; **2:** 841–8.

Press OW, Eary JF, Appelbaum FR et al, Phase II trial of 131-I-B1 (anti-CD20) antibody therapy with autologous stem cell transplantation for relapsed B cell lymphomas. *Lancet* 1995; **346**: 336–40.

Price CGA, Merrabux J, Murtagh S et al, The significance of circulating cells carrying t(14;18) in long remission from follicular lymphoma. *J Clin Oncol* 1991; **9:** 1527–34.

Romaguera JE, McLaughlin P, North L et al, Multivariate analysis of prognostic factors in stage IV follicular low-grade lymphoma: a risk model. *J Clin Oncol* 1991; **9:** 762–9.

Sander CA, Yano T, Clark HM et al, p53 mutation is associated with progression in follicular lymphomas. *Blood* 1993; **82:** 1994–2004.

Solal-Celigny P, Lepage E, Brousse N et al, Recombinant interferon alfa-2b combined with a regimen containing doxorubicin in patients with advanced follicular lymphoma. *N Engl J Med* 1993; **329:** 1608–14.

Wendum D, Sebban C, Gaulard P et al, Follicular large-cell lymphoma treated with intensive chemotherapy: an analysis of 89 cases included in the LNH87 trial and comparison with the outcome of diffuse large B-cell lymphoma. Groupe d'Etude des Lymphomes de l'Adulte. *J Clin Oncol* 1997; **15:** 1654–63.

Follicular lymphoma – Grades 1–3*

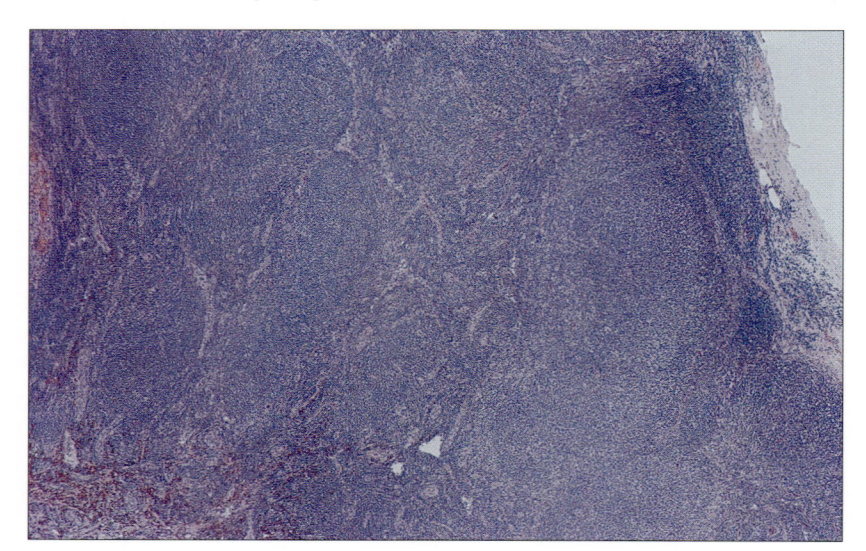

Figure 3.3

Follicular lymphoma – Grade I of III:

(a) Low power shows a lymph node with distortion of the normal architecture by a proliferation of crowded, somewhat poorly circumscribed follicles. (H&E stain)

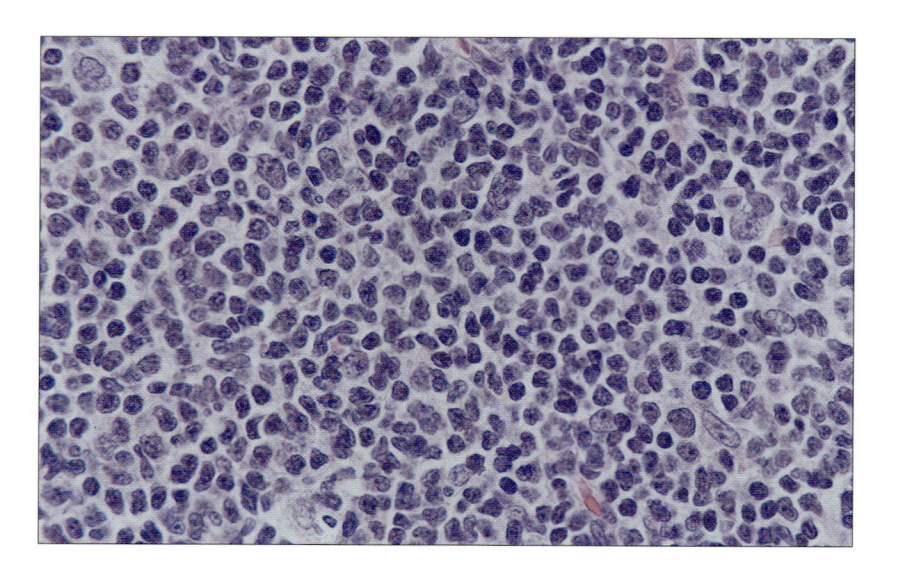

(b) Neoplastic follicles contain predominantly centrocytes (small cleaved lymphoid cells), with only a few large cells. (H&E stain)

*Clinicians refer to these entities as 'follicular lymphoma' on the basis of their growth patterns in nodes. Some diffuse large B-cell lymphomas (see Chapter 2) are derived from follicle center B cells; thus, not all tumors of follicle center B-cell origin grow in a follicular pattern. In the WHO classification, three grades of follicular lymphoma are recognized, the entity in the Working Formulation called follicular small cleaved cell lymphoma is follicular lymphoma, grade I in the WHO classification; follicular mixed lymphoma is follicular lymphoma, grade II; and follicular large cell lymphoma is follicular lymphoma, grade III.

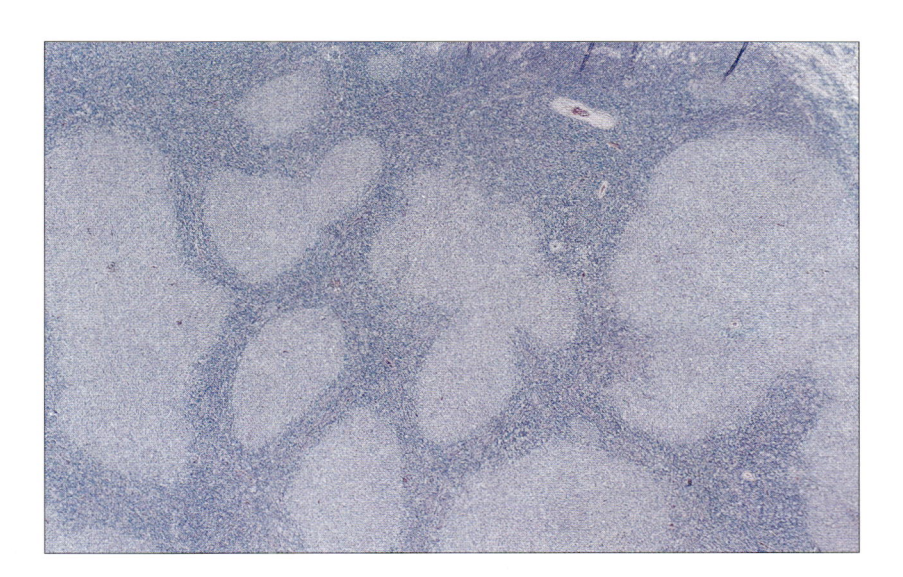

Figure 3.4

Follicular lymphoma – Grade II of III:

(a) Much of the lymph node is occupied by large, pale, somewhat irregularly shaped follicles. (H&E stain)

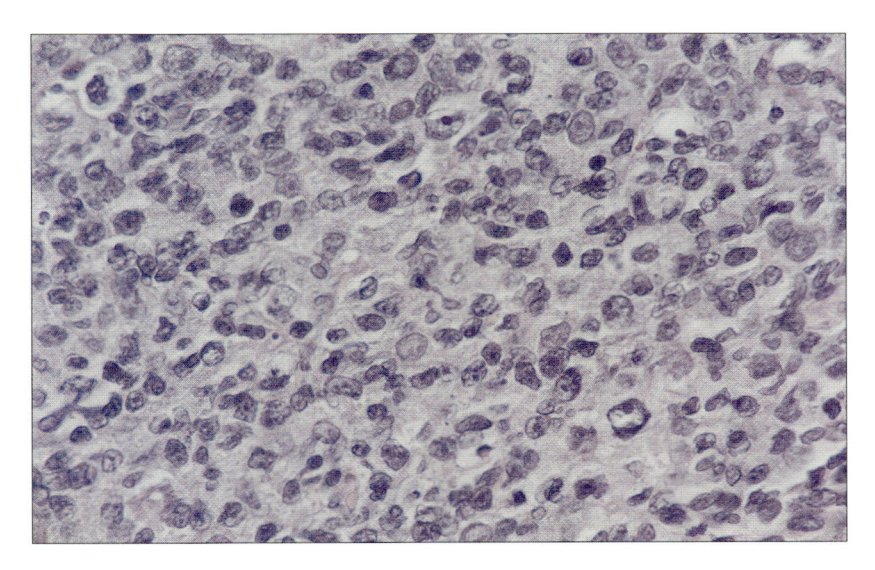

(b) Higher power shows a mixture of centrocytes and centroblasts. (H&E stain)

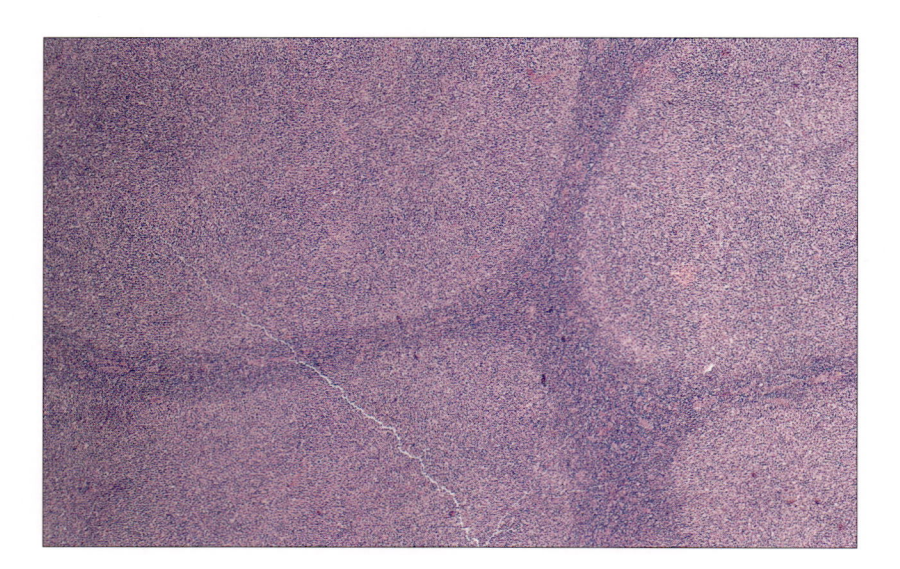

Figure 3.5

Follicular lymphoma – Grade III of III:

(a) Most of the lymph node is replaced by very large follicles. (H&E stain)

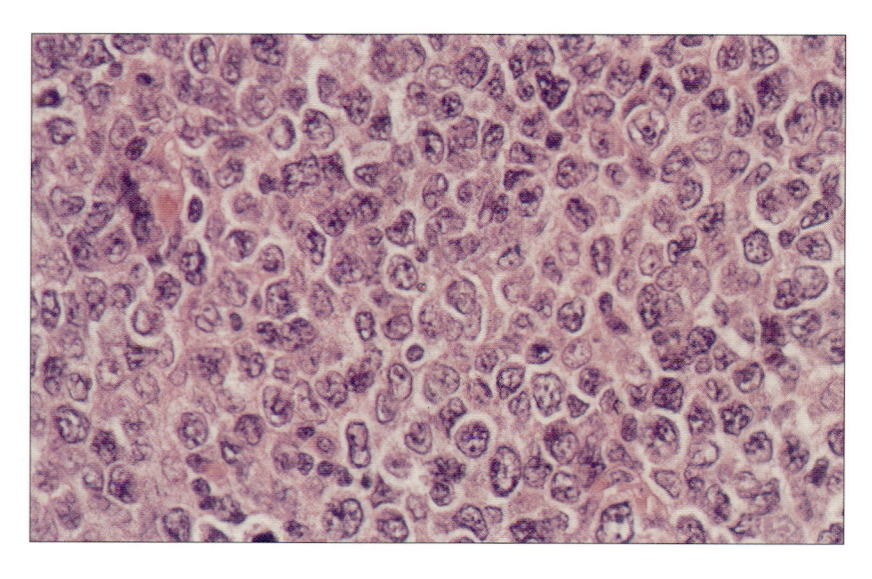

(b) Most cells in the follicles are centroblasts. (H&E stain)

Follicular lymphoma – Immunohistochemistry

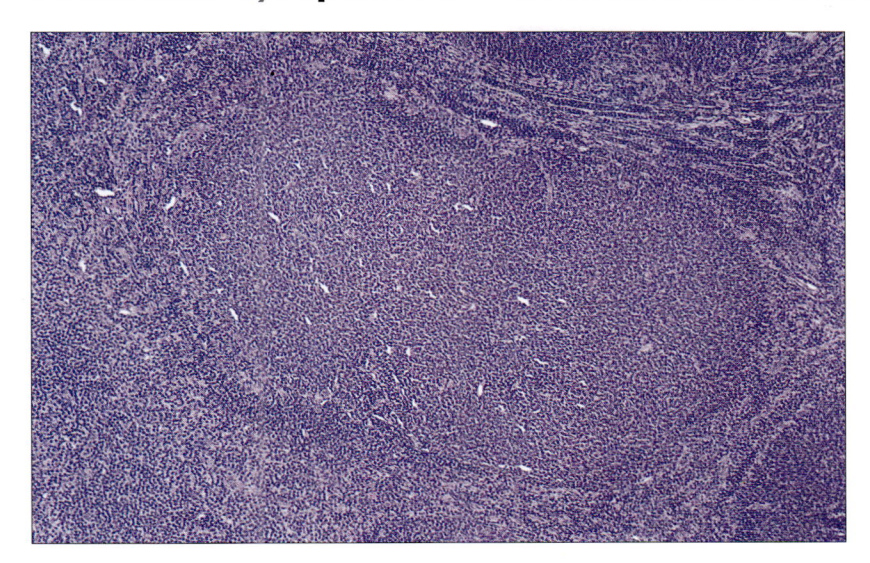

Figure 3.6

Follicular lymphoma – Immunohistochemistry used in the differential diagnosis with follicular hyperplasia:

(a) This lymph node contains an atypical lymphoid proliferation, with follicular hyperplasia and follicular lymphoma included in the differential diagnosis. (H&E stain)

(b) High power shows predominantly centrocytes with scattered centroblasts. (H&E stain)

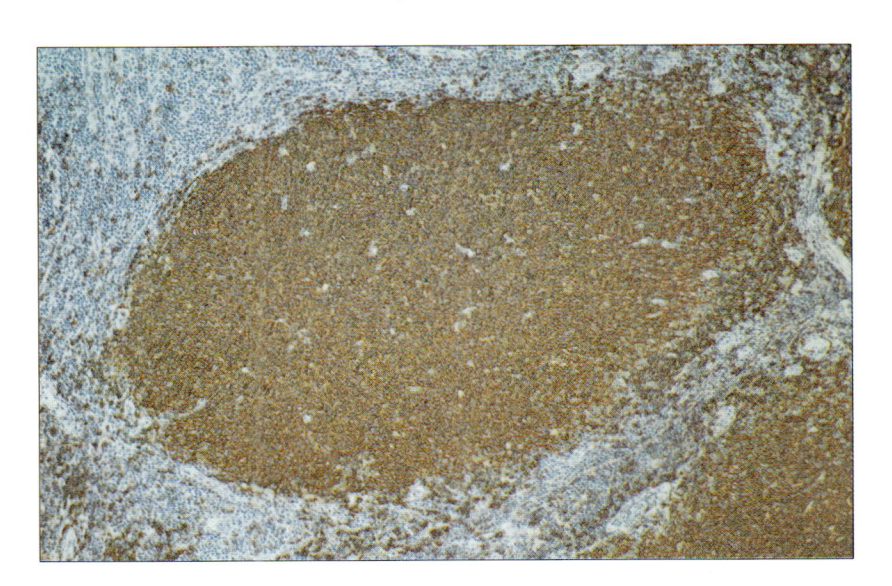

(c) Most cells in the follicles are B cells (L26⁺). (Immunoperoxidase technique on paraffin sections)

Contd

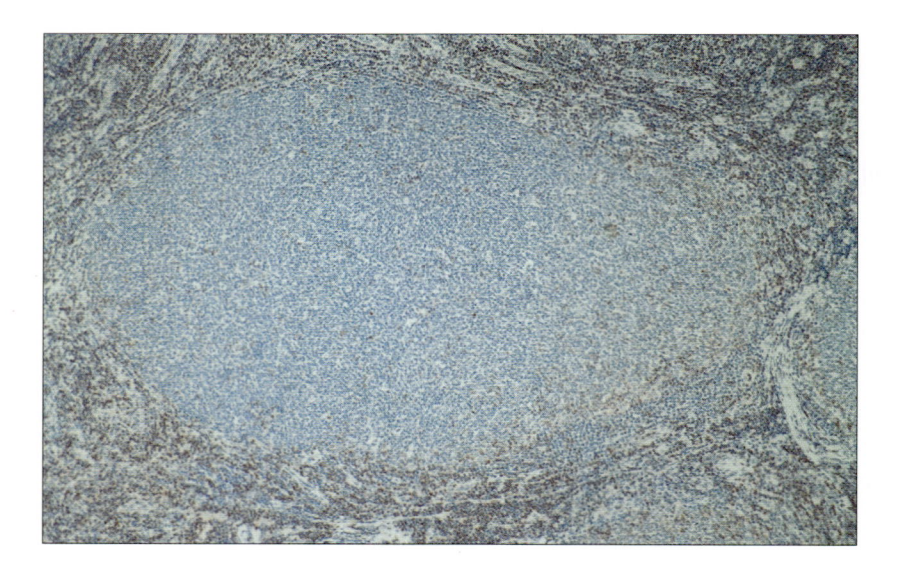

Figure 3.6 *continued*

(**d**) Interfollicular cells are predominantly T cells (CD3$^+$). (Immunoperoxidase technique on paraffin sections)

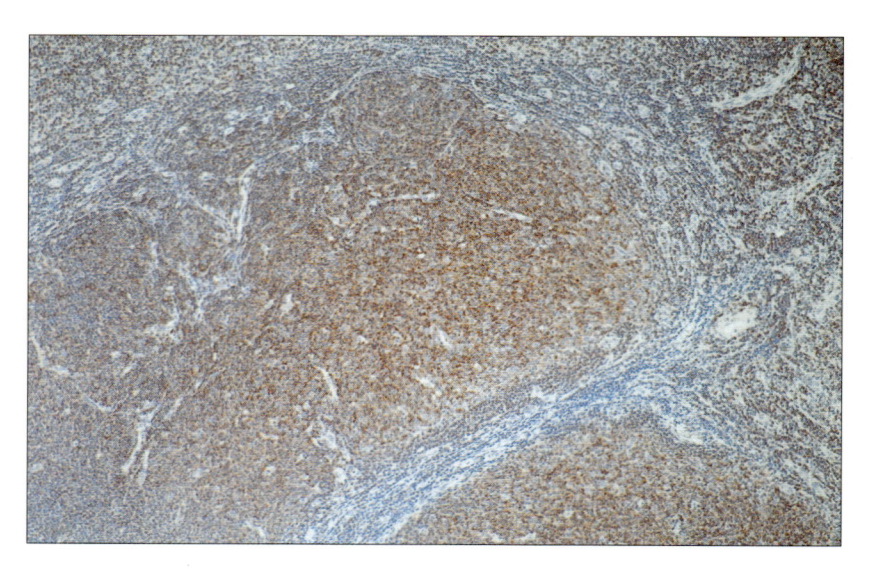

(**e**) Most B cells express BCL2 protein, confirming a diagnosis of follicular lymphoma and excluding follicular hyperplasia. (Immunoperoxidase technique on paraffin sections)

Follicular lymphoma – Marrow involvement

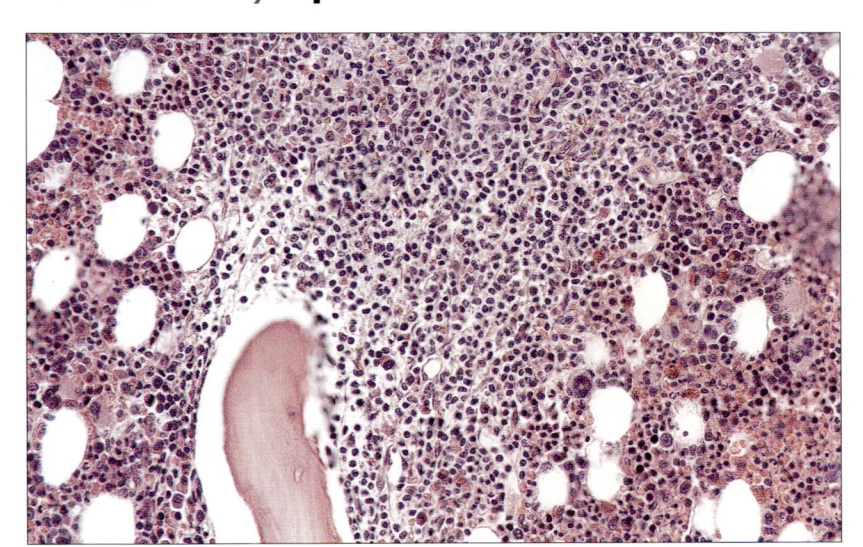

Figure 3.7

Follicular lymphoma – Marrow involvement:

There is a prominent paratrabecular aggregate, consistent with marrow involvement by follicular lymphoma. (H&E stain)

4 Peripheral T-cell lymphomas

Peripheral T-cell lymphoma, unspecified type

Definition and classification

The term 'peripheral T-cell lymphoma' has been used both in a general context to refer to all neoplasms of T cells that express a mature, post-thymic T-cell phenotype ('peripheral' here is used to distinguish mature cells from precursor or thymic immature T cells) and in a specific context to refer to a subset of diffuse aggressive lymphomas that express T-cell markers. In the latter context, peripheral T-cell lymphomas account for about 25% of all diffuse aggressive lymphomas; these include most of the tumors formerly called (in the Working Formulation) diffuse mixed lymphoma, about 33% of tumors formerly called immunoblastic lymphomas, and about 15% of diffuse large cell lymphomas. In the Kiel classification, these tumors were subdivided into tumors of medium-sized cells, large cells, or mixed medium and large cells. Because of the difficulty in reproducibly dividing these lymphomas into three groups and the questionable prognostic value of doing so, the REAL classification and the WHO classification do not cytologically grade peripheral T-cell lymphomas.

In addition to the peripheral T-cell lymphomas not further defined, five peripheral T-cell lymphomas fit into discrete clinicopathologic entities: angioimmunoblastic T-cell lymphoma, adult T-cell leukemia/lymphoma, angiocentric T/NK-cell lymphoma, intestinal T-cell lymphoma and anaplastic large cell lymphoma. T-cell chronic lymphocytic leukemia, large granular lymphocyte leukemia and mycosis fungoides are also tumors of peripheral T cells. Anaplastic large cell lymphoma is discussed in Chapter 9; T-cell chronic lymphocytic leukemia and large granular lymphocyte leukemia are discussed in Chapter 5; and angiocentric lymphoma and intestinal T-cell lymphoma are discussed in Chapter 14. Angioimmunoblastic T-cell lymphoma and adult T-cell leukemia/lymphoma are discussed in separate sections of this chapter.

Frequency

About 15% of all lymphomas are of T-cell origin. Geographic differences are noted in the incidence of T-cell lymphomas: T-cell lymphomas are more common than B-cell lymphomas in Japan and in other Asian countries. A significant fraction of the T-cell lymphomas in Japan are related to HTLV-I infection. In the 1400 cases analyzed by the Non-Hodgkin's Lymphoma Classification Project, 7% were peripheral T-cell lymphomas. The breakdown was as follows: peripheral T-cell lymphoma not further specified, 3.7%; angiocentric, 1.4%; angioimmunoblastic, 1.2%; while intestinal, hepatosplenic and adult T-cell leukemia/lymphoma together account for less than 1% of cases.

Pathology

Histology

Peripheral T-cell lymphomas, unspecified, may show preferential involvement of paracortical regions of lymph nodes, which are normally T-cell-rich. Occasionally, the lymphoid follicles will be spared. In most cases, the architecture of the node is effaced by sheets of atypical cells of various sizes. The tumor cells have a moderate amount of pale cytoplasm. A mixed inflammatory cell background is often present, composed of eosinophils, plasma cells and histiocytes. In some tumors, the histiocytes resemble epithelial cells in some ways, and they are called epithelioid histiocytes. If these cells are numerous and clustered together, the lymphoma is sometimes called 'Lennert's lymphoma'; however, most experts agree that the criteria for making this diagnosis are not sufficiently well developed and the biologic features of the tumor are not sufficiently well characterized to preserve the distinct designation.

Immunophenotype

The diagnosis of peripheral T-cell lymphoma, unspecified type, relies on immunophenotype data. Regardless of the skill of the pathologist, light-microscopic analysis is insufficient to make this diagnosis definitively in a large fraction of the cases. In most cases, one or more pan-T-cell antigens are expressed, including CD7, CD5, CD2 and CD3. In about 60% of cases, one of these will be non-detectable, most frequently CD7. CD2 is the last to be lost, and thus is the most reliable pan-T marker in this setting. The phenotype of the cells is $CD4^+$ in about 65% of cases and $CD8^+$ in 15% of cases, with double-positive and double-negative tumors each accounting for about 10% of cases. In most cases, one or more activation markers are expressed, including HLA-DR, CD25 (low-affinity IL-2 receptor) or CD71 (transferrin receptor). Antigen expression may change over time. The phenotypes of peripheral T-cell lymphomas are heterogeneous, and the phenotypic diversity does not have an obvious clinical correlation.

More specific phenotypes are characteristic of some of the named entities among the peripheral T-cell lymphomas. For example, anaplastic large cell lymphomas are $CD30^+$, and angiocentric T/NK-cell lymphoma, nasal type, is $CD56^+$ and contains clonal Epstein–Barr virus genomes.

Genetics

The genetic heterogeneity is similar to the immunophenotypic heterogeneity, and here, too, clinical correlations are not strong. As would be expected for mature T cells, the T-cell antigen receptor genes (*TCR*) are rearranged in about two-thirds of cases. Assessment of clonality is based upon assessment of the structure of the *TCR* genes, but the gene examined varies depending upon the technique being employed. Using restriction fragment analysis (Southern blotting), *TCRβ* is the locus that is usually analyzed, because it is rearranged in most T-cell lymphomas and appropriate probes are available to detect the altered size of rearranged fragments. Using PCR analysis, the *TCRγ* locus is more commonly analyzed. The *TCRγ* gene has a smaller number of variable regions than the *TCRβ* gene, and the construction of consensus primers is easier. Clonality determination is important not only to confirm the neoplastic (clonal) nature of the tumor, but also to aid in differential diagnosis. Mature T cells may be the predominant cells in an enlarged node in T-cell-rich B-cell lymphoma, but the neoplastic cell is a clonal B cell in that disease, and analysis of the *TCR* genes will reveal the T cells to be polyclonal reactive cells. However, genetic analysis of clonality may be less critical in tumors that have lost expression of one of the pan-T-cell markers; the alteration in phenotype has been strongly correlated with *TCRβ* rearrangements. Therefore clonal analysis may not be necessary in such cases.

Numerical and structural changes are noted in many cases of peripheral T-cell lymphoma, unspecified type, but no individual alteration is common. Breaks involving the *TCR* loci (especially *TCRα,δ*–14q11 and *TCRβ*–7q35) are often seen. The chromosomes most frequently altered in structure are 1, 6, 2, 4, 11, 14 and 17. Breakpoints at 6q23 are common. Aneuploidy typically involves trisomies of 3 or 5 and an extra X chromosome. At present, the diversity of genetic findings has not allowed a consistent model of molecular pathogenesis to be constructed.

Clinical characteristics

For most patients, it is not possible to determine on the basis of clinical presentation alone whether the diffuse aggressive lymphoma that has been diagnosed is of B-cell or T-cell origin. The most common presentation for peripheral T-cell lymphoma, unspecified type, is generalized lymphadenopathy (80%) and/or extranodal disease (liver, bone marrow, skin). On a population basis, the median age is higher (around 60 years), and a higher frequency of extranodal disease, spleen involvement and systemic symptoms (60%) is noted in those with T-cell lymphomas; however, patients with T-cell lymphomas are less likely to have bulky disease and involvement of the gastrointestinal tract (intestinal T-cell lymphoma is a distinct entity – see Chapter 14). A very wide range of clinical symptoms may be noted, and the presence of some syndromes is a hint of the T-cell nature of the tumor. For example, profound anemia and the hemophagocytic syndrome nearly always suggest T-cell lymphoma (most common in angiocentric lymphoma). Specific named entities produce more well-recognized clinical syndromes, such as necrotic facial or nasal lesions (angiocentric NK-cell lymphoma), or hypercalcemia and skin lesions (HTLV-I-induced adult T-cell leukemia/lymphoma). In most instances, little about peripheral T-cell lymphomas, unspecified type, is peculiar to that type of lymphoma.

Hemograms may show mild anemia or thrombocytopenia. Hypereosinophilia is noted on occasion. About 85% of patients have lactate dehydro-genase (LDH) elevations. Some patients present with systemic illness without localizing symptoms, abnormal liver function tests, and infiltration of unusual organs by lymphoma cells. It is hypothesized that many of the systemic manifestations of T-cell lymphoma are paraneoplastic syndromes related to the production of cytokines by the tumor. Some patients have had previous medical illnesses such as a prior lymphoma or a prior diagnosis of an autoimmune disease such as vasculitis or arthritis.

Treatment

Peripheral T-cell lymphoma, unspecified type, is usually in advanced stage at diagnosis, and is treated in the same fashion as advanced-stage diffuse large B-cell lymphoma (see Chapter 2). Whether T-cell phenotype alone influences prognosis is not completely clear. In several studies, patients with T-cell lymphomas have had a significantly poorer prognosis than patients with aggressive-histology B-cell lymphomas treated similarly; in some studies, no significant differences have been noted. In the studies where a difference has been found, the difference is usually in remission duration rather than complete response rate. Only one of the published studies has analyzed the results based upon the International Prognostic Index (IPI). The Groupe d'Etudes des Lymphomes de l'Adulte (GELA) examined their results with the LNH87 protocol, analyzing whether immunophenotype was an independent prognostic factor. They found that anaplastic large cell lymphoma had a good prognosis with this treatment. However, the peripheral T-cell lymphomas other than anaplastic large cell lymphoma had a poorer treatment outcome than either anaplastic large cell lymphoma or the diffuse large B-cell lymphomas. The peripheral T-cell lymphomas also had more patients with poor prognostic factors. When patients of the same IPI prognostic category with B-cell lymphoma and T-cell lymphoma were compared, those with 0–1 factor had similar outcome. When patients with three poor prognostic factors were compared, those with T-cell tumors fared worse. Thus, at least for some forms of treatment, T-cell phenotype is itself a prognostic factor. In the view of the present author (DLL), it is probable that the importance of phenotype will diminish with improvements in treatment. The nucleoside analogues seem to have greater toxicity for neoplastic T cells than for neoplastic B cells, and these agents are being worked into new multiagent regimens. Furthermore, some evidence that treatment can be an equalizer has already been obtained. The use of high-dose therapy with autologous bone marrow transplantation as salvage treatment of relapsed patients achieved similar results in both T-cell and B-cell lymphoma (30–35% long-term survival).

In addition, Karakas and colleagues have used the VACPE regimen in 27 patients with aggressive-histology T-cell lymphoma and in 55 patients with aggressive-histology B-cell lymphoma:

- V, vincristine 2 mg on day 1;
- A, doxorubicin 25 mg/m^2 on days 1–3;
- C, cyclophosphamide 800 mg/m^2 on day 1;
- P, prednisone 60 mg/m^2 on days 1–7;
- E, etoposide 120 mg/m^2 on days 1–3.

The complete response rate for patients with T-cell lymphoma was 77%; that for B-cell lymphoma was 84%. Seventy-five percent of the complete responders with T-cell lymphoma and 70% of the complete responders with B-cell lymphoma remain in their initial complete response at four years of follow-up. The five-year overall survival for the two groups was similar: around 62%.

We have seen other instances in which prognostic factors have changed with improvements in therapy. It is not yet clear that the differences related to immunophenotype need to be addressed by developing completely distinct regimens. The results obtained in Burkitt's and lymphoblastic lymphoma with more recently developed regimens attest to the fact that aggressive tumors of different lineages can be treated with the same regimen, and similar excellent outcomes can be obtained.

Angioimmunoblastic T-cell lymphoma

Definition and classification

Recognition that this disease is a malignant T-cell disorder came relatively recently. Early reports in the 1970s described a systemic illness with diffuse adenopathy, fevers, skin rash, hypergammaglobulinemia and a benign diagnosis on histopathology. The disease was called 'angioimmunoblastic lymphadenopathy with dysproteinemia' (abbreviated AILD), and was felt to be an abnormal immune reaction to an unknown stimulus. However, the median survival for this benign condition was about 18 months. Some cases were called 'angioimmunoblastic lymphadenopathy-like lymphoma' based on cellular atypia, but the recognition that this was a peripheral T-cell lymphoma came with molecular studies demonstrating clonal rearrangements of *TCR* genes. The lymphomas were most commonly called 'diffuse mixed' or 'large cell immunoblastic' in the Working Formulation. The designation of this entity in the REAL classification has also been adopted by the WHO classification. The disease is now called 'angioimmunoblastic T-cell lymphoma' (AILD – the D stands for 'dysproteinemia', which is no longer an official part of the name).

Frequency

Angioimmunoblastic T-cell lymphoma is the most common T-cell lymphoma in the Western world. It accounts for about half of all peripheral T-cell lymphomas.

Pathology

Histology

The lymph node architecture is effaced by a polymorphous cellular infiltrate that may extend beyond the node and into the surrounding fat. The peripheral sinuses of the node are open or dilated. The postcapillary venules are richly arborized, and the overall cellularity of the node may appear to be decreased at low power. The neoplastic cells vary in morphology, but are present in clusters and demonstrate abundant pale or clear cytoplasm and round or slightly irregular nuclei with condensed chromatin. Normal cells of a variety of types are part of the infiltrate, including proliferating vessels, normally appearing lymphocytes, plasma cells, immunoblasts, eosinophils, epithelioid histiocytes, and hyperplastic clusters of follicular dendritic cells. Any residual follicles appear 'burned out' in that they lack the usual lymphocyte populations and consist mainly of vessels and dendritic cells.

Immunophenotype

The abnormal cells are usually CD4$^+$ T cells that also express CD3. The clusters of follicular dendritic cells can be more readily detected by performing immunohistology using an antibody to CD21, which is expressed on these dendritic cells. In 10–15% of cases, immunoglobulin genes are *also* clonally rearranged.

Genetics

No specific genetic lesion has been identified, but genetic abnormalities are present in the neoplastic cells. Genetic lesions include trisomy 3 and/or an extra X chromosome. Trisomy 5 has also been reported. In many cases, clones with genetic lesions unrelated to the major cytogenetic changes were also found, suggesting oligoclonal proliferations as part of these disorders.

Clinical characteristics

AILD is a disease of adults; the median age is 60 years and the male-to-female ratio is 3–6:1. Patients present with a systemic illness characterized by fevers, weight loss, skin rash, generalized lymphadenopathy and polyclonal hypergammaglobulinemia. About half of the patients have hepatosplenomegaly, and many patients have evidence of autoimmunity, including Coombs' positive hemolytic anemia. Additional clinical problems include bone marrow involvement, pulmonary infiltrates, pleural effusions and circulating immune complexes. Infections are the cause of death in a majority of patients. The pathogenesis of the disease remains unknown. However, cytokines are felt to play a role. The hypergammaglobulinemia has been correlated with the levels of IL-4 produced by the tumor cells.

Treatment

The most effective treatment approach is the use of combination chemotherapy such as that used to treat diffuse aggressive-histology lymphoma (see Chapter 2). Some patients are curable with primary combination chemotherapy. Small numbers of patients have been reported to respond to chronic low-dose interferon treatment or to cyclosporine. Some authors begin treatment with prednisone alone, followed by interferon, with chemotherapy being reserved for patients in whom these treatments no longer work.

Adult T-cell leukemia/lymphoma

Definition and classification

Adult T-cell leukemia/lymphoma (ATL) was first recognized as a distinct clinical entity by Uchiyama and his colleagues in Japan in 1977. The causative agent, the human T-lymphotropic virus, type I (HTLV-I), was isolated by Poiesz and Ruscetti in the Gallo laboratory in 1979. An international collaboration rapidly demonstrated that the virus caused the clinical syndrome both in its endemic form in Japan and the Caribbean and in its sporadic form in Europe and the USA. ATL is a rapidly progressive systemic illness associated with circulating malignant cells, diffuse adenopathy, hypercalcemia, and an accompanying immunologic defect characteristic of CD4$^+$ T-cell dysfunction. The nodal pathology could be classified in many categories in the Working Formulation, including diffuse small cleaved cell, diffuse mixed, diffuse large cell, large cell immunoblastic, and diffuse small non-cleaved cell non-Burkitt's lymphoma. However, the clinicopathologic syndrome is readily identifiable, and is now known as ATL. Because of the features of the malignant cell, the disease is classified as a peripheral T-cell lymphoma.

Frequency

ATL accounts for about half of the lymphoid malignancies in endemic areas such as southwestern Japan, the Caribbean, central Africa, and Central and South America. Over one million people in Japan are infected with the virus, but only 400–500 new cases of ATL are diagnosed each year. The virus is transmitted mainly from mother to child, especially by breast milk. Sexual transmission and blood transfusion are minor routes of infection, and the risk of developing ATL from these exposures is lower because of the very long latency (20–60 years) between infection and disease. The lifetime risk of developing ATL is 0.5–7%, with the highest risk associated with neonatal infection. The annual risk among infected individuals is about 0.6–1.5/1000 carriers/year. Because the incidence of infection is higher in females but the incidence of ATL is higher in males, it is felt that females have a lower risk of progression than males. Tropical spastic paraparesis/HTLV-I-associated myelopathy (TSP/HAM) is another disease caused by HTLV-I in endemic areas. The disease is an inflammation of the pyramidal tract, and occurs with a much shorter latency than ATL.

Pathology

Histology

Lymph nodes and involved organs show a pleomorphic infiltrate of tumor cells that vary greatly in size. The cells have fluted nuclei that give the impression of flower petals, and so they are often called 'flower' cells. They are routinely observed on peripheral blood smear. In some cases, the malignant cells can mimic Reed–Sternberg cells. The involvement of the bone marrow with tumor is considerably less impressive given the high white blood cell counts that are often seen. Even when bone is involved with lytic lesions, these are usually free of tumor cells and represent the activation of osteoclasts by tumor-derived cytokines.

Immunophenotype

The malignant cells are peripheral T cells that express CD2, CD3 and CD4, but not CD7 or CD8. They express (and shed into the serum) large amounts of CD25, which can be used as a tumor marker. The cells also express other activation markers such as HLA-DR. However, the amount of CD3/TCR expressed is lower than on normal T cells.

Genetics

The T cells show a clonal integration of the HTLV-I provirus and clonal rearrangements of the *TCRβ* locus. The viral infection in the tumor cells is largely latent. Intact virions are not usually produced, and only the viral Tax protein is routinely detected, often in very small amounts. However, Tax can induce the expression of many genes that regulate cell proliferation, and it is thought that the viral-induced proliferation is necessary for the cells to accumulate additional genetic hits, only some of which are defined. About 30% of cases have mutant *p53*. Cytogenetic abnormalities may be present, though no signature alteration has been found. Structural changes in chromosome 14, especially 14q11, deletion of 6q, loss of an X or Y chromosome, and trisomy of 3, 7 and 21 have been noted.

Clinical characteristics

The median age of onset if 57 years in Japan; the male-to-female ratio is about 1.4. Among Caribbean Blacks, the median age of onset is about 45 years, with a male-to-female ratio of 0.6. The disease occurs in four different recognized forms (see Table 4.1). About 5% of patients have smouldering disease with low tumor volume and few stigmata of malignancy; five-year survival is about 70%. About

> **Table 4.1**
> **Diagnostic criteria for clinical subtypes of ATL**
>
> **Smoldering type**
> - ≤ 5% abnormal T cells in the peripheral blood
> - Normal total lymphocyte count
> - Normal serum calcium; LDH ≤ 1.5 times normal
> - No adenopathy, liver, spleen, CNS, bone or GI-tract involvement; no ascites or effusion
> - Skin and pulmonary lesions may be present (biopsy-documented)
>
> **Chronic type**
> - Absolute lymphocytosis ≥ 400/μl with flower cells
> - Normal serum calcium; LDH ≤ 2 times normal
> - No CNS, bone, GI-tract involvement; no ascites or effusion
> - Involvement of skin, spleen, liver, lung and nodes may be present
>
> **Lymphoma**
> - No lymphocytosis, with ≤ 1% abnormal lymphocytes
> - Histologically positive nodes
>
> **Acute type**
> - Everyone else
> - Usually with leukemia, adenopathy, hypercalcemia
>
> CNS, central nervous system; GI, gastrointestinal; LDH, lactate dehydrogenase.

hypercalcemia, weakness, poor performance status and a skin rash. On laboratory examination, the peripheral white blood cell count is high owing to the presence of many 'flower' cells. Shortness of breath may be accompanied by diffuse bilateral pulmonary infiltrates. The differential diagnosis includes opportunistic infection with *Pneumocystis carinii* or other pathogens or leukemic infiltration. Infection and leukemic infiltration each affect about half of the patients with respiratory problems. The skin lesions are variable, ranging from a localized papular eruption to a generalized erythroderma. However, unlike the erythroderma of cutaneous T-cell lymphoma/ Sézary syndrome, the rash of ATL usually does not itch. The stomach wall may be infiltrated with tumor cells, and diarrhea and malabsorption may reflect small-bowel involvement. Gastrointestinal tract involvement is unusual in other forms of peripheral T-cell lymphoma, but may be seen in about 25% of ATL patients. Leptomeningeal involvement of the central nervous system occurs in about 10% of patients, and is more common in the lymphoma-type presentation. Unlike other forms of neoplastic meningitis, cerebrospinal fluid (CSF) protein is often normal in patients with ATL involvement of the central nervous system; therefore a normal CSF protein level does not rule out the diagnosis. Usually 'flower' cells are detectable on cytocentrifuge specimens.

19% of patients have chronic-type disease. They have greater numbers of circulating tumor cells, and can have involvement of skin, liver, spleen, lung and lymph nodes, but no involvement of the central nervous system, bone or gastrointestinal tract, and no effusions or ascites can be present. The five-year survival of this group is about 25%. About 19% of patients present with mainly nodal disease (this presentation may be somewhat more common in the West), and the majority of patients (57%) present with acute-type disease. The prognosis of these two groups is similar and dismal; long-term survival is very rare.

The most common form, the acute type, usually presents with a short prodrome of no more than two weeks. Patients present with fever, infection,

Treatment

Given the relationship between the disease and infection with HTLV-I, the best approach is to prevent the infection, which will prevent the disease. The most effective preventive measure is to keep HTLV-I-seropositive mothers from nursing their newborn babies. Blood bank screening has greatly reduced the risk of transmission through blood products, and sexual transmission of the virus is inefficient.

If the disease develops, treatments are largely unsatisfactory. No standard approach has been developed. All patients should be treated as a part of a clinical trial aimed at making systematic observations about treatment response.

Bibliography

Armitage JO, Greer JP, Levine AM et al, Peripheral T-cell lymphoma. *Cancer* 1989; **63:** 158–63.

Armitage JO, Vose JM, Linder J et al, Clinical significance of immunophenotype in diffuse aggressive non-Hodgkin's lymphoma. *J Clin Oncol* 1989; **9:** 1426–31.

Coiffier B, Brousse N, Peuchmaur M et al, Peripheral T-cell lymphomas have a worse prognosis than B-cell lymphomas: a prospective study of 361 immunophenotyped patients treated with the LNH84 regimen. *Ann Oncol* 1990; **1:** 45–50.

Falini A, Pileri S, DeSolas I et al, Peripheral T-cell lymphoma associated with hemophagocytic syndrome. *Blood* 1990; **75:** 434–44.

Gill PS, Harrington W Jr, Kaplan MK et al, Treatment of adult T-cell leukemia/lymphoma with a combination of interferon-alpha and zidovudine. *N Engl J Med* 1995; **332:** 1744–8.

Gisselbrecht C, Gaulard P, Lepage E et al, Prognostic significance of T-cell phenotype in aggressive non-Hodgkin's lymphomas. *Blood* 1998; **92:** 76–82.

Henni T, Gaulard P, Divine M et al, Comparison of genetic probe with immunophenotype analysis in lymphoproliferative disorders: a study of 87 cases. *Blood* 1988; **72:** 1937–43.

Hsu SM, Waldron JW, Hsu PL et al, Cytokines in malignant lymphomas: review and prospective evaluation. *Hum Pathol* 1993; **24:** 1040–57.

Jaffe E, Blattner W, Blayney D et al, The pathologic spectrum of adult T-cell leukemia/lymphoma in the United States. *Am J Surg Pathol* 1984; **8:** 263–75.

Kamada N, Sakurai M, Miyamoto K et al, Chromosome abnormalities in adult T-cell leukemia/lymphoma: a Karyotype Review Committee report. *Cancer Res* 1992; **52:** 1481–93.

Karakas T, Bergmann L, Stutte HJ et al, Peripheral T-cell lymphomas respond well to vincristine, Adriamycin, cyclophosphamide, prednisone, and etoposide (VACPE) and have a similar outcome as high-grade B-cell lymphomas. *Leuk Lymphoma* 1996; **24:** 121–9.

Kwak LW, Wilson M, Weiss LM et al, Similar outcome of treatment of B-cell and T-cell diffuse large-cell lymphomas: the Stanford experience. *J Clin Oncol* 1991; **9:** 1426–31.

Poiesz B, Ruscetti F, Gazdar A et al, Detection and isolation of type C retrovirus particles from fresh and cultured lymphocytes of a patient with cutaneous T-cell lymphoma. *Proc Natl Acad Sci USA* 1980; **77:** 7415–19.

Rodriguez J, Pugh WC, Cabanillas F, T-cell rich B-cell lymphoma. *Blood* 1993; **82:** 1586–9.

Schlegelberger B, Himmler A, Godde E et al, Cytogenetic findings in peripheral T-cell lymphomas as a basis for distinguishing low-grade and high-grade lymphomas. *Blood* 1994; **83:** 505–11.

Schlegelberger B, Zhang Y, Weber-Matthiesen K et al, Detection of aberrant clones in nearly all cases of angioimmunoblastic lymphoadenopathy with dysproteinemia-type T-cell lymphoma by combined interphase and metaphase cytogenetics. *Blood* 1994; **84:** 1640–8.

Shimoyama M, Takatsuki K, Araki K et al, Major prognostic factors of patients with adult T-cell leukemia/lymphoma: a cooperative study. *Leuk Res* 1991; **15:** 81–90.

Siegert W, Agthe A, Griesser H et al, Treatment of angioimmunoblastic lymphadenopathy (AILD)-type T-cell lymphoma using prednisone with or without the COP-BLAM/IMVP-16 regimen. A multicenter study. Kiel Lymphoma Study Group. *Ann Intern Med* 1992; **117:** 364–70.

Uchiyama T, Yodoi J, Sagawa K et al, Adult T-cell leukemia: clinical and hematologic features of 16 cases. *Blood* 1977; **50:** 481–92.

Vose JM, Peterson C, Bierman PJ et al, Comparison of high-dose therapy and autologous bone marrow transplantation for T-cell and B-cell non-Hodgkin's lymphomas. *Blood* 1990; **76:** 424–31.

Weiss LM, Strickler JG, Dorfman RF et al, Clonal T-cell populations in angioimmunoblastic lymphadenopathy and angioimmunoblastic lymphadenopathy-like lymphoma. *Am J Pathol* 1986; **122:** 392–7.

Peripheral T-cell lymphoma, unspecified type

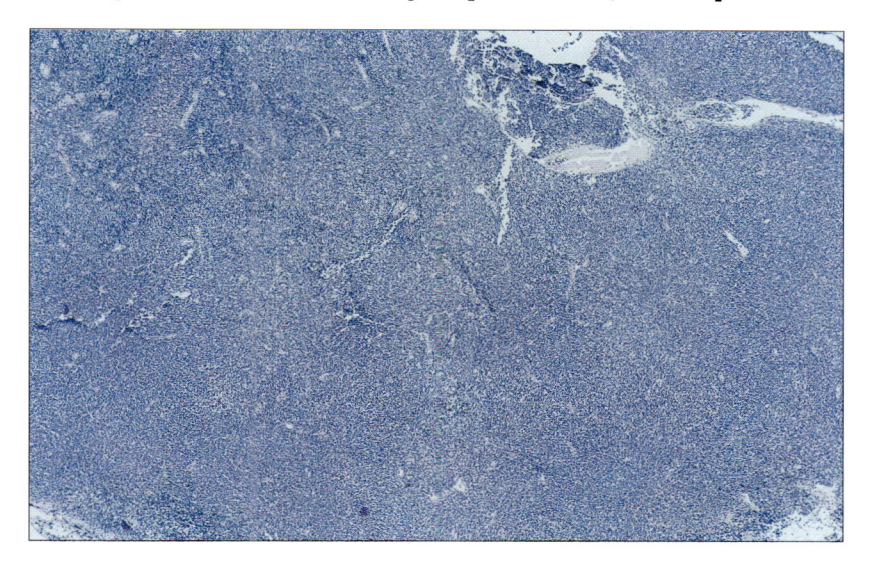

Figure 4.1

Peripheral T-cell lymphoma, unspecified type:

(a) This lymphoma involves the nose, but lacks the distinctive features of angiocentric (nasal/nasal-type T/NK-cell) lymphoma, and is thus classified as peripheral T-cell lymphoma, unspecified. There is a dense diffuse infiltrate of atypical lymphoid cells. (H&E stain)

(b) A very thin layer of residual squamous epithelium overlies the lymphoma in some areas. (H&E stain)

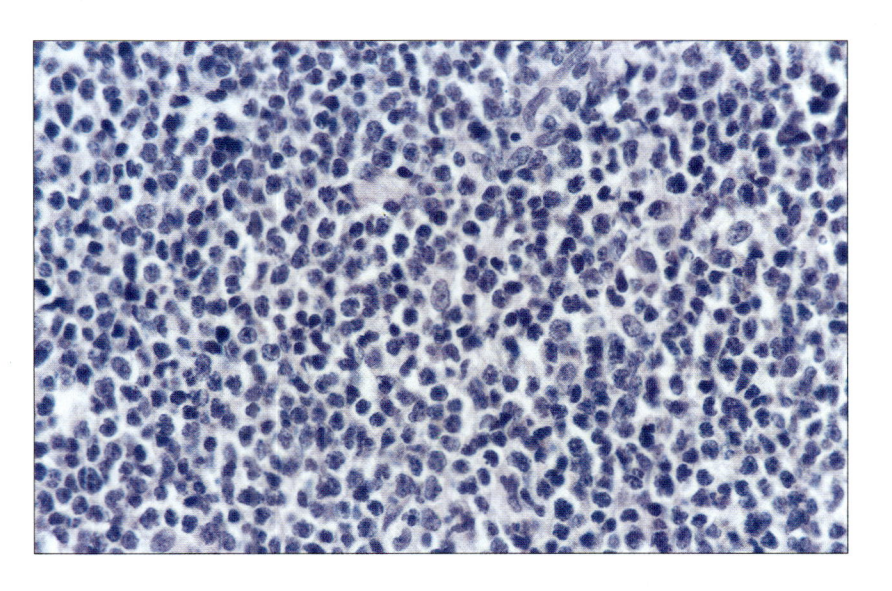

(c) The neoplastic cells are slightly larger than small lymphocytes, and have irregular nuclei. This case would fall into the 'medium-sized cell' category (H&E stain)

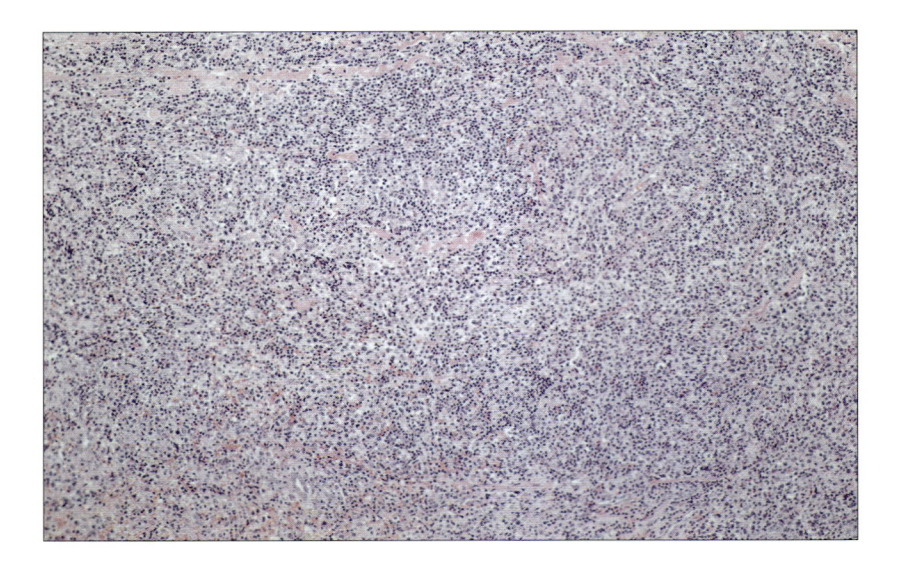

Figure 4.2

Peripheral T-cell lymphoma, unspecified type:

(a) This lymphoma involves a lymph node. There is diffuse obliteration of the nodal architecture. (H&E stain)

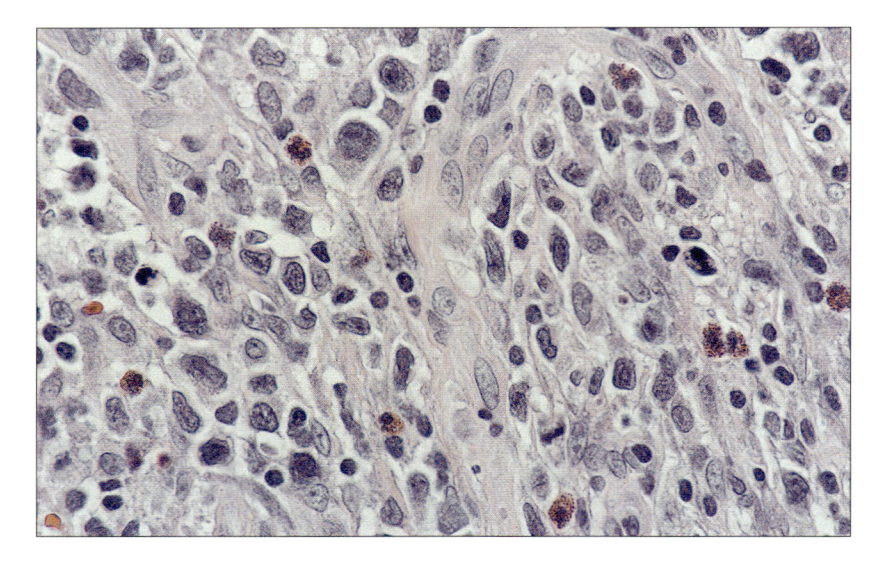

(b) High-power examination shows intermediate- and large-sized atypical lymphoid cells. This case would be subclassified in the 'medium and large cell' category. (H&E stain)

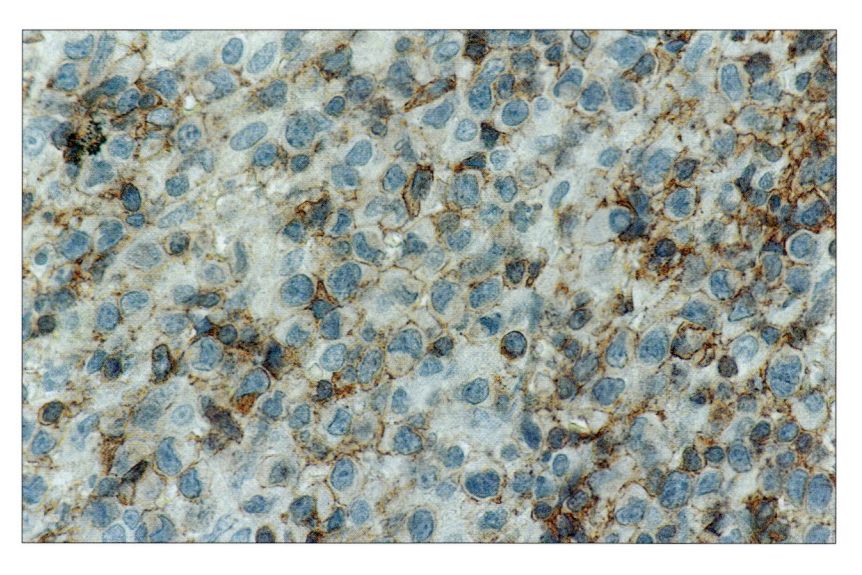

(c) The neoplastic cells express T-cell-associated antigens (CD3 shown here). (Immunoperoxidase technique on paraffin sections)

Angioimmunoblastic T-cell lymphomas

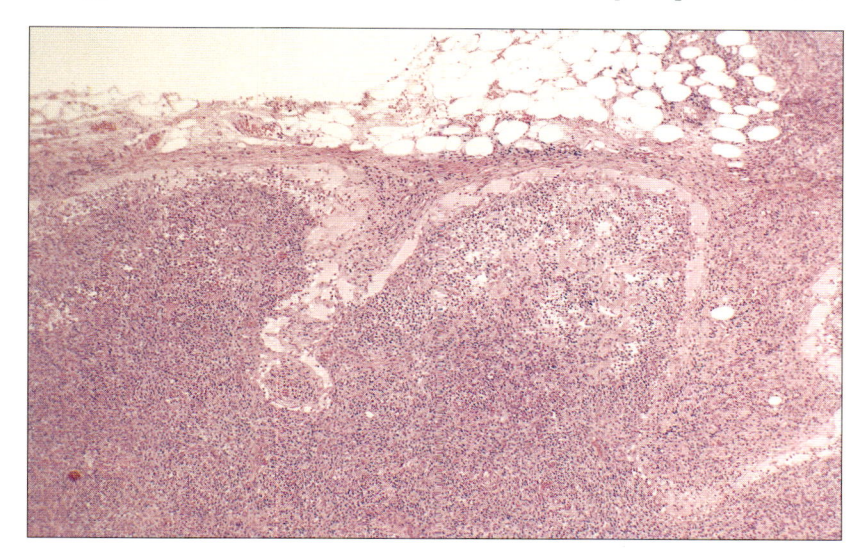

Figure 4.3

Angioimmunoblastic T-cell lymphoma:

(a) The lymphoma obliterates the normal nodal architecture and extends into perinodal fat. The subcapsular sinus, however, remains widely patent. (H&E stain)

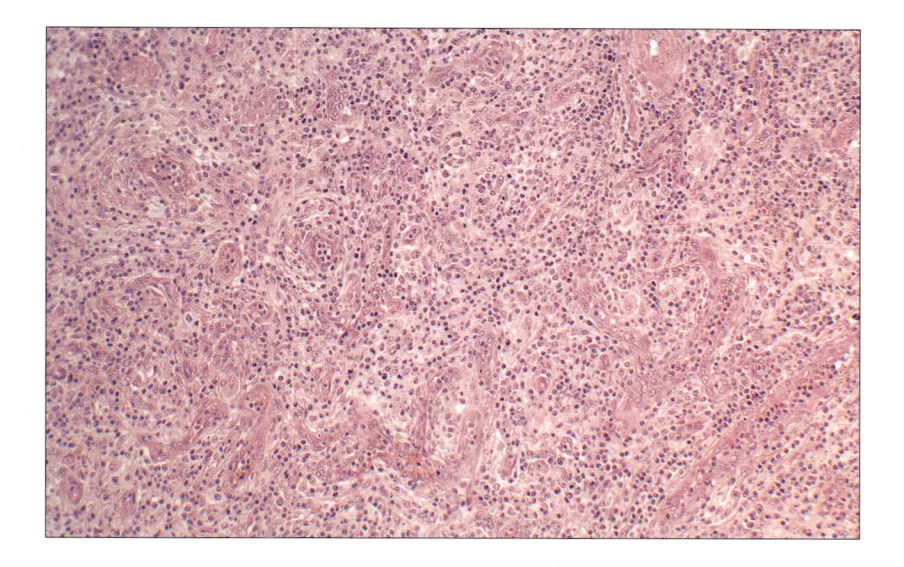

(b) Numerous small blood vessels course through the lymphoma. (H&E stain)

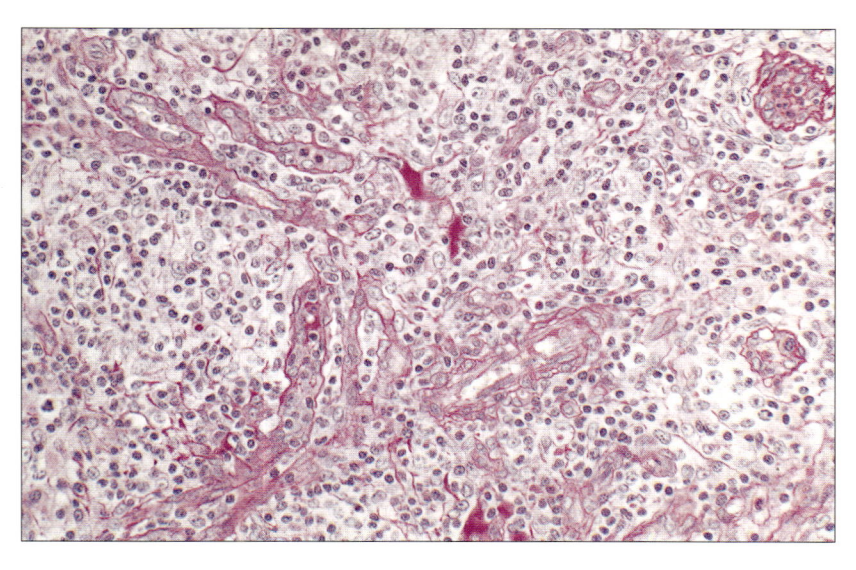

(c) A PAS stain highlights the basement membranes of the blood vessels.

Contd

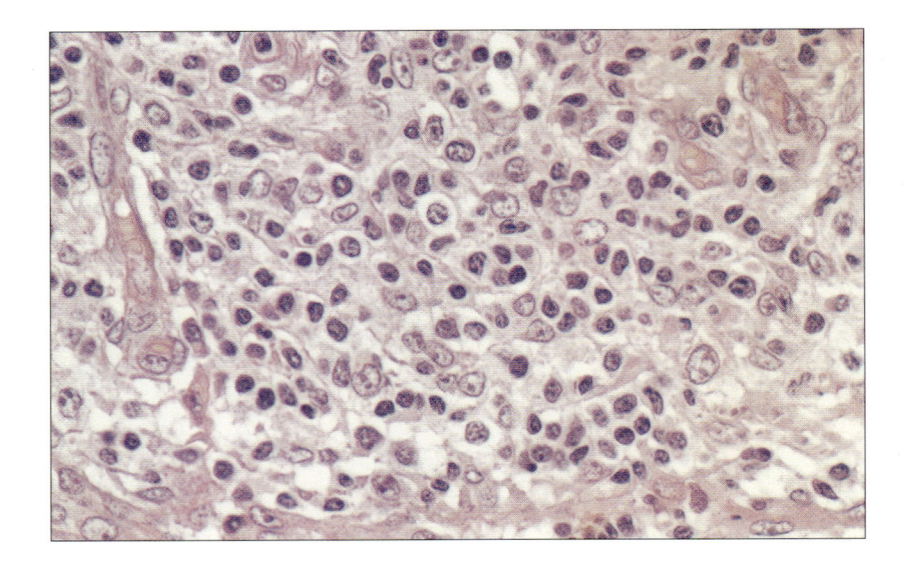

Figure 4.3 *continued*

(d) The neoplastic cells are predominantly intermediate-sized lymphoid cells with oval to slightly irregular nuclei and abundant clear cytoplasm. (H&E stain)

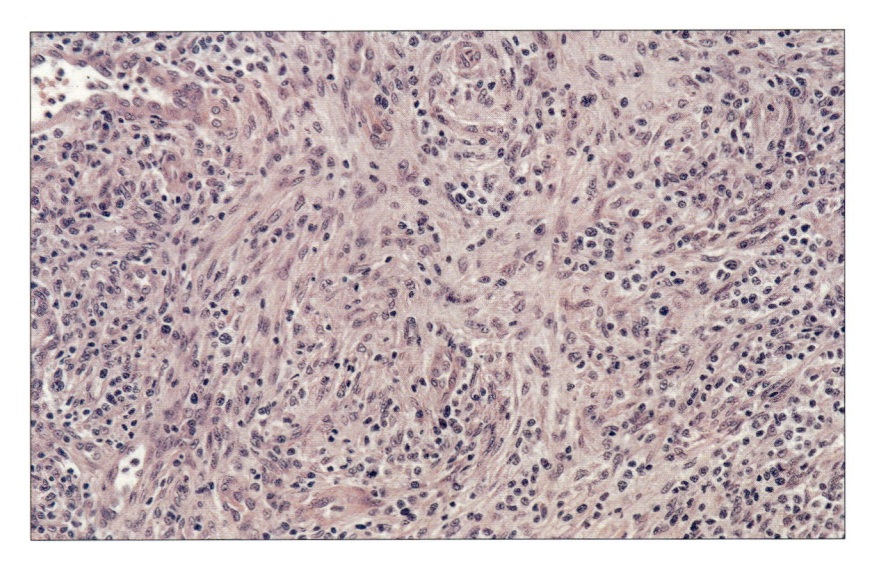

(e) In areas, aggregates of follicular dendritic cells resembling 'burnt-out' follicular centers are seen. (H&E stain)

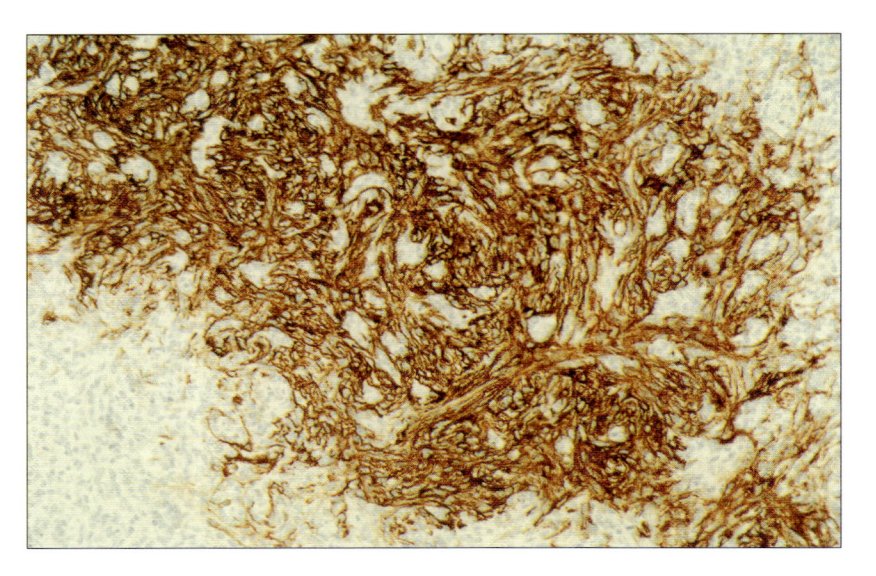

(f) There is an extensive network of CD21+ follicular dendritic cells. (Immunoperoxidase technique on paraffin sections)

Adult T-cell leukemia/lymphoma

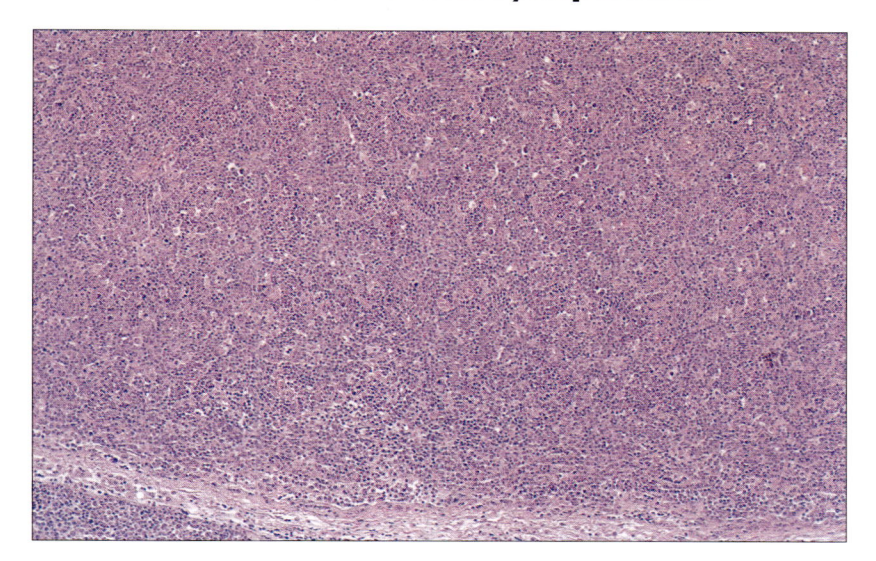

Figure 4.4

Adult T-cell leukemia/lymphoma:

(a) The normal architecture of the lymph node is obliterated. (H&E stain)

(b) Higher power shows intermediate- and large-sized atypical lymphoid cells. (H&E stain)

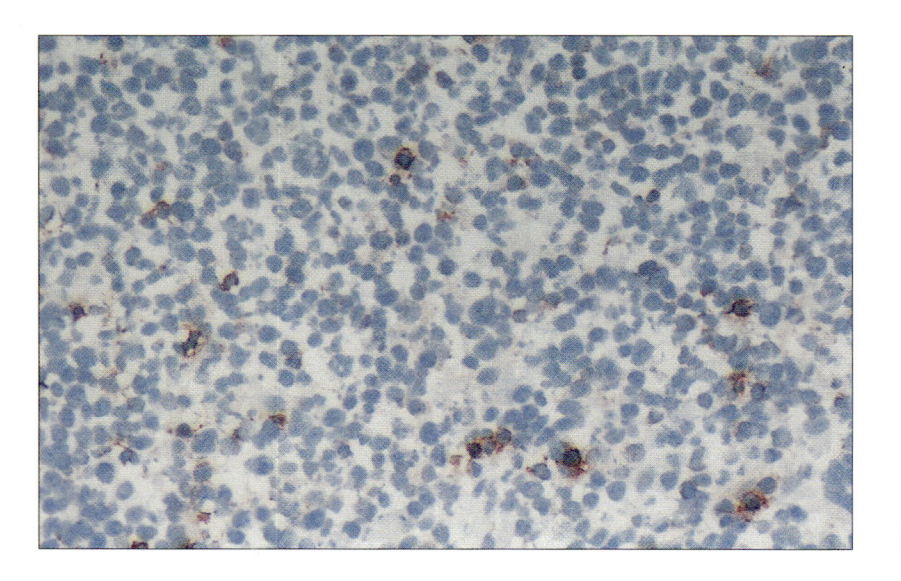

Neoplastic cells lack CD8 (**c**) but express CD4 (**d**). (Immunoperoxidase technique on frozen sections)

(c)

Contd

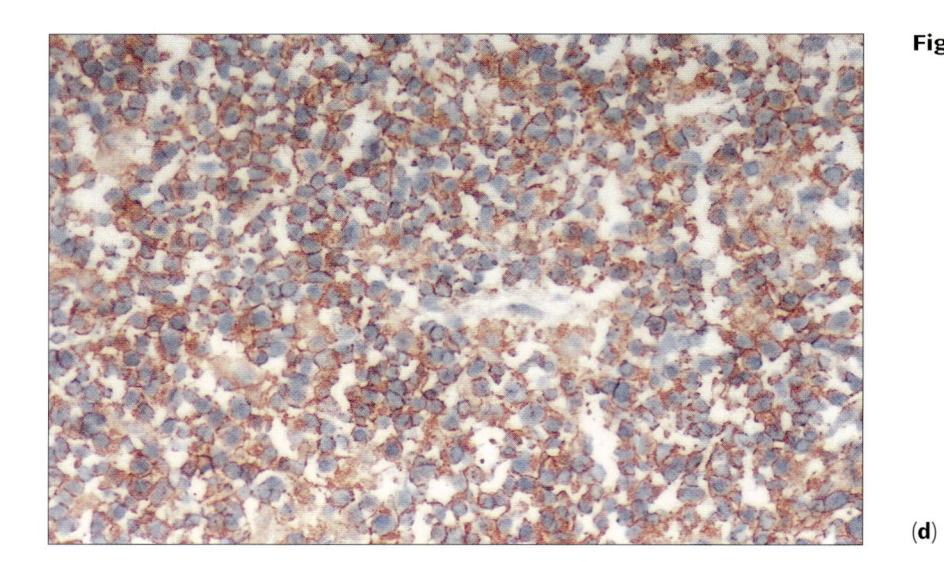

Figure 4.4 *continued*

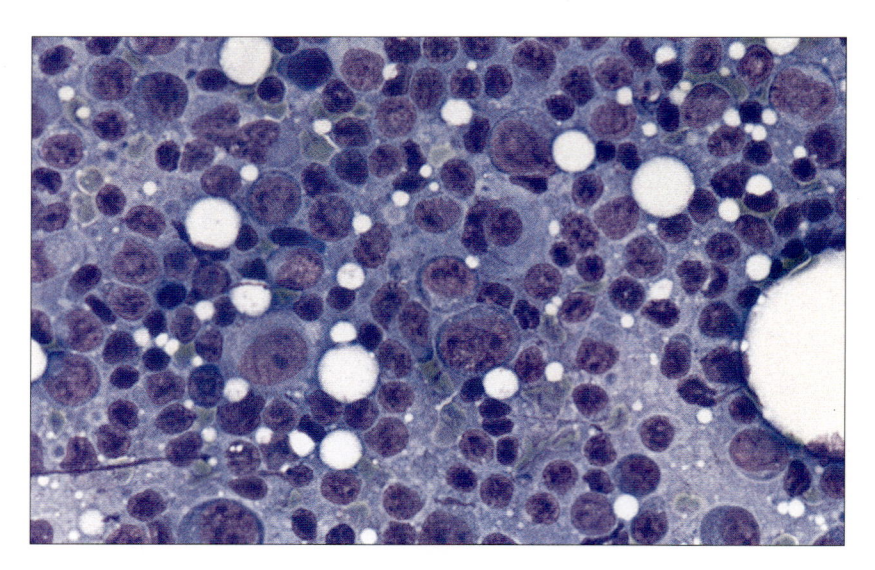

(d)

(e) A Wright-stained aspirate of a lymph node shows a similar population of small-, intermediate- and large-sized atypical lymphoid cells.

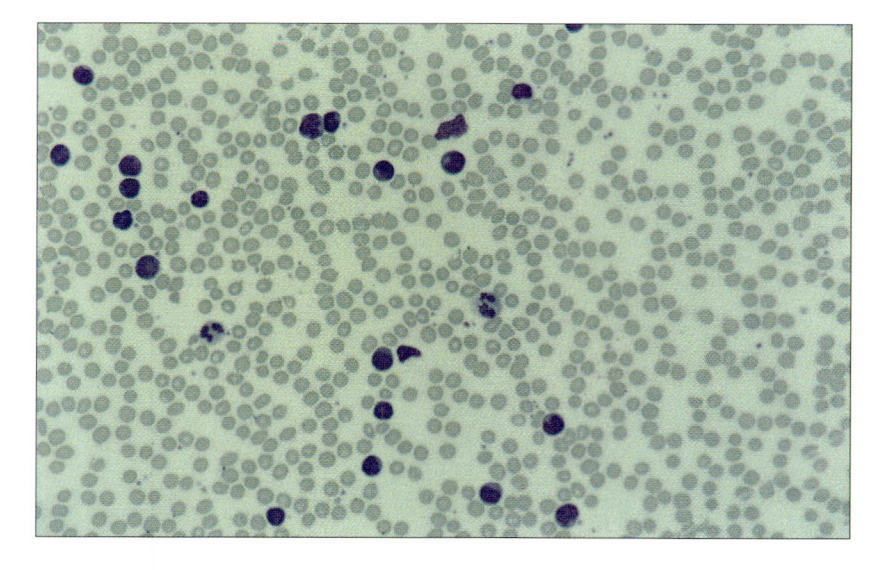

(f) The peripheral blood shows a lymphocytosis. (Wright stain)

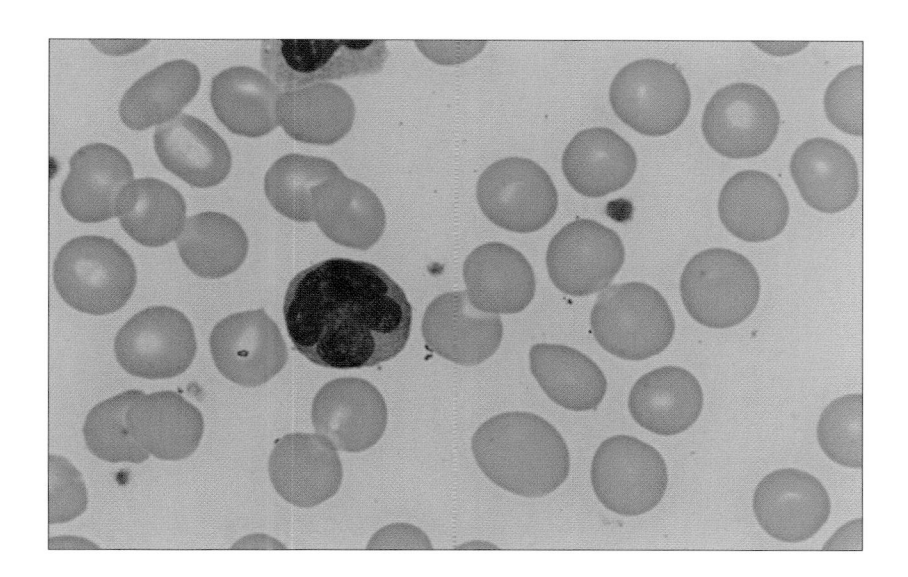

Figure 4.4 *continued*

(g) The circulating cells are atypical lymphoid cells with lobated nuclei (flower cells). (Wright stain)

5 Small lymphocytic lymphoma/Chronic lymphocytic leukemia

Definition and classification

Chronic lymphocytic leukemia and small lymphocytic lymphoma form a single disease entity derived from a common lymphocyte population. The vast majority of cases are of B-cell origin, and, in particular, the disease emerges from the CD5+ B-cell subset, which generally responds to antigenic stimulation without the help of T cells that recognize the same antigen (so-called cognate T-cell help). Most commonly, patients have both bone marrow involvement and peripheral adenopathy. When adenopathy dominates the clinical picture and the peripheral white blood cell count is less than 15 000/μl (or the absolute lymphocyte count is less than 4000/μl), the disease is often designated 'small lymphocytic lymphoma'. The distribution of the tumor cells in the body may depend on the expression of particular adhesion molecules on the cell surface. In the Rappaport scheme, small lymphocytic lymphoma was designated 'diffuse well-differentiated lymphocytic lymphoma'; this reflected the diffuse pattern of growth and the normal cytology of the malignant cells. However, like other lymphomas, this is a clonal malignancy.

Rarely, chronic lymphocytic leukemia is derived from peripheral T cells. In these instances, the cells are usually somewhat larger than small lymphocytes, the natural history of the disease is more aggressive, and patients develop very high white blood cell counts with little adenopathy. The vast majority of these cases represent a small cell variant of T-cell prolymphocytic leukemia.

Frequency

About 12 500 cases are diagnosed in the USA each year. Chronic lymphocytic leukemia is the most common form of leukemia in the Western world, accounting for 25% of cases. The incidence is declining; it fell from 3.3 per 100 000 in 1973 to 2.3 per 100 000 in 1990. The disease is more common in Whites than in African–Americans, and is extremely uncommon in Asia. This entity accounted for 6.7% of the 1400 cases that were reviewed by the Non-Hodgkin's Lymphoma Classification Project, drawn from nine centers worldwide.

Pathology

Histology

Lymph node architecture is effaced and the nodes are usually diffusely infiltrated with sheets of small lymphocytes. Occasionally, involved nodes demonstrate the presence of naked germinal centers. A similar pattern may be present in mantle-cell lymphoma; however, the cells are usually distinguishable on the basis of differences in cell morphology (see Chapter 6). In small lymphocytic lymphoma, the cells are usually about the size of normal resting lymphocytes; the nuclear chromatin is clumped and the cytoplasm is sparse and basophilic. Some variation in nuclear contour is seen, but this feature has no prognostic significance.

In addition to the small lymphocytes, aggregates of larger cells called proliferation centers are present. Because of their shape and the presence of cells of various sizes, these growth centers may be called pseudofollicles. At least three cell types are present in proliferation centers: small lymphocytes, larger cells called prolymphocytes, and (the largest cells) paraimmunoblasts. The prolymphocytes and paraimmunoblasts have more dispersed nuclear chromatin, usually with a prominent central nucleolus, and more abundant cytoplasm than small lymphocytes, which is also lighter-staining.

Bone marrow involvement with small lymphocytic lymphoma can be patchy (nodular), interstitial (lacy) or diffuse. Nodular or interstitial involvement generally has a better prognosis and reflects a lower tumor burden. The malignant cells are fragile, and peripheral blood smears frequently show 'smudge cells' or 'Gumprecht's shadows', cell remnants destroyed in the process of making the smear.

Similarly to follicular lymphoma, small lymphocytic lymphoma can progress to diffuse large B-cell lymphoma, but it does so at a much lower rate than does follicular lymphoma. This histologic transformation is called Richter's syndrome. The change in histology is accompanied by an acceleration in the natural history of the disease. In addition to the fact that transformation is more unusual in small lymphocytic lymphoma (about 10–15%), sometimes the large cell lymphoma appears to be derived from a different B cell than the original tumor – a feature that is exceedingly rare in follicular lymphoma. In addition, the transformation of small lymphocytic lymphoma may lead to a cell that resembles the Reed–Sternberg cell of Hodgkin's disease. The Hodgkin's-like transformation is often associated with Epstein–Barr virus infection of the malignant cell.

Immunophenotype

The malignant cell is a mature B cell derived from the B1 subset of cells. The cells express fewer numbers of surface immunoglobulin molecules (IgM) than follicular center cells, and the expression of CD20 and CD22 is also weaker than in mantle cells or follicular center cells. Small lymphocytic lymphoma cells are $CD5^+$ and are usually $CD23^+$; mantle-cell lymphoma cells are $CD5^+$ and $CD23^-$. Antigens expressed on these cells that are detectable in paraffin sections include CD43, CD20 and CD79a. The B1 subset of B cells does not develop immunologic memory (probably because of the absence of T-cell help), and the antibody repertoire produced by this cell subset is not capable of undergoing affinity maturation (a process that occurs in follicular centers). Furthermore, many autoantibodies are derived from this subset of cells, with each antibody recognizing antigens on multiple normal tissues. The B1 subset of cells is generally long-lived and circulates freely throughout the body. These cells populate the mantle zones of lymph nodes, but mantle-cell lymphoma has different genetic lesions and different clinical manifestations than small lymphocytic lymphoma.

Genetics

About 30% of cases show trisomy of chromosome 12, and this alteration is said to convey a more aggressive natural history. About 25% of cases have deletions involving the retinoblastoma gene product on chromosome 13q. The development of a 14q+ abnormality (often with the breakpoint at the site of the immunoglobulin heavy-chain gene at 14q32) may be a harbinger of progression either to a more aggressive prolymphocytic variant of small lymphocytic lymphoma or to Richter's syndrome.

Clinical characteristics

The disease increases in frequency with age (median age 61 years), and is twice as common in men as in women. Leukemia is a more common presentation than lymphoma. Many patients are discovered to have chronic lymphocytic leukemia incidentally when a complete blood count documents absolute small lymphocytosis. Yet even patients with peripheral blood involvement usually have diffuse adenopathy (80%). Similarly, when adenopathy is the presenting feature of the illness, the bone marrow is nearly always also involved, and a careful examination of the peripheral blood usually demonstrates the presence of circulating monoclonal CD5+ B cells. As the disease progresses, patients develop splenomegaly and hepatomegaly. About half of the patients have a palpable spleen at presentation. Extranodal involvement may occur in a minority of patients.

B symptoms are highly unusual. A patient presenting with fevers most likely has an infection. This disease is associated with hypogammaglobulinemia as well as cellular immune defects. Thus infection is a major cause of morbidity and mortality in these patients. Patients also have an increased risk of autoimmune phenomena. Autoimmune hemolytic anemia and immune thrombocytopenic purpura are the most common, but pure red cell aplasia and autoimmune neutropenia may also occur. Most often, the pathogenesis of the autoimmune phenomena is the production of autoantibody by a cell other than the malignant B cell clone. However, some tumor cells produce autoreactive antibodies.

Patients may develop anemia or thrombocytopenia during the course of disease, and the etiology may be complex. When the mechanism is increased destruction by an autoantibody or by hypersplenism, appropriate treatment can completely reverse the problem, and the natural history of the disease is relatively unaffected. When the mechanism is decreased production due to marrow infiltration with tumor cells, the prognosis is poor.

Two staging systems are in widespread use for chronic lymphocytic leukemia: the Rai system and the Binet system (see Table 5.1). These systems relate prognosis to the development of progressive marrow failure, and are more accurate at predicting the natural history of disease than the Ann Arbor staging classification for lymphoma. In the Ann Arbor staging system, nearly all the patients have stage IVA disease.

Table 5.1
Staging systems for small lymphocytic lynphoma/chronic lymphocytic leukemia

Rai clinical staging system[a]

Stage	Clinical features at diagnosis	Median survival (months)
0	Blood and marrow lymphocytosis	>150
I	Lymphocytosis and enlarged nodes	101
II	Lymphocytosis and large spleen and/or liver	>71
III	Lymphocytosis and anemia (<11 g/dl)	19
IV	Lymphocytosis and thrombocytopenia (<100 000/μl)	19

[a]This system has been simplified to three stages by grouping I and II together and III and IV together

Binet clinical staging system

Stage	Clinical features at diagnosis	Median survival (years)
A	Blood and marrow lymphocytosis and less than three areas of palpable lymphoid tissue enlargement	>7
B	Blood and marrow lymphocytosis and three or more areas of palpable lymphoid tissue enlargement	<5
C	Same as B with anemia (hgb < 11 g/dl in men; < 10 g/dl in women) or thrombocytopenia (plts < 100 000/μl)	<2

Treatment

Supportive care is very important in the management of patients with chronic lymphocytic leukemia/small lymphocytic lymphoma. Patients who develop a serious infection in the face of hypogammaglobulinemia should receive monthly intravenous injections of immunoglobulin. Patients who develop autoimmune anemia or thrombocytopenia should receive prednisone 1 mg/kg/day, with doses tapered to the minimum necessary to control the autoimmunity. For those who develop pure red cell aplasia, cyclosporine plus prednisone appears to be more effective than prednisone alone. Patients with hypersplenism should undergo splenectomy.

Randomized clinical trials have demonstrated that treatment of early-stage disease does not improve survival. In general, antitumor therapy is withheld until one or more of the following symptoms or signs develops: anemia or thrombocytopenia related to marrow replacement, disease-related symptoms, symptomatic adenopathy (nodes compressing a hollow viscus like bowel or ureter or putting pressure on a nerve), blood lymphocyte doubling time shorter than 4–6 months, or transformation either to a prolymphocytic variant or to Richter's syndrome (diffuse large B-cell lymphoma). Elevated white blood cell count alone is not an indication for treatment. Patients do not experience any untoward effects from peripheral blood count elevations as high as 800 000/µl from chronic lymphocytic leukemia lymphocytes, but above that level hyperviscosity may become a problem.

Perhaps 2% of patients may present with localized nodal disease, and careful examination of the bone marrow and peripheral blood does not detect involvement. For these rare patients, radiation therapy may be curative. No therapy currently available is considered curative for the 98% of patients who do not have localized disease; however, many agents are capable of producing significant antitumor effects. The most powerful of these are the nucleosides, particularly fludarabine (25 mg/m^2 daily × 5 every 4 weeks) and cladribine (0.1 mg/kg daily × 7 every 4 weeks). Pentostatin is also highly active. Oral alkylating agents such as chlorambucil and cyclophosphamide induce responses in the majority of patients when used as initial therapy, and the response is improved by addition of a glucocorticoid. Because the nucleosides are myelotoxic and lymphotoxic, their use is associated with an increased risk of infection, and so glucocorticoids should not be given together with nucleosides. However, rational combinations of nucleosides with alkylating agents and with cytosine arabinoside are currently being tested. The advantage of nucleosides is that a large fraction of patients achieve clinical complete remissions; fewer patients treated with alkylating agents achieve complete remission, but the acute toxicity is less than that seen with nucleosides.

For younger patients and those who have more aggressive disease, experimental approaches employing high-dose therapy with either autologous or allogeneic stem cell transplantation may offer advantages over conventional-dose therapy. The graft-versus-tumor effects seen in allogeneic transplantation have led to prolonged remissions in the highly selected small subset of patients who have received this treatment approach.

Older patients may die of intercurrent illness or of infection before the chronic lymphocytic leukemia/small lymphocytic lymphoma progresses to life-threatening status. These patients have an increased risk of second malignancies, including melanoma, lung cancer, colorectal cancer and soft tissue sarcomas. Multiple myeloma is 10 times more frequent in patients with chronic lymphocytic leukemia/small lymphocytic lymphoma than in the general population.

Patients who do not die of infection or second neoplasm may die from progressive marrow failure as tumor cells replace the hematopoietic elements. In addition, the disease may transform into more aggressive disease in three ways: to prolymphocytic leukemia (10%), Richter's syndrome (10%) or acute lymphoblastic leukemia (rare). The survival after each type of transformation is only a few months unless the disease is successfully treated.

Other small lymphocytic leukemia/lymphomas

In addition to B-cell chronic lymphocytic leukemia/small lymphocytic lymphoma, five other entities either have a chronic course or are derived from cells that resemble small lymphocytes. All together, they are about 10% as frequent as B-cell chronic lymphocytic leukemia/small lymphocytic lymphoma.

B-prolymphocytic leukemia

Rare patients present with high peripheral white blood cell counts (>100 000/µl) and neoplastic B cells that are somewhat larger than those seen in chronic lymphocytic leukemia, but marker studies are similar, though only half express CD5. The cells frequently have a 14q+ defect, and deletions in chromosome 6q and rearrangements of chromosomes 1 and 12 are occasionally seen. The patients are often over 70 years old, and fatigue, weakness, weight loss and splenomegaly are more prominent features of the disease. Nucleosides are moderately active, but the median survival is only three years.

Hairy cell leukemia

This rare B-cell tumor produces symptoms from splenomegaly and pancytopenia. The pancytopenia is related to reversible marrow fibrosis and the production of cytokines that inhibit hematopoiesis. The malignant B cells are strongly surface-immunoglobulin-positive, and they express CD11c, CD19, CD20, CD22 and CD25 in increased amounts. Soluble CD25 levels can act as a tumor marker. The cells express a tartrate-resistant alkaline phosphatase that can be detected histochemically. CD103 is said to be more or less specific for hairy cell leukemia. Circulating leukemic cells usually do not exceed 5000/µl. Nucleosides are highly effective at treating this disease; long-term remissions are usually obtained. Interferon-α is also effective, but remissions are not as durable.

T-chronic lymphocytic leukemia

This is a disease of small lymphocytes that express CD3 and either CD4 or CD8 but not both. Patients have adenopathy, marked lymphocytosis, diffuse marrow infiltration, and skin involvement. The distinction of this disease from cutaneous T-cell lymphoma/Sézary syndrome is based on the absence of Pautrier's microabscesses in T-chronic lymphocytic leukemia and the presence of more convoluted nuclear contour in Sézary syndrome. Survival with this disease is usually less than two years.

T-prolymphocytic leukemia

This disease of prominently nucleolated larger lymphocytes is characterized by distinctive chromosomal rearrangements and inversions involving the long arm of chromosome 14. The three most common changes are inv(14)(q11;q32.1), a balanced translocation t(14;14)(q11;q32.1), and translocations with inverted duplication of the region 14q32–14qter. These changes all involve activation of the TCL1 locus at 14q32.1 by juxtaposition with a T-cell antigen receptor gene locus, usually *TCRα* at 14q11. It is not clear what TCL1 does, but transgenic mice overexpressing this protein develop T-prolymphocytic leukemia. The malignant cells express CD2 and CD3; about 75% express CD4, 20% express CD8, and some express both. The CD7 antigen, which is usually present on thymocytes, is also expressed on these cells. The disease is more common in people with ataxia telangiectasia, a genetic disorder of DNA repair. The disease is rapidly progressive, with high white blood cell counts, diffuse rapidly progressive adenopathy, diffuse skin lesions, and splenomegaly. Median survival is about six months.

Large granular lymphocytic leukemia

Two types of malignant cells give rise to large granular lymphocytic leukemia: one is a $CD3^+CD8^+$ T cell and the other is a $CD56^+CD3^-$ natural killer (NK) cell. Patients often present with immune abnormalities such as recurrent infections (40%), rheumatoid arthritis (30%), splenomegaly (50%) and hepatomegaly (25%), and the bone marrow is infiltrated with large granular lymphocytes. Patients usually present with anemia and neutropenia. Morbidity and mortality are usually related to neutropenia. The T-cell disorder is more common and more chronic in its natural history; the NK-cell variant is rapidly progressive, with death occurring within two to three months from multiorgan failure.

Bibliography

Ben Ezra J, Burke JS, Swartz WG et al, Small lymphocytic lymphoma: a clinicopathologic analysis of 268 cases. *Blood* 1989; **73:** 579–87.

Byrd JC, Flinn IW, Grever MR (eds), Chronic lymphocytic leukemia. *Semin Oncol* 1998; **25:** 4–125.

Chikkappa G, Pasquale D, Zarrabi MH et al, Cyclosporine and prednisone therapy for pure red cell aplasia in patients with chronic lymphocytic leukemia. *Am J Hematol* 1992; **41:** 5–11.

DiGhiero G, Maloum K, Desablens B et al, Chlorambucil in indolent chronic lymphocytic leukemia. French Cooperative Group on Chronic Lymphocytic Leukemia. *N Engl J Med* 1998; **338:** 1506–14.

Dreger P, von Neuhoff N, Kuse R et al, Early stem cell transplantation for chronic lymphocytic leukaemia: a chance for cure? *Br J Cancer* 1998; **77:** 2291–7.

Galton DAG, Goldman JM, Wiltshaw E et al, Prolymphocytic leukemia. *Br J Haematol* 1974; **27:** 7–23.

Gatti RA, McConville CM, Taylor AMR, Sixth International Workshop on Ataxia-Telangiectasia. *Cancer Res* 1994; **54:** 6007–10.

Hoyer JD, Ross CW, Li CY et al, True T-cell chronic lymphocytic leukemia: a morphologic and immunophenotypic study of 25 cases. *Blood* 1995; **86:** 1163–9.

Jurlander J, The cellular biology of B-cell chronic lymphocytic leukemia. *Crit Rev Oncol Hematol* 1998; **27:** 29–52.

Keating MJ, O'Brien S, Kantarjian H et al, Long-term follow-up of patients with chronic lymphocytic leukemia treated with fludarabine as a single agent. *Blood* 1993; **81:** 2878–84.

Khouri IF, Przepiorka D, van Besien K et al, Allogeneic blood or marrow transplantation for chronic lymphocytic leukaemia: timing of transplantation and potential effect of fludarabine on acute graft-vs-host disease. *Br J Haematol* 1997; **97:** 466–73.

Lilliemark J, Porwit A, Juliusson G, Intermittent infusion of cladribine in previously treated patients with low grade non-Hodgkin's lymphoma. *Leuk Lymphoma* 1997; **25:** 313–18.

Loughran TP Jr, Clonal diseases of large granular lymphocytes. *Blood* 1993; **82:** 1–14.

Momose H, Jaffe ES, Shin SS et al, Chronic lymphocytic leukemia/small lymphocytic lymphoma with Reed–Sternberg-like cells and possible transformation to Hodgkin's disease. Mediation by Epstein Barr virus. *Am J Surg Pathol* 1992; **16:** 859–67.

O'Brien S, Kantarjian H, Beran M et al, Fludarabine and granulocyte colony-stimulating factor in patients with chronic lymphocytic leukemia. *Leukemia* 1997; **11:** 1631–5.

Rai KR, Cladribine for the treatment of hairy cell leukemia and chronic lymphocytic leukemia. *Semin Oncol* 1998; **25**(Suppl 7): 19–22.

Robertson LE, Pugh W, O'Brien S et al, Richter's syndrome: a report on 39 patients. *J Clin Oncol* 1993; **11:** 1985–9.

Tallman MS, Hakimian D, Variakojis D et al, A single cycle of 2-chlorodeoxyadenosine results in complete remission in the majority of patients with hairy cell leukemia. *Blood* 1992; **80:** 2203–9.

Van Dongen JJM, Hooijkaas H, Michiels JJ et al, Richter's syndrome with different immunoglobulin light chains and different heavy chain gene rearrangements. *Blood* 1984; **84:** 571–5.

B-cell chronic lymphocytic leukemia

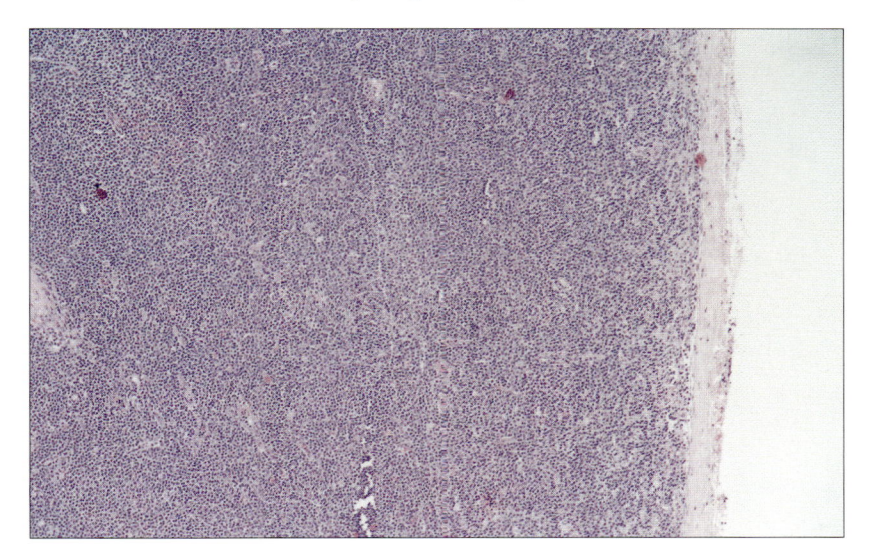

Figure 5.1

B-cell chronic lymphocytic leukemia:

(a) Low power shows a diffuse cellular infiltrate obliterating the normal architecture of this lymph node. (H&E stain)

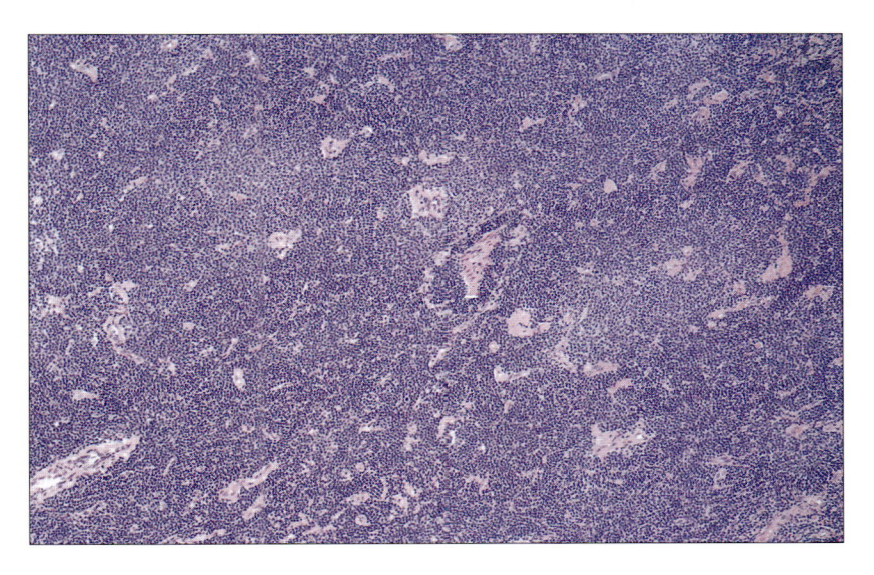

(b) Pseudofollicles, appearing as ill-defined, slightly paler areas, are present. (H&E stain)

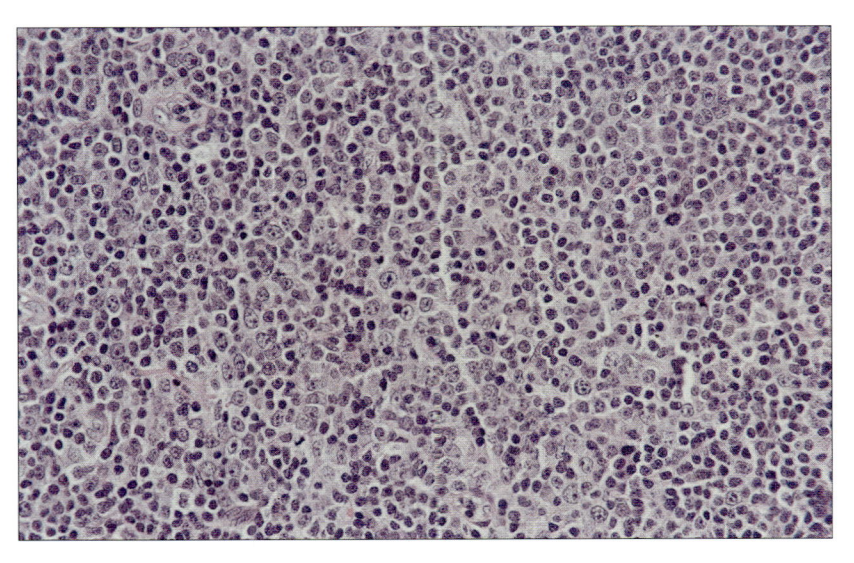

(c) Slightly higher power of a pseudofollicle shows larger, pale cells admixed with numerous small lymphocytes. (H&E stain)

Contd

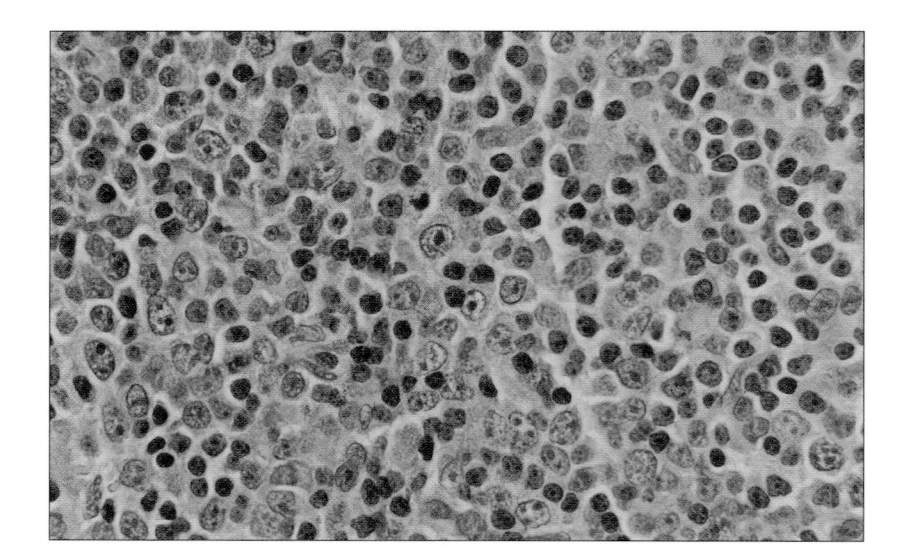

Figure 5.1 *continued*

(d) High power shows that the pseudofollicle consists of intermediate-sized prolymphocytes and large paraimmunoblasts in a background of small lymphocytes. (H&E stain)

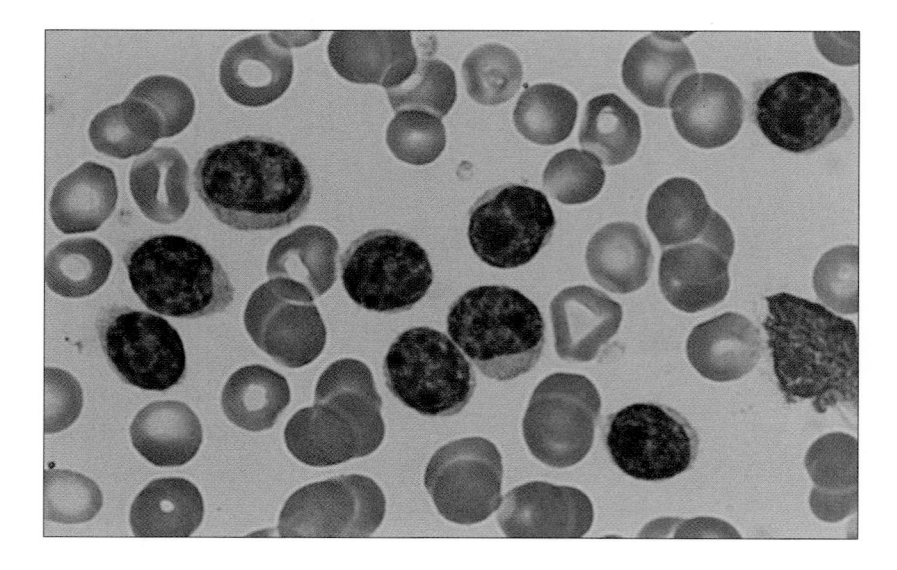

(e) The peripheral blood in this case shows a marked increase in small lymphocytes. (Wright stain)

Hairy cell leukemia

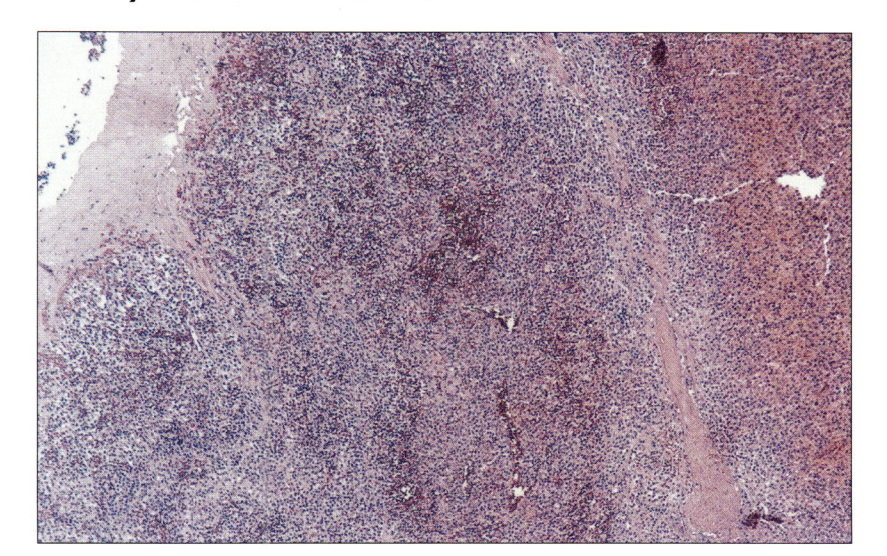

Figure 5.2

Hairy cell leukemia – Spleen:

(a) There is diffuse red pulp involvement by hairy cell leukemia: white pulp is inconspicuous. (H&E stain)

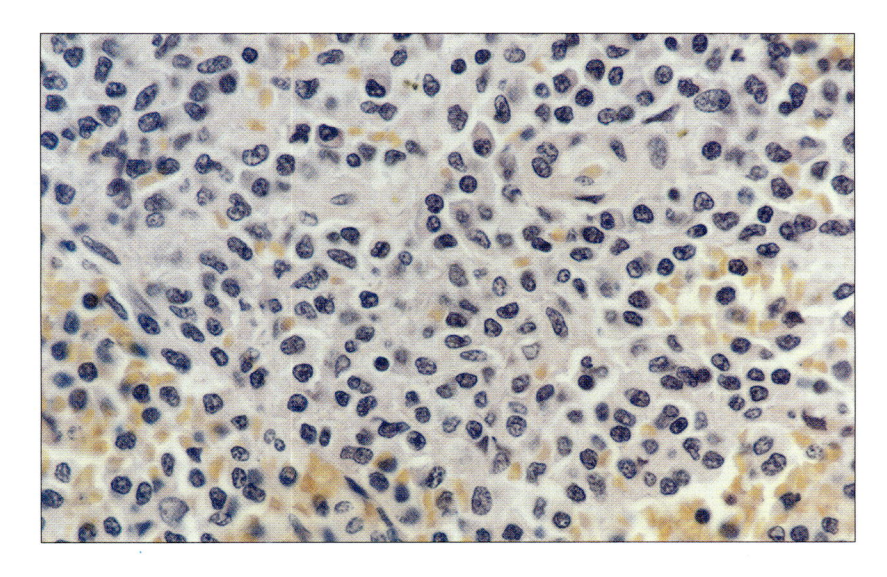

(b) Higher power shows lymphoid cells with oval or bean-shaped nuclei and abundant pale pink cytoplasm. (H&E stain)

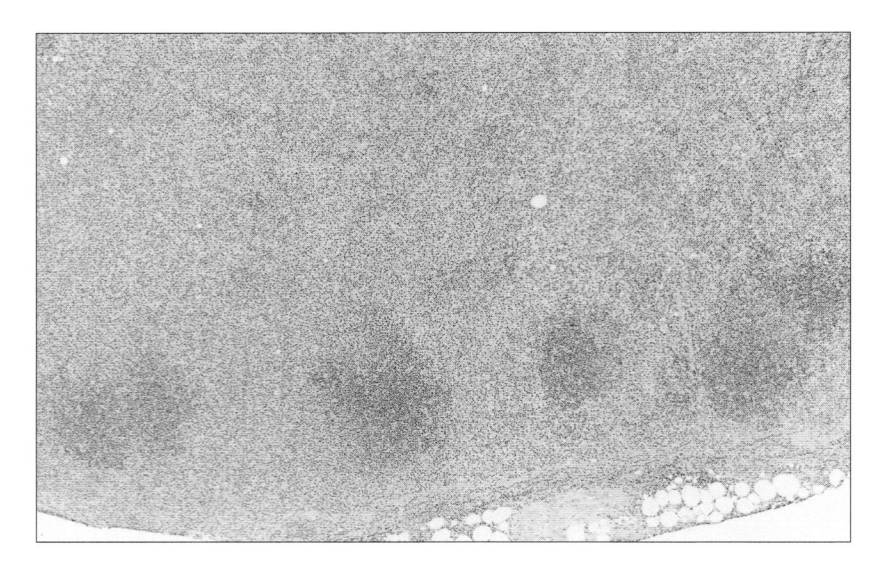

Figure 5.3

Hairy cell leukemia – Abdominal lymph node:

(a) Hairy cell leukemia has replaced much of the node, with sparing of a few primary follicles at the periphery of the node. (H&E stain)

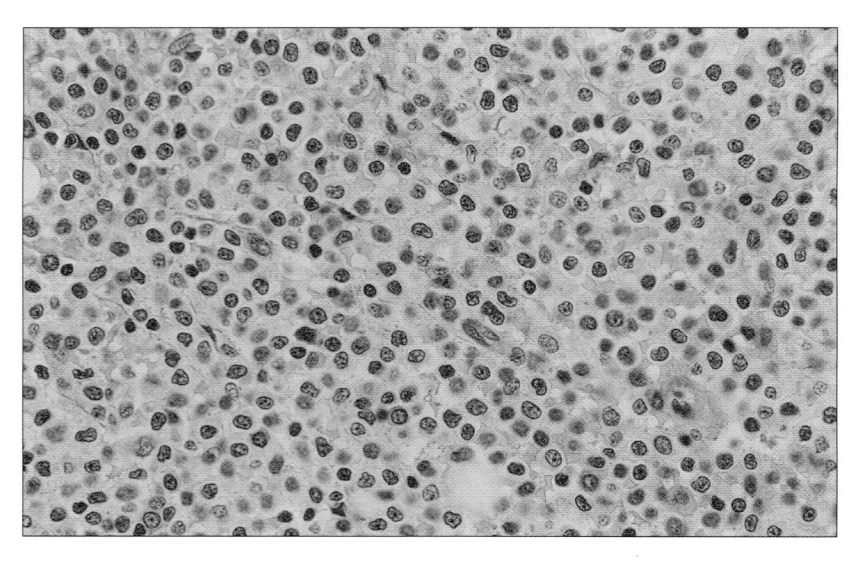

(b) Higher power shows atypical lymphoid cells similar to those found in the spleen. (H&E stain)

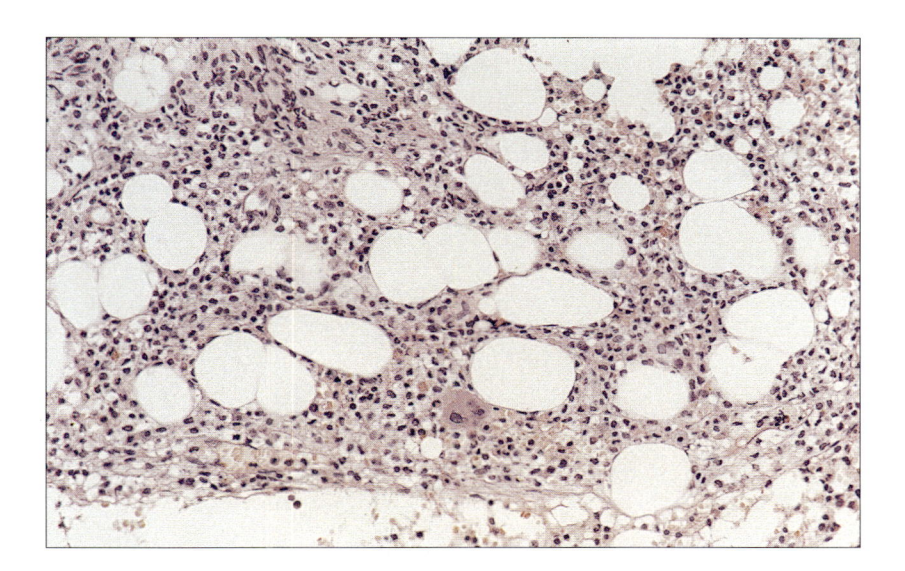

Figure 5.4

Hairy cell leukemia – Bone marrow:

The interstitial pattern of infiltration characteristic of hairy cell leukemia is shown. (H&E stain)

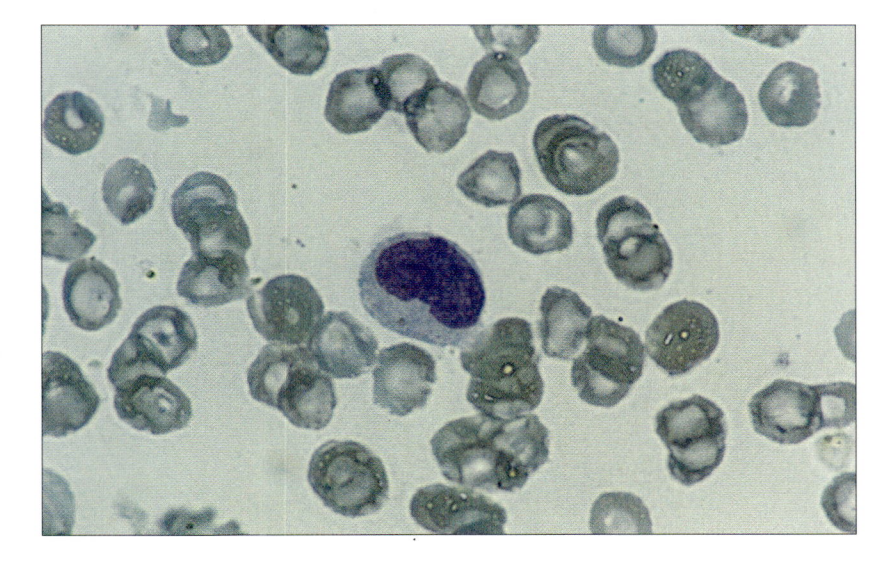

Figure 5.5

Hairy cell leukemia – Peripheral blood:

This circulating hairy cell has a bean-shaped nucleus with evenly dispersed chromatin and abundant pale cytoplasm. (Wright stain)

T-chronic lymphocytic leukemia and T-prolymphocytic leukemia

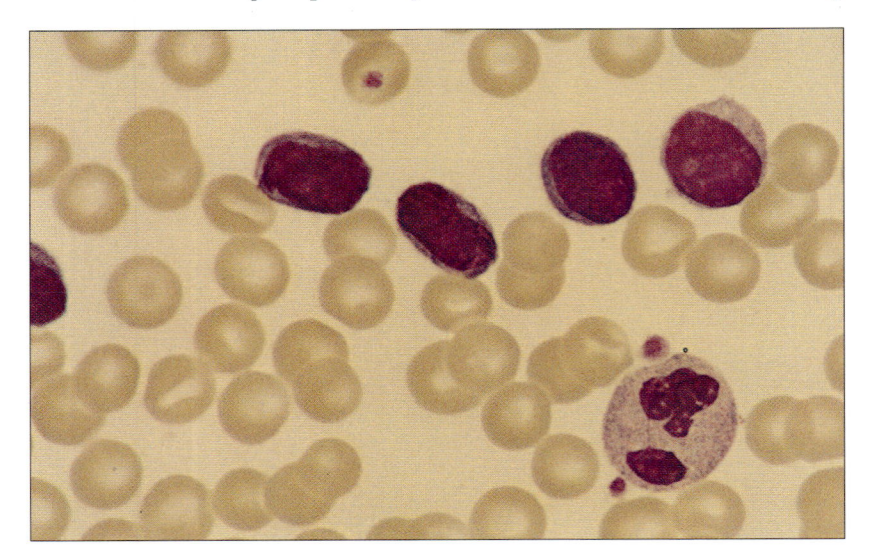

Figure 5.6

T-chronic lymphocytic leukemia:

In this case, neoplastic cells are similar to, or slightly larger than normal lymphocytes. (Wright stain)

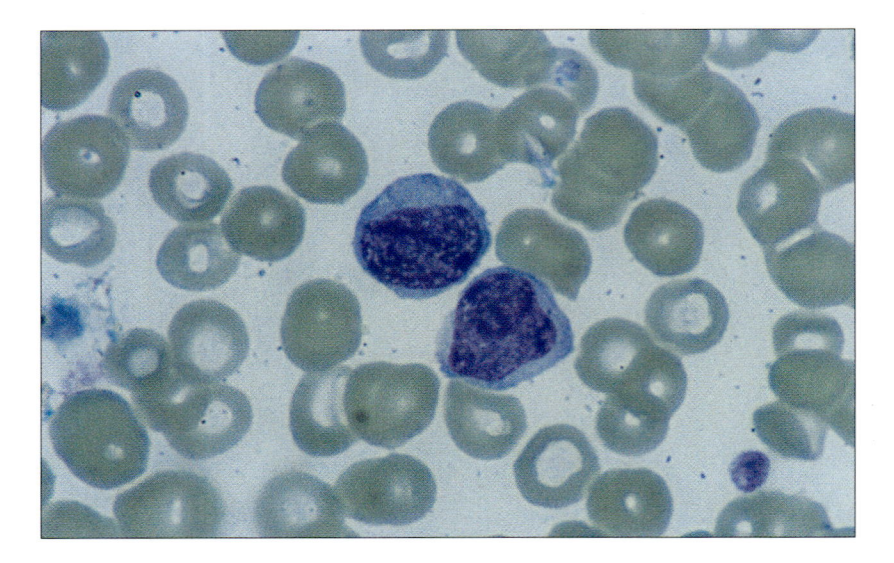

Figure 5.7

T-prolymphocytic leukemia:

Neoplastic cells are larger and more variable in size and shape than small lymphocytes (**a,b**). Cytoplasm is abundant and occasionally vacuolated. (Wright stain)

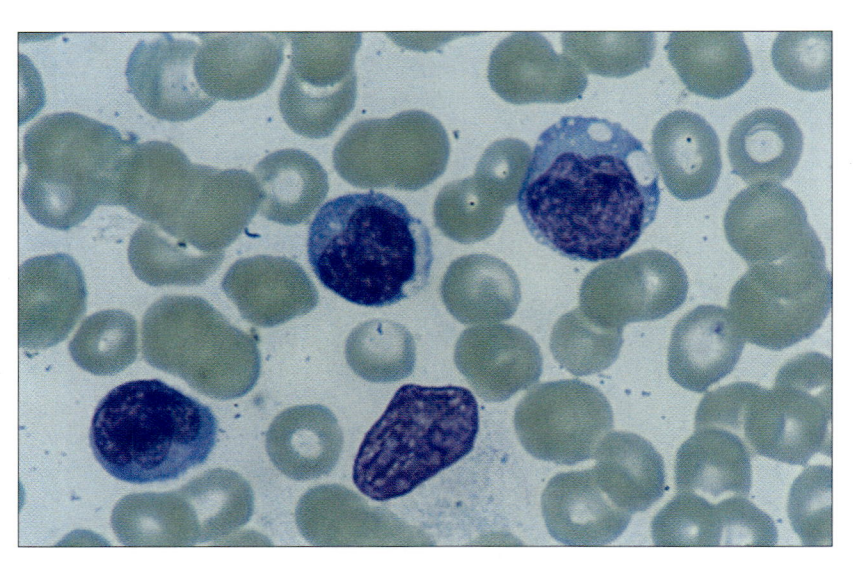

(a)

(b)

Large granular lymphocytic leukemia

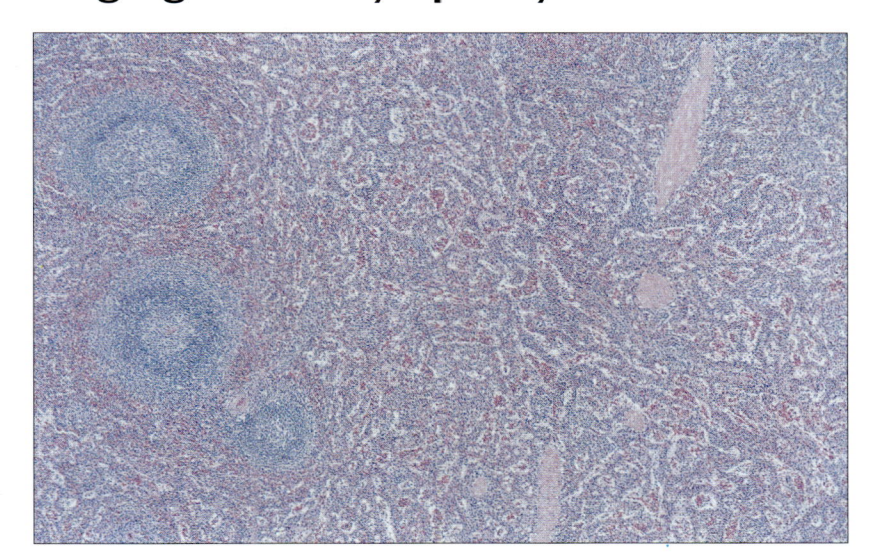

Figure 5.8

Large granular lymphocytic leukemia – T-cell type, spleen:

(a) Low power shows expanded red pulp with increased numbers of lymphoid cells. The white pulp is normal. (H&E stain)

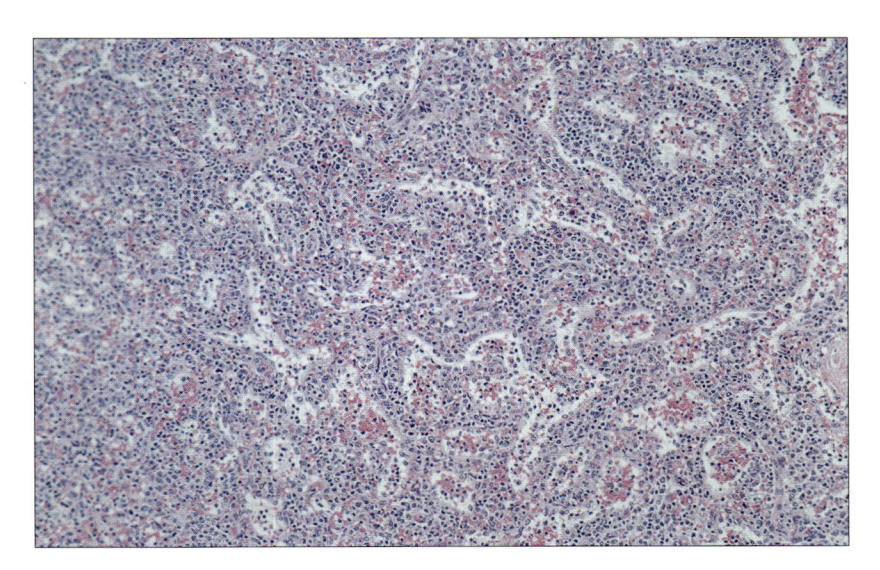

(b) Lymphoid cells are predominantly within splenic cords. (H&E stain)

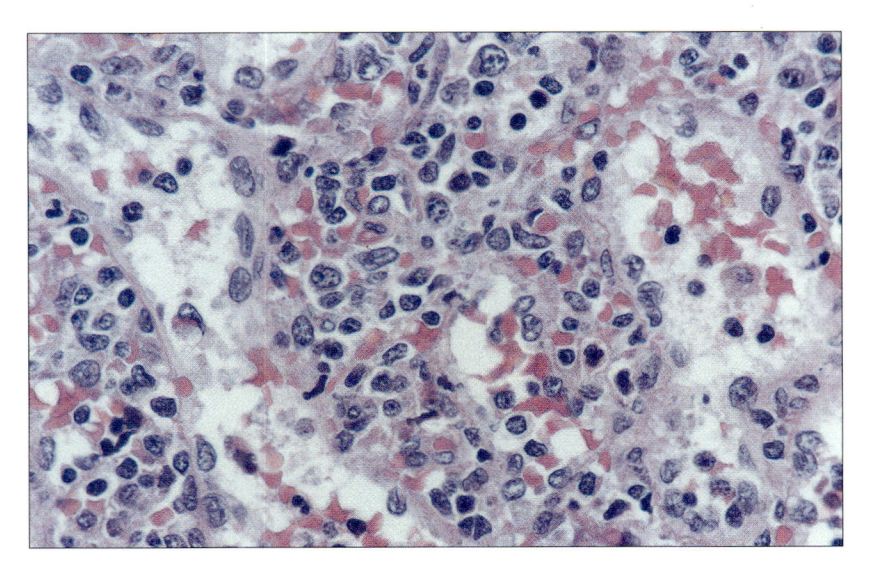

(c) The neoplastic cells are intermediate to large lymphoid cells with irregular nuclei and relatively abundant cytoplasm. (H&E stain)

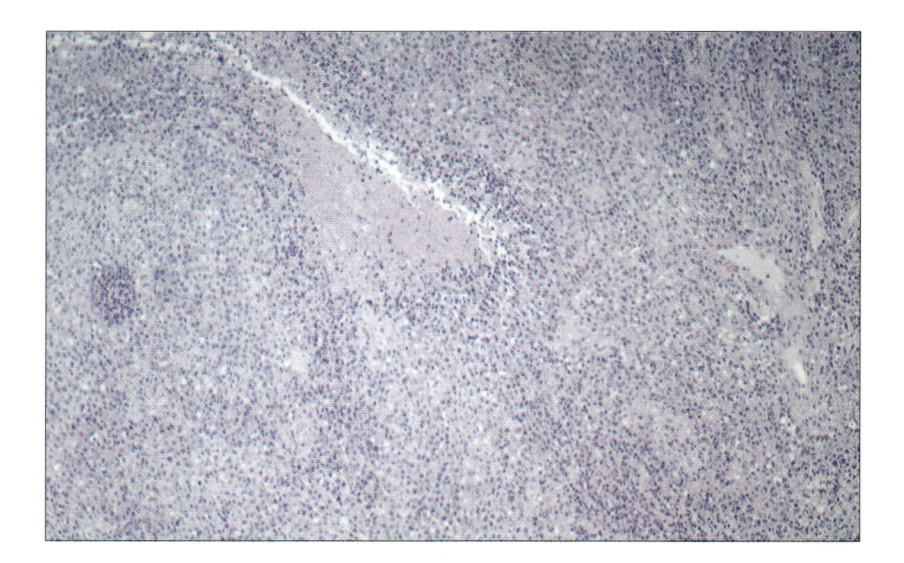

Figure 5.9

Large granular lymphocytic leukemia – NK-cell type:

(a) This neoplasm arose in an Asian patient. There were multiple small extranodal deposits of tumor, with a diffuse infiltrate of neoplastic cells with small foci of necrosis. (H&E stain)

(b) Neoplastic cells are large, and have oval to irregular nuclei, with a high mitotic rate. (H&E stain)

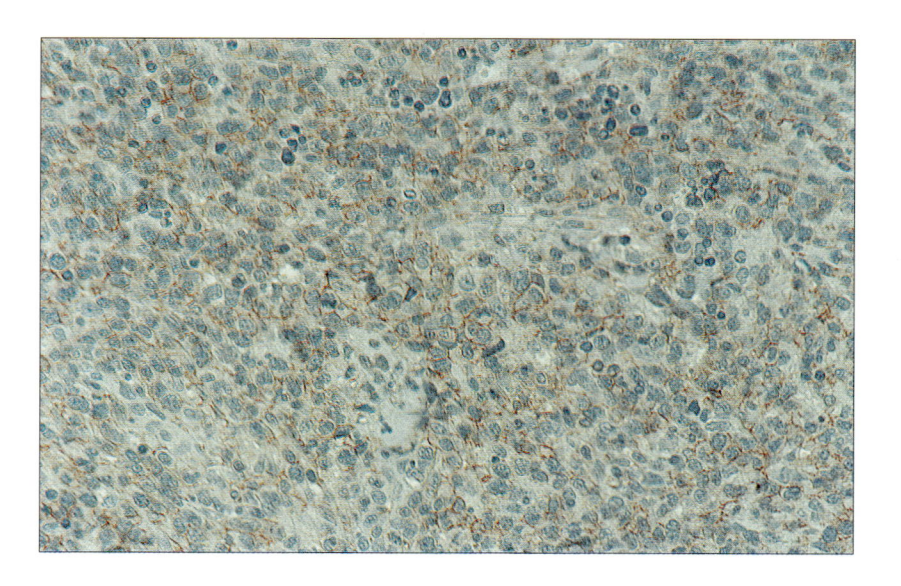

Neoplastic cells expressed T- and NK-cell-associated antigens such as CD43 (c), as well as CD56 (d), but lacked B-cell antigens (e). (Immunoperoxidase technique on paraffin sections)

(c)

Small lymphocytic lymphoma/Chronic lymphocytic leukemia

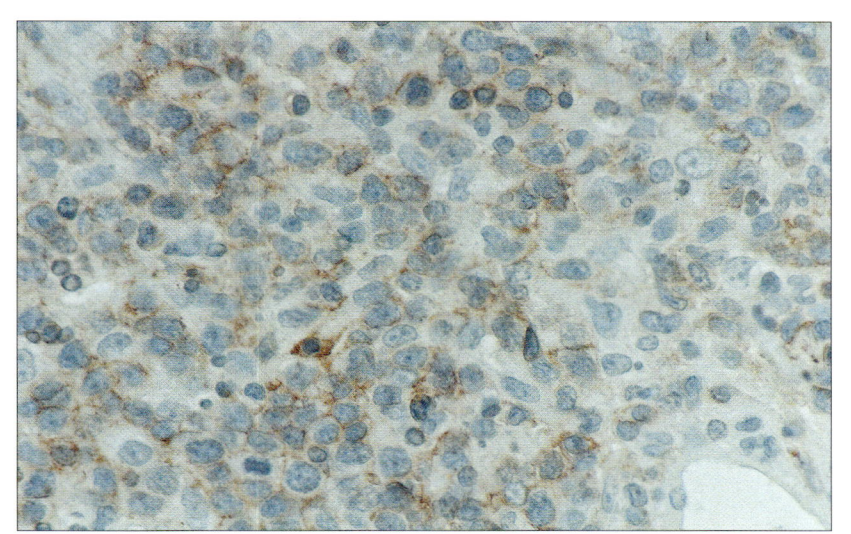

(d)

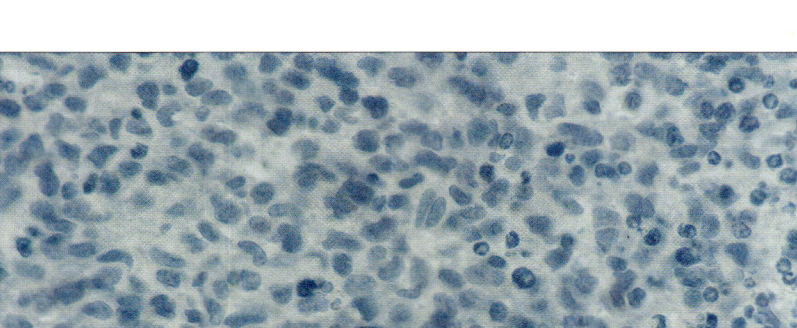

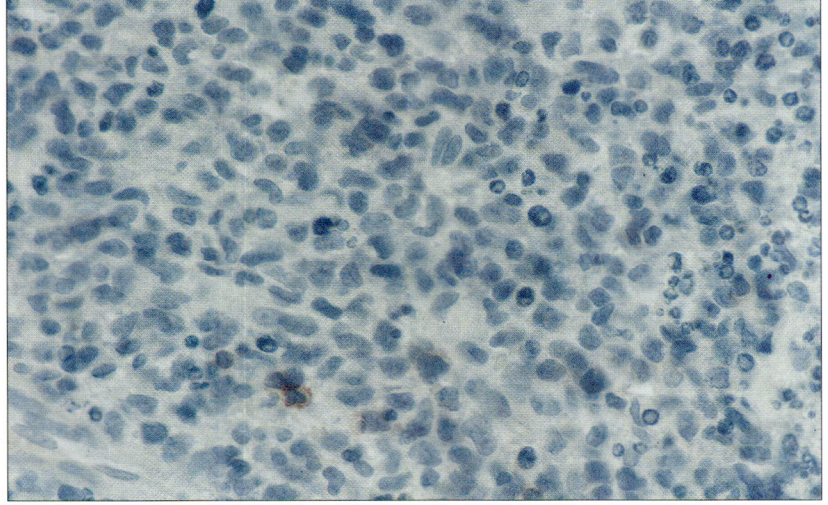

(e)

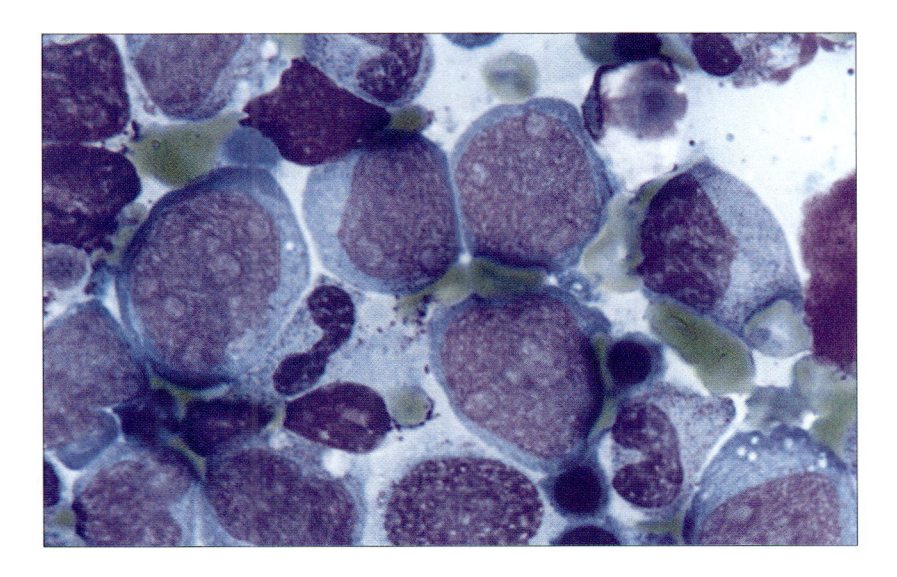

(f) The bone marrow aspirate shows many large blast cells, some with cytoplasmic granules. The patient died within a month of diagnosis. (Wright stain)

Figure 5.9 *continued*

6 Mantle-cell lymphoma

Definition and classification

The existence of mantle-cell lymphoma (MCL) as a distinct clinico-pathologic entity was eventually formalized only in 1994 in the REAL classification. MCL had previously been referred to by a variety of names. In the Kiel classification, it was called 'centrocytic lymphoma' to distinguish it from the lymphoma arising from follicular center cells. The International Working Formulation failed to recognize MCL as a distinct entity, and therefore pathologists categorized most of these patients as having diffuse small cleaved cell lymphoma (in 50–60% of cases) and follicular small cleaved lymphoma (in approximately 33% of cases).

Later, some pathologists in the USA designated it 'lymphocytic lymphoma of intermediate differentiation' or 'intermediate cell lymphoma'. The terminology 'mantle-cell lymphoma' was proposed at an international consensus conference in 1992; however, it was only with the REAL classification that this entity, which had formerly been believed to be a rather low-grade malignant lymphoma, was finally defined and the aggressiveness of its course recognized. MCL is currently considered to be one of the non-Hodgkin's lymphoma subtypes with the worst prognosis.

Frequency

Because of these recent developments, it is difficult to ascertain the exact incidence of MCL. In a recent evaluation of the clinical significance of the REAL classification in a survey of more than 1400 cases of non-Hodgkin's lymphoma from nine institutions in the USA, Canada, Europe, South Africa and Hong Kong, MCL accounted for 6% of all lymphoma cases.

Pathology

Histology

MCL is characterized histologically by neoplastic expansion of the mantle zone surrounding lymph node germinal centers, with a homogeneous population of small- to medium-sized lymphoid cells with irregular nuclei, inconspicuous nucleoli, and scant, pale cytoplasm. The size of the malignant cells is between those of small lymphocytic lymphoma and follicular lymphoma cells. At least at diagnosis, only a few large cells are admixed. However, the presence of blastic or blastoid large cells is more frequent in relapsing patients. MCL initially infiltrates the mantle zone surrounding normal germinal centers, generating a pattern that some authors designate 'mantle-zone lymphoma': on other occasions, however, the pattern may resemble pseudofollicles, and may therefore be called 'nodular'. As the disease progresses, the germinal centers are destroyed by the neoplastic infiltrate, generating the diffuse variant. MCL is sometimes characterized by slightly larger cells with a high mitotic index, and is then therefore termed a blastoid variant. Although the prognostic significance of the different variants of MCL remains controversial, most authors believe that the mantle-zone variant is the most benign and the blastoid variant the most aggressive in a continuous spectrum. In contrast to follicular lymphomas, MCL in fact does not show an abrupt transformation from indolent to aggressive disease.

Immunophenotyping (Table 6.1)

MCL has a monoclonal B-cell phenotype with a typical positivity for surface immunoglobulins and for pan-B antigens (CD19, CD20 and CD22), Generally, there is also a reversal of the normal λ:κ ratio. The pan-T-cell antigen CD5 is also expressed on the cell surface, while the CD10 antigen is absent. MCL cells are usually negative for CD23 antigen. The immunophenotypic characteristics might be helpful, especially in differential diagnosis with other 'small round cell lymphomas' such as small lymphocytic lymphoma and follicular lymphoma. Sometimes, however, molecular examination will be necessary to eventually establish the diagnosis of MCL.

Genetics

The majority of MCL harbor the t(11;14)(q13;q32) translocation. This abnormality, which is only rarely found in other types of non-Hodgkin's lymphoma, juxtaposes the enhancer element of the immunoglobulin heavy-chain J_H region on chromosome 14 with the *BCL1* (or *PRAD1*) proto-oncogene that codes for the cyclin D1 protein on chromosome 11. The translocation causes the *BCL1* gene to become deregulated, and the cyclin D1 protein is consequently overexpressed. It is possible that this overexpression of cyclin D1 promotes progression of cells from the G_1 phase of the cell cycle to the S phase, causing excessive proliferation.

Because of the extensive breakpoint heterogeneity of the t(11;14) translocation, the polymerase chain reaction (PCR) can detect only 50–60% of cases. Polyclonal and monoclonal antibodies, which detect cyclin D1 overexpression,

Table 6.1
Immunophenotype of mantle-cell lymphoma

Surface marker	Mantle-cell lymphoma	Follicular lymphoma	Small lymphocytic lymphoma
CD5	++	–	++
Surface immuno-globulin	++	+++	+
CD19	++	++	++
CD20	+++	++	+
CD10	–	+	–
CD23	–	±	+

have been shown to be highly specific for MCL, and are likely to become standard diagnostic tools once they are commercially available. A weak expression of cyclin D1 is often seen in hairy cell leukemias, but without the presence of t(11;14).

Clinical characteristics (Table 6.2)

MCL occurs in older patients (the median age in most series is 60 years) and shows a striking male predominance. Generalized adenopathy, splenomegaly and bone marrow involvement are common. Limited-stage disease is rare, with stage I and non-bulky stage II disease found in fewer than 15% of patients. Extranodal sites in addition to marrow are frequently involved, particularly Waldeyer's ring and the gastrointestinal tract. There is peripheral blood involvement in 20–40% of cases, but absolute lymphocyte counts above 20 000/l are uncommon. A distinctive form of gastrointestinal involvement in which polypoid lesions are seen over long segments of bowel has been termed 'multiple lymphomatous polyposis'. In contrast to other non-Hodgkin's lymphomas, large-bowel involvement is often seen during the course of the disease. Patients may then present with melena, abdominal pain, diarrhea or a palpable mass. Since gastrointestinal involvement is already

Table 6.2
Mantle-cell lymphoma: clinical features at presentation

Generalized adenopathies	90%
Splenomegaly	55%
Hepatomegaly	35%
Bone marrow infiltration	75%
Peripheral blood lymphocytosis	25%
Gastrointestinal involvement	15%
Waldeyer's ring involvement	10%
Ann Arbor stage III–IV	90%
B symptoms	35%
Bulky disease	30%
Poor performance status	20%
Elevated LDH	40%
Elevated β_2-microglobulin	50%

present at diagnosis in approximately 25% of cases, staging must include a careful endoscopic evaluation, including the ear, nose and throat region.

The clinical course is often moderately aggressive at diagnosis, with small disseminated lymph nodes, a good performance status, and few or no systemic symptoms. With time, lymph nodes increase in volume, blood involvement becomes more pronounced, further extranodal sites appear, and the lymphoma shows its full aggressiveness. Adversed prognostic factors, such as poor performance status, B symptoms, high lactate dehydrogenase (LDH) level or high β_2-microglobulin level, are seen in more than 50% patients at this more advanced and aggressive stage of the disease. The International Lymphoma Prognostic Index can be useful in MCL patients, but it discriminates less well between good-risk and poor-risk patients than in diffuse large cell or follicular lymphomas.

Treatment and outcome (Table 6.3)

Multiple clinical series have reported a median survival of three to four years for patients with MCL. These data have been confirmed by the International Lymphoma Study Group classification project, in which MCL patients had the shortest median time to progression and the shortest median survival of all lymphoma subtypes. The pattern of response to chemotherapy is unique among the lymphomas: while MCL is 'almost normally' sensitive to chemotherapy at diagnosis (although in most series partial responses are more common than complete responses), this sensitivity rapidly declines at first and second relapse. The

Table 6.3
Response to treatment and survival of mantle-cell lymphoma patients in the most representative retrospective analyses published[a]

	Meusers	Norton	Argatoff	Teodorovic	Zucca	Coiffier
n	63	66	80	64	65	119
Response to treatment						
CR (%)	48	9		45	51	26
PR (%)	38	62		25	35	33
Relapse after CR (%)	11				48	84
DFS (months)	9	10		21	44	22
EFS (months)		13		20		16
Survival (months)	34	36	43	45	42	40

CR, complete response; PR, partial response; DFS, disease-free survival; EFS, event-free survival.
[a]Modified, with permission, from Coiffier B, Which treatment for mantle-cell lymphoma patients in 1998? *J Clin Oncol* 1998; **16**: 3–5.

reduced complete response rate is mainly dependent on the great difficulty in obtaining a complete clearance of the bone marrow in marrow-positive patients.

Thus far, there has been no convincing evidence from the numerous studies that any conventional chemotherapy regimen would be curative. While the median progression-free survival time of the responding patient will be on the order of 15–18 months, 6–8% of patients will be relapse-free after 10 years. These data point to a subset of patients with an indolent disease course: as yet, however, there are no prognostic factors by which these cases could prospectively be recognized.

There has been only one randomized, prospective trial analyzing the treatment of MCL: this rather old German study randomized 63 patients with 'centrocytic lymphoma' to receive either CVP (cyclophosphamide, vincristine and prednisone) or CHOP (cyclophosphamide, doxorubicin, vincristine and prednisone) chemotherapy. No statistically significant difference was noted between the two groups with respect to response rate, relapse-free survival, or median overall survival time (32 versus 37 months).

Recently, the South West Oncology Group (SWOG) and the European Organization for Research and Treatment of Cancer (EORTC) examined retrospectively some of their previous studies. In these retrospective analyses, there was no hint of a plateau in the survival curve of patients treated with an anthracycline-containing regimen, and no significant survival advantage emerged, on an historical comparison, for doxorubicin-based treatments over the CVP regimen. However, at least two retrospective single-centre studies suggest that MCL patients may survive longer if treated with an anthracycline-containing regimen. Purine analogues, such as fludarabine, seem to be of only limited value in the treatment of these patients. Preliminary data indicate a 33% response rate with the anti-CD20 antibody Rituximab. Thus far, intensive chemotherapy associated with total-body irradiation and followed by autologous stem cell transplantation or purged bone marrow has yielded mixed and generally rather disappointing results. These rather negative results are consistent in relapsing patients, while treatment might hold greater benefits in first-line responding patients.

Outside clinical trials, for the time being, it seems appropriate that patients with a good performance status and who are below the age of 70 can be treated with a doxorubicin-containing regimen. Patients with a poor performance status and/or age greater than 70 might still be treated more appropriately with chlorambucil alone or with CVP.

Bibliography

Banks PM, Chan J, Cleary ML et al, Mantle-cell lymphoma: a proposal for unification of morphologic, immunologic and molecular data. *Am J Surg Pathol* 1992; **16:** 637–40.

Coiffier B, Which treatment for mantle-cell lymphoma patients in 1998? *J Clin Oncol* 1998; **16:** 3–5.

de Boer CJ, Schuring E, Dreef E et al, Cyclin D1 protein analysis in the diagnosis of mantle-cell lymphoma. *Blood* 1995; **86:** 2715–23.

Decaudin D, Bosq J, Tertian G et al, Phase II trial of fludarabine monophosphate in patients with mantle-cell lymphomas. *J Clin Oncol* 1198; **16:** 13–18.

Fisher RI, Dahlberg S, Nathwani BN et al, A clinical analysis of two indolent lymphoma entities: mantle-cell lymphoma and marginal zone lymphoma (including the mucosa-associated lymphoid tissue and monocytoid B-cell sub-categories): a Southwest Oncology Group study. *Blood* 1995; **85:** 1075–82.

Freedman AS, Neuberg D, Gribben JG et al, High-dose chemotherapy and anti-B-cell monoclonal antibody-purged autologous bone marrow transplantation in mantle-cell lymphoma: evidence for long-term remission. *J Clin Oncol* 1998; **16:** 13–18.

Harris NL, Jaffe ES, Stein H et al, A revised European–American classification of lymphoid neoplasms: a proposal from the International Lymphoma Study Group. *Blood* 1994; **84:** 1361–92.

Hiddeman W, Unterhalt M, Herrmann R et al, Mantle-cell lymphomas have more widespread disease and a slower response to chemotherapy compared with follicle-center lymphomas: results of a prospective comparative analysis of the German Low-Grade Lymphoma Study Group. *J Clin Oncol* 1998; **16:** 1922–30.

Ketterer N, Salles G, Espinouse D et al, Intensive therapy with peripheral stem cell transplantation in 16 patients with mantle-cell lymphoma. *Ann Oncol* 1997; **8:** 701–4.

Louie DC, Offit K, Jaslow R et al, p53 overexpression as

a marker of poor prognosis in mantle-cell lymphomas with t(11;14)(q13;q32). *Blood* 1995; **86:** 2892–9.

Meusers P, Engelhard M, Bartels H et al, Multicentre randomized therapeutic trial for advanced centrocytic lymphoma: anthracycline does not improve the prognosis. *Hematol Oncol* 1989; **7:** 365–80.

Non-Hodgkin's Lymphoma Classification Project, A clinical evaluation of the International Lymphoma Study Group classification of non-Hodgkin's lymphoma. *Blood* 1997; **89:** 3909–18.

Norton AJ, Matthews J, Pappa V et al, Mantle-cell lymphoma: natural history defined in a serially biopsied population over a 20-year period. *Ann Oncol* 1995; **6:** 249–56.

Segal GH, Masih AS, Fox AC et al, CD5-expressing B-cell non Hodgkin's lymphomas with bcl-1 gene rearrangement have a relatively homogeneous immunophenotype and are associated with an overall poor prognosis. *Blood* 1995; **85:** 1570–9.

Teodorovic I, Pittaluga S, Kluin-Nelemans JC et al, Efficacy of four different regimens in 64 mantle-cell lymphoma cases: clinicopathologic comparison with 498 other non-Hodgkin's lymphoma subtypes. *J Clin Oncol* 1995; **13:** 2829–6.

Williams ME, Nichols GE, Swerdlow SH et al, In situ hybridization detection of cyclin D1 mRNA in centrocytic/mantle-cell lymphoma. *Ann Oncol* 1995; **6:** 297–9.

Williams ME, Swerdlow SH, Rosenberg CL et al, Characterization of chromosome 11 translocation breakpoints at the bcl-1 and PRAD 1 loci in centrocytic lymphoma. *Cancer Res* 1992; **52**(Suppl 19): 5541s–4s.

Zucca E, Roggero E, Pinotti G et al, Patterns of survival in mantle-cell lymphoma. *Ann Oncol* 1995; **6:** 257–62.

Zucca E, Stein H, Coiffier B, European Lymphoma Task Force (ELTF): report of the Workshop on Mantle-Cell Lymphoma (MCL). *Ann Oncol* 1994; **5:** 507–11.

Mantle-cell lymphoma

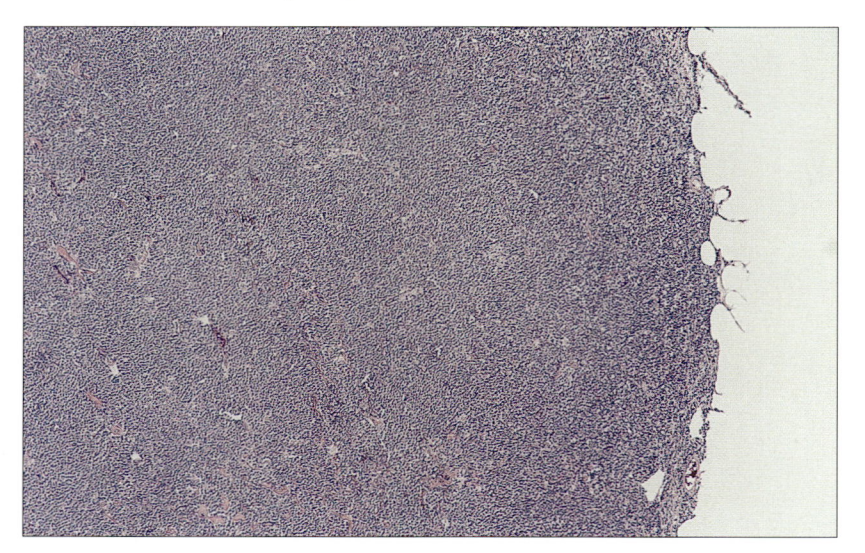

Figure 6.1

Mantle-cell lymphoma:

(a) The normal architecture of the lymph node is obliterated by a diffuse infiltrate of lymphoid cells. (H&E stain)

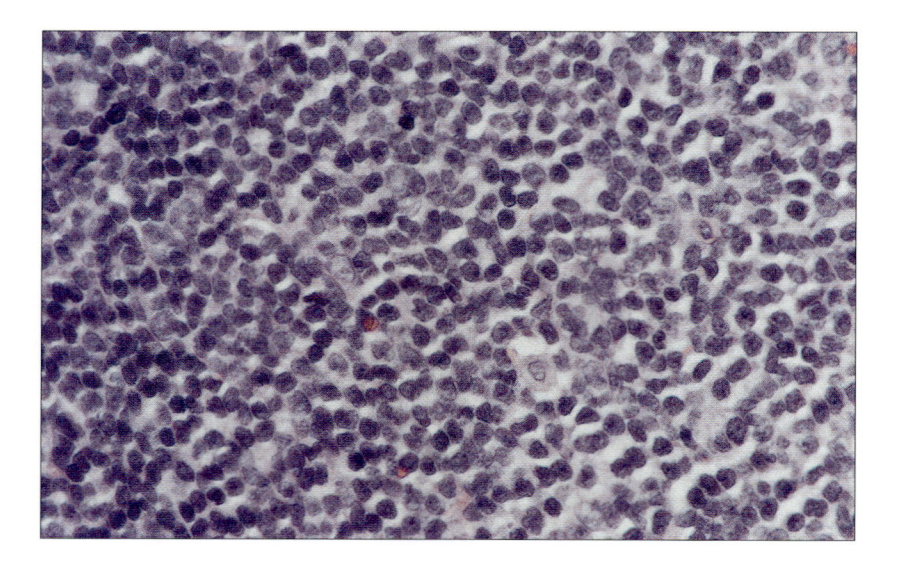

(b) High-power examination shows a monomorphous population of small lymphoid cells with slightly irregular nuclei and scant cytoplasm; centroblasts (large non-cleaved cells) are absent. (H&E stain)

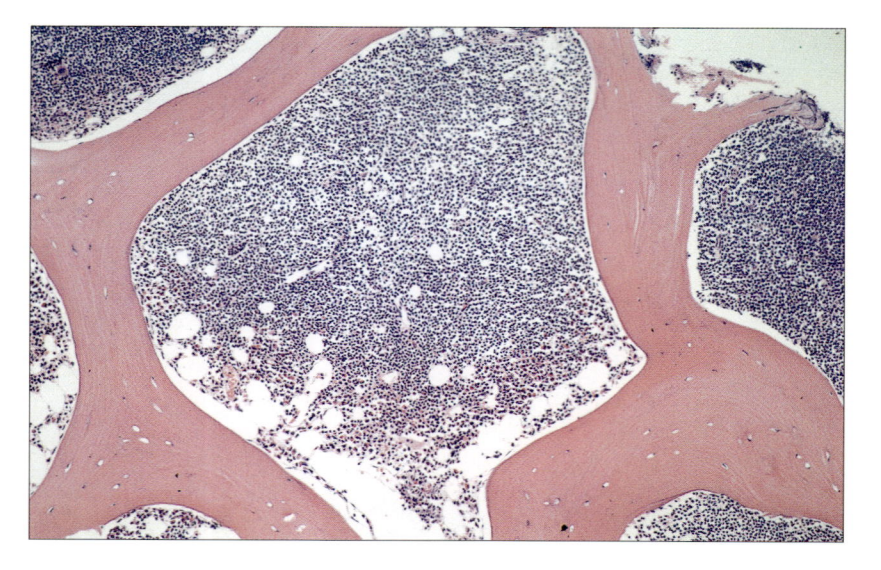

(c) Lymphoma occupies the majority of the bone marrow in this case. (H&E stain)

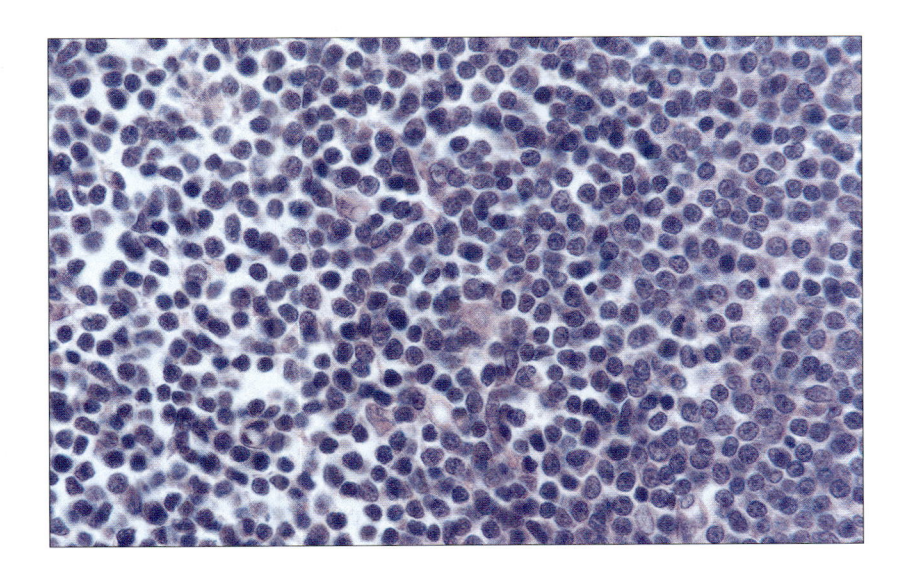

Figure 6.1 *continued*

(d) The neoplastic population in the marrow consists of lymphoid cells that are only slightly larger and more irregular than normal lymphocytes. (H&E stain)

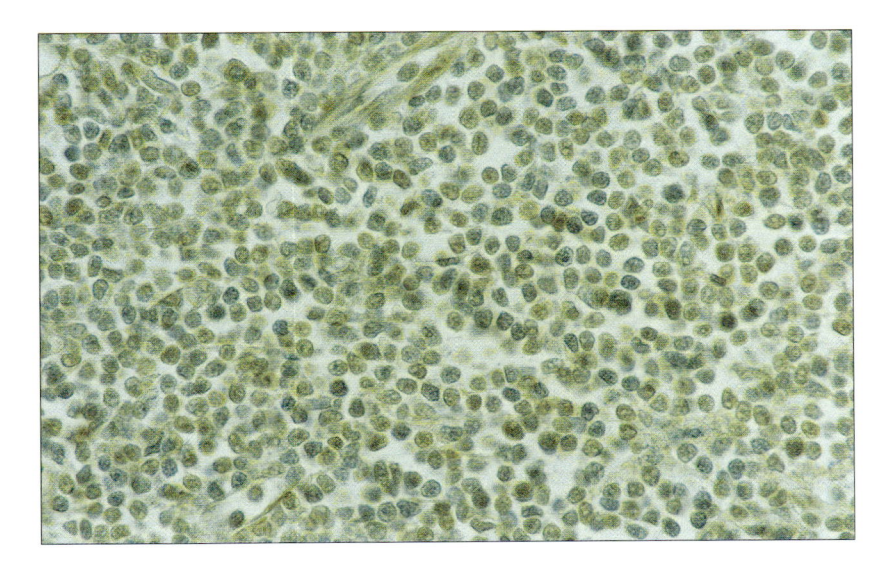

(e) The neoplastic cells express nuclear cyclin D1, confirming the diagnosis of mantle-cell lymphoma. (Immunoperoxidase technique on paraffin sections)

7 MALT lymphoma (extranodal marginal-zone B-cell lymphoma)

Definition and classification

The group of MALT (mucosa-associated lymphoid tissue) lymphomas comprises a number of low-grade extranodal B-cell lymphomas that share similar clinical, pathologic, immunologic and molecular features (Table 7.1). This condition has been widely accepted only in recent years, and has been included in the REAL classification as a specific entity: extranodal marginal-zone B-cell lymphoma. In the past, many MALT lymphomas, particularly those arising in the stomach, may have been misinterpreted as 'pseudolymphomas'; however, a number of features contribute to their definition as a malignant condition: monoclonality is usually demonstrable, non-random chromosomal aberration can be detected, and histologic transformation into a high-grade lymphoma is possible, as well as dissemination to the regional lymph nodes and sometimes to the bone marrow. At least in some instances, they may also have been recognized as malignant lymphomas in the past and included in any of the subtypes from A to F in the Working Formulation.

In addition to MALT lymphomas, the REAL classification includes two other provisional entities among the lymphomas of postulated marginal-zone derivation: nodal marginal-zone B-cell lymphoma (monocytoid lymphoma) and splenic marginal-zone B-cell lymphoma with circulating villous lymphocytes. Despite the fact that all types of marginal-zone lymphoma appear to share many morphologic, immunophenotypic and cytogenetic features, whether or not they represent a unique entity is still controversial.

Paradoxically, MALT lymphoma usually arises in the context of pre-existing prolonged lymphoid reactive proliferations in mucosal sites where

---

Table 7.1
Typical features of MALT lymphoma

Histological features
- Centrocyte-like cells (small- to medium-sized B lymphocytes with abundant cytoplasm and irregularly shaped nuclei)
- Variable degree of plasma cell differentiation
- Scattered transformed blasts (large cells)
- Lymphoepithelial lesions (invasion and partial destruction of mucosal glands or crypts by aggregates of tumor cells)
- Non-neoplastic reactive follicles and follicular colonization

Immunophenotype of centrocyte-like cells
- Surface immunoglobulins, usually IgM
- $CD19^+$, $CD20^+$, $CD22^+$
- $CD5^-$, $CD10^-$, $CD23^-$
- BCL1 (PRAD1) protein expression always negative
- BCL2 protein expression usually positive

Genetic characteristics
- Trisomy 3 in approximately 60% of cases
- t(11;18)(q21;p21) in approximately 35% of cases
- BCL1, BCL2 and c-MYC usually not rearranged

lymphocytes are not normally present. These pre-existing disorders can be due either to infectious conditions such as *Helicobacter pylori* gastritis, or to autoimmune processes such as myoepithelial sialadenitis (MESA), usually due to Sjögren's syndrome, and Hashimoto's thyroiditis. There are several lines of evidence suggesting that antigen stimulation is critical to the development and growth of MALT lymphomas.

MALT lymphomas are particularly common in the gastrointestinal tract, but have been described in most extranodal sites (salivary glands, thyroid, lung, ocular adnexa, and even in leptomeninges). The gastric localization is by far the most common and best-studied localization; hence it can be taken as representative of the group as a whole.

The onset of MALT lymphomas in the stomach is preceded by the acquisition of MALT as a result of *H. pylori* infection. The microorganism can be found in the gastric mucosa in nearly all instances, with several lines of evidence suggesting a link between *H. pylori* chronic gastritis and MALT lymphoma of the stomach. This close association of *H. pylori* with gastric MALT lymphoma has led to the hypothesis that the microorganism may provide the antigenic stimulus for sustaining the growth of the lymphoma in the stomach.

Frequency

In a recent evaluation of the clinical significance of the REAL classification in a survey of more than 1400 non-Hodgkin's lymphomas from nine institutions in the USA, Canada, the UK, Switzerland, France, Germany, South Africa and Hong Kong, marginal zone B-cell MALT lymphomas represented 7.6% of the total number of cases, including both the most common gastrointestinal and the less usual non-gastrointestinal localizations. Some additional information is available regarding primary MALT lymphomas of the stomach: the highest prevalence has been reported in northeastern Italy (13.2:100 000/year, which is 13 times higher than in corresponding UK communities) suggesting the existence of important geographic variations. The incidence in the USA has been estimated to be between 1: 30 000 and 1:80 000.

Pathology

Histology

The histologic features of low-grade B-cell lymphomas of MALT type are similar regardless of the site of origin.

The tumor cells are usually small- to medium-sized lymphocytes with moderately abundant cytoplasm and irregularly shaped nuclei resembling those of follicular center centrocytes, and have been termed centrocyte-like (CCL) cells. Resemblance to centrocytes is the general rule – however, the morphologic pattern of the neoplastic cells covers a quite large spectrum, and in some cases they can be similar to so-called monocytoid cells (abundant pale cytoplasm and well-defined cell borders) or to small lymphocytes, sometimes with lymphoplasmacytic features. Any of these cytologic aspects can predominate, or they can coexist to various degrees in the same case. Scattered transformed blasts (large cells) can also be found. Some degree of plasma cell differentiation is often present. The lymphoma cells infiltrate diffusely in the lamina propria and grow around reactive follicles. These reactive follicles are a characteristic feature of MALT lymphomas. Another non-neoplastic component is represented by a reactive, often abundant, T-cell population.

A pivotal feature of low-grade MALT lymphoma is the presence of a variable number of lymphoepithelial lesions defined by evident invasion and partial destruction of mucosal glands or crypts by aggregates of tumor cells. Lymphoepithelial lesions are of striking relevance for the diagnosis of low-grade gastric MALT lymphoma, and are typically seen in MALT lymphomas of the thyroid, salivary glands and lungs. However, they can be less numerous or not well developed in other extranodal sites (e.g. the lacrimal glands or the skin), and, moreover, they can be sometimes be seen in the context of florid chronic gastritis, and can also be present in other MALT sites.

Within the stomach, low-grade MALT lymphoma is often multifocal. Microscopic lymphoma foci can be present at sites distant from the main tumor, and may explain the frequent reports of relapses in the gastric stump after surgical excision. MALT lymphoma usually remains localized at the initial site, but can sometimes present with involvement of multiple mucosal sites.

Some diagnostic difficulties can arise in the presence of an increased number of large cells – a finding that may suggest histologic progression to a high-grade lymphoma. This problem has been studied in particular in the stomach, where a small component of low-grade MALT lymphoma can be identified in a significant proportion of high-grade lymphomas, and, conversely, foci of high-grade (large cell) lymphoma can be seen in low-grade gastric MALT lymphoma, suggesting transition from one to the other, analogous to other low-grade lymphomas. The prevalence and time interval of the histologic transformation of MALT lymphomas are unknown. It has been proposed that the presence of compact confluent clusters or sheets of large cells can be used as the criterion for the high-grade transformation, but thus far there has been no general agreement.

The prognostic significance of the presence of focal areas of high grade within a low-grade specimen still needs clarification. In recent studies, the presence of a large cell component at diagnosis or of a diffusely distributed increased number of blasts has been found to be predictive of a less favorable long-term outcome in gastric MALT lymphoma patients, but not in those with MALT lymphoma presenting in non-gastrointestinal sites.

Immunophenotype

There is an almost complete phenotype homology between MALT lymphoma B cells and marginal-zone B cells (of the spleen, Peyer's patches and lymph nodes), with typical positivity for surface immunoglobulins and pan-B antigens (CD19, CD20 and CD79a) and a lack of CD5, CD10, CD23 and BCL1 (PRAD1) expression. Immunostaining for CD21 (follicular dendritic cells), for Ki-67, and for BCL2 and BCL6 proteins may contribute to the identification of residual reactive follicles. A search for surface immunoglobulins may be essential for distinguishing between a suspicious reactive lymphoid infiltrate and a MALT lymphoma in cases where the morphologic pattern is equivocal. The demonstration of a clear-cut restriction of light chains (κ:λ ratio > 10:1, or vice versa) strongly supports the diagnosis of B-cell lymphoma. Immunostaining with the pan-B-cell CD20 antibody may help to distinguish CCL cells from plasma cells and to identify lymphoepithelial lesions. These latter can be highlighted with antibodies to cytokeratin.

Genetics

Karyotype studies of gastric MALT lymphoma present technical difficulties, and a limited number of cases have been published. The most frequent abnormality appears to be trisomy 3, which has been reported to be detectable in approximately 60% of both low-grade and high-grade MALT lymphomas. The chromosomal translocation t(11;18)(q21;p21) has been described in approximately one-third of low-grade MALT lymphomas, and it may represent an important pathogenetic event. Less frequently, trisomies of chromosomes 18, 12 and 7, and the chromosomal translocation t(1;14) have also been reported. The *BCL1*, *BCL2* and c-*MYC* oncogenes are usually not rearranged.

Clinical characteristics

The disease affects both sexes, with a median age at presentation in the sixth decade, the signs and symptoms depending on the involved extranodal site. The most common presenting symptoms of low-grade gastric MALT lymphomas are non-specific dyspepsia or epigastric pain. Endoscopy usually reveals non-specific gastritis or peptic ulcer, with massive lesions being unusual. Most often, the disease is localized in the antrum or is multifocal (Table 7.2). Unlike most low-grade B-cell lymphomas of peripheral lymph nodes, low-grade MALT lymphoma is usually a very indolent disease, often remaining localized for a prolonged period, with some cases showing no progression for several years with no treatment.

The lack of uniformity in the criteria adopted for histologic classification make it difficult to find clear information in the historical literature about survival. Long-term overall survival for low-grade MALT lymphoma of the stomach seems to be

Table 7.2
Clinical and endoscopic characteristics at presentation in a series of 93 patients with low-grade MALT lymphoma[a]

Clinical features	n	%	Laboratory abnormalities	n	%	Endoscopic features	n	%
Median age: 63 years (range: 21–89)								
Sex								
Female	46	49						
Male	47	51						
Stage:			*LDH:*			*Endoscopic appearance:*		
I	84	88	Normal	54	58	Ulcers	44	47
II	4	4	Elevated	1	1	Gastritis	28	30
IV	7	8	Not assessed	38	41	Erosions	21	23
Bone marrow involvement:			β_2-*microglobulin:*			*Gastric localization:*		
Yes	7	8	Normal	46	50	Antrum	38	41
No	79	84	Elevated	4	4	Body	11	12
Not assessed	7	8	Not assessed	43	46	Fundus	10	11
Main symptoms:						Multifocal	31	33
Abdominal pain	49	53				Gastric stump	3	3
Dyspepsia	30	32				*H. pylori infection:*		
Nausea/vomiting	7	8				Present (histology)	67	72
Bleeding	2	2				Present (serological)	4	4
No symptoms	5	5				Not assessed (no test)	22	24
B symptoms:								
Absent (A)	92	99						
Present (B)	1	1						
Performance status (ECOG):								
0 (normal activity)	80	86						
1 (treatment for symptoms, but ambulatory)	13	14						

[a]Modified, with permission, from Pinotti G, Zucca E, Roggero E et al, Clinical features, treatment and outcome in a series of 93 patients with low-grade gastric MALT lymphoma. *Leuk Lymphoma* 1997; **26:** 527–37.

approximately 85%. Survival might be different in other sites. Some very recent studies, however, suggest that there can be a very favorable outcome when the disease is localized, but cases with disseminated disease at presentation or unfavorable prognostic index may have a particularly poor prognosis. Cases with primary gastrointestinal involvement may have a longer survival than the non-gastrointestinal ones.

Treatment and outcome

There is increasing evidence that eradication of *H. pylori* with antibiotics can be effectively employed as the sole initial treatment for low-grade gastric MALT lymphomas. Patients not responding to the eradication of *H. pylori* may harbor high-grade lesions that were not initially appreciated. The use of antibiotics as first-line therapy may avert or at

Table 7.3 Antibiotic regimens for *H. pylori* eradication in low-grade MALT lymphoma currently in use at the Servizio Oncologico Cantonale, Bellinzona[a]		
First-line treatment		
Omeprazole	20 mg	b.i.d. for 10 days
Amoxicillin	1000 mg	b.i.d. for 10 days
Clarithromycin	500 mg	b.i.d. for 10 days
Second-line treatment		
Omeprazole	20 mg	b.i.d. for 7 days
Metronidazole	400 mg	b.i.d. for 7 days
Clarithromycin	500 mg	b.i.d. for 7 days

[a]The aim is to eradicate *H. pylori* infection, and any regimen can be employed. At least thus far, no regimen has been proven to be superior in inducing lymphoma regression, which depends on the successful eradication of *H. pylori*. The schemes reported here showed eradication rates of about 90%.

least postpone the necessity for surgical resection in the majority of patients, and the current procedure at the Servizio Oncologico Cantonale, Belinzona is to eradicate *H. pylori* before considering further therapeutic options (Table 7.3). However, a strict onco-hematological and endoscopic follow-up of the antibiotic-treated patients is needed since whether treatment for *H. pylori* will definitely cure the lymphoma is still unknown. Chemotherapy with single-agent chlorambucil and local radiotherapy have been shown capable of inducing complete remissions in most cases, and can therefore be used in patients who do not respond to antibiotics. The need for surgical resection should be redefined. Surgery has been widely used in the past, with excellent results for localized disease. However, follow-up endoscopy may reveal, in the remaining gastric mucosa, the reappearance of lymphoepithelial lesions that can result in a local recurrence. Indeed, the fact that MALT lymphoma is often a multifocal disease suggests that clear excision margins are not necessarily a guarantee of radical resection. No statistically significant difference has been found in either overall survival or event-free survival between gastric low-grade MALT lymphoma patients who received different initial treatments (chemotherapy alone, surgery alone, surgery with additional chemotherapy or radiation therapy, or antibiotics against *H. pylori*).

It is more difficult to give therapeutic guidelines for non-gastric MALT lymphomas, because of the variety of organ-specific problems that can be found. In general, local radiation can be used successfully for localized lesions; chemotherapy is usually mandatory for advanced or disseminated disease. Surgery has only a diagnostic role (biopsy).

Bibliography

Auer IA, Gascoyne R, Connors JM et al, t(11;18)(q21;q21.1) is the most common translocation in MALT lymphomas. *Ann Oncol* 1997; **8:** 979–85.

Bayerdörffer E, Neubauer A, Rudolph B et al, Regression of primary gastric lymphoma of mucosa associated lymphoid tissue type after cure of *Helicobacter pylori* infection. *Lancet* 1995; **345:** 1591–4.

Harris NL, Jaffe ES, Stein H et al, A revised European–American classification of lymphoid neoplasms: a proposal from the International Lymphoma Study Group. *Blood* 1994; **84:** 1361–92.

Isaacson PG, The MALT lymphoma concept updated. *Ann Oncol* 1995; **6:** 319–20.

Isaacson PG, Spencer J, Malignant lymphoma of mucosa-associated lymphoid tissue. *Histopathology* 1987; **11:** 445–62.

Neubauer A, Thiede C, Morgner A et al, Cure of *Helicobacter pylori* infection and duration of remission of low-grade gastric MALT lymphoma. *J Natl Cancer Inst* 1997; **89:** 1350–5.

Non-Hodgkin's Lymphoma Classification Project, A clinical evaluation of the International Lymphoma Study Group classification of non-Hodgkin's lymphoma. *Blood* 1997; **89:** 3909–18.

Pinotti G, Zucca E, Roggero E et al, Clinical features, treatment and outcome in a series of 93 patients with low-grade gastric MALT lymphoma. *Leuk Lymphoma* 1997; **26:** 527–37.

Roggero E, Zucca E, Cavalli F, Gastric mucosa-associated lymphoid tissue lymphomas: more than a fascinating model. *J Natl Cancer Inst* 1997; **89:** 1328–30.

Roggero E, Zucca E, Pinotti G et al, Eradication of *Helicobacter pylori* infection in primary low-grade gastric lymphoma of mucosa associated lymphoid tissue. *Ann Intern Med* 1995; **122:** 767–9.

Thieblemont C, Bastion Y, Berger F et al, Mucosa-associated gastrointestinal and nongastrointestinal lymphoma behavior: analysis of 108 patients. *J Clin Oncol* 1997; **15:** 1624–30.

Wotherspoon AC, Doglioni C, Diss TC et al, Regression of primary low-grade B-cell gastric lymphoma of mucosa associated lymphoid tissue type after eradication of *Helicobacter pylori. Lancet* 1993; **342:** 575–7.

Zucca E, Roggero E, Biology and treatment of MALT lymphoma: the state of the art in 1996. A workshop at the 6th International Conference on Malignant Lymphoma. *Ann Oncol* 1996; **7:** 787–92.

Zucca E, Pinotti G, Roggero E et al, High incidence of other neoplasms in patients with low-grade gastric MALT-lymphoma. *Ann Oncol* 1995; **6:** 726–8.

Zucca E, Roggero E, Pileri S, B-cell lymphoma of malt type: a review with special emphasis on diagnostic and management problems of low-grade gastric tumours. *Br J Haematol* 1998; **100:** 3–14.

Zucca E, Bertoni F, Roggero E et al, Molecular analysis of the progression from *Helicobacter pylori*-associated chronic gastritis to mucosa-associated lymphoid tissue lymphoma of the stomach. *N Engl J Med* 1998; **338:** 804–10.

MALT lymphoma

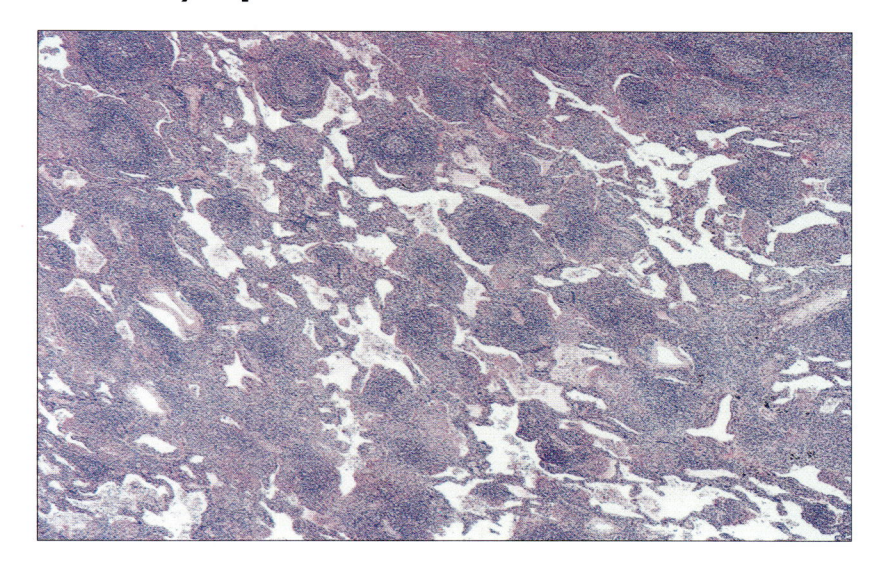

Figure 7.1

MALT lymphoma (extranodal marginal-zone B-cell lymphoma) – Lung:

(a) There is a dense interstitial infiltrate with formation of multiple small nodules. (H&E stain)

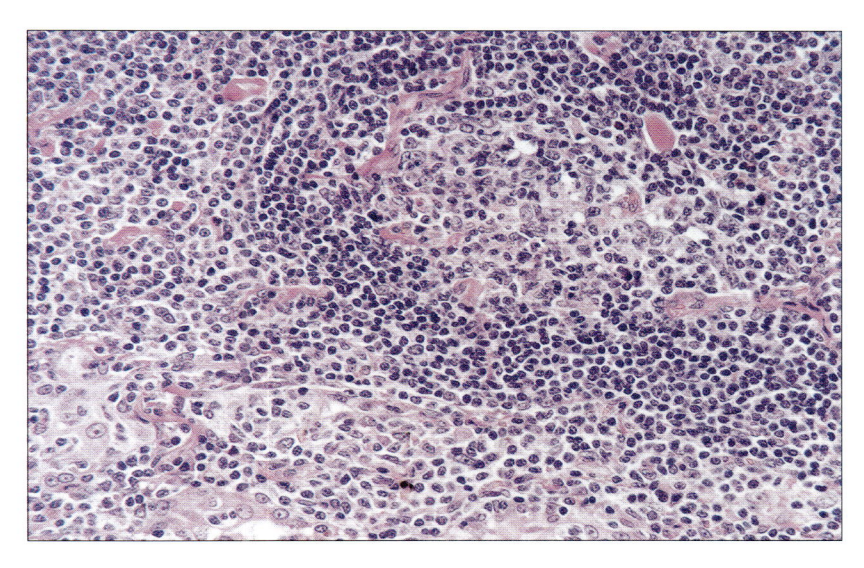

(b) Higher power shows that the nodules consist of reactive lymphoid follicles surrounded by pale marginal-zone B cells. (H&E stain)

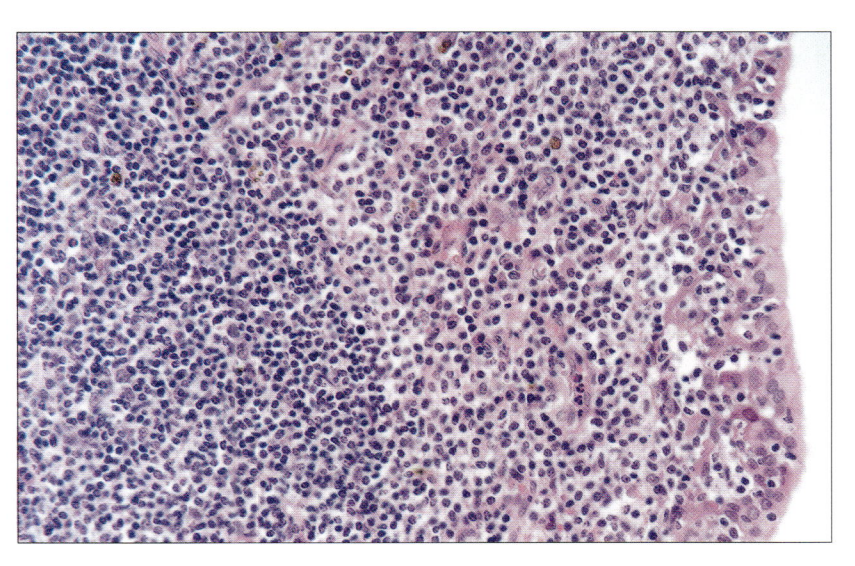

(c) In this area, lymphoma involves a bronchiole. A band of pale marginal-zone B cells is seen just beneath the epithelium, while darker small lymphocytes are seen adjacent to the pale cells. (H&E stain)

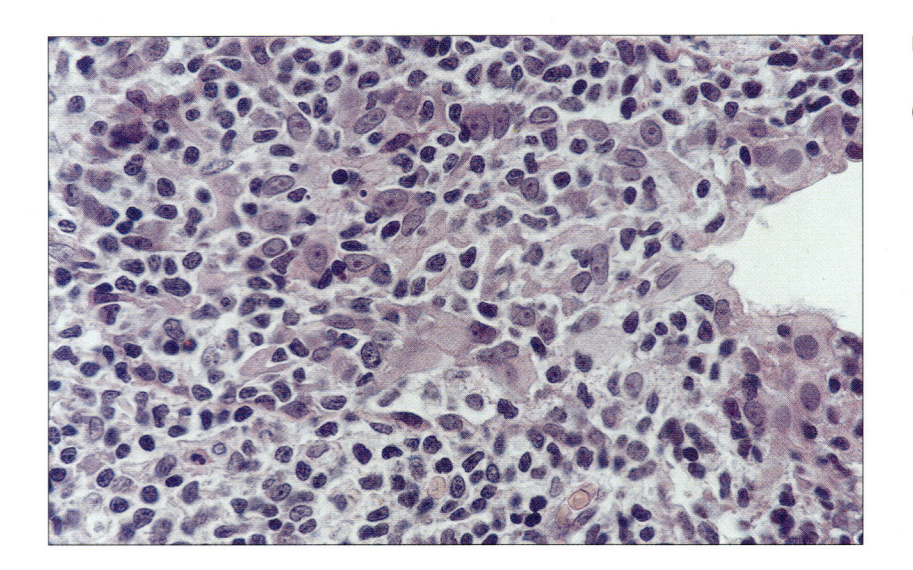

Figure 7.1 *continued*

(**d**) Invasion of bronchiolar epithelium by the lymphoma. (H&E stain)

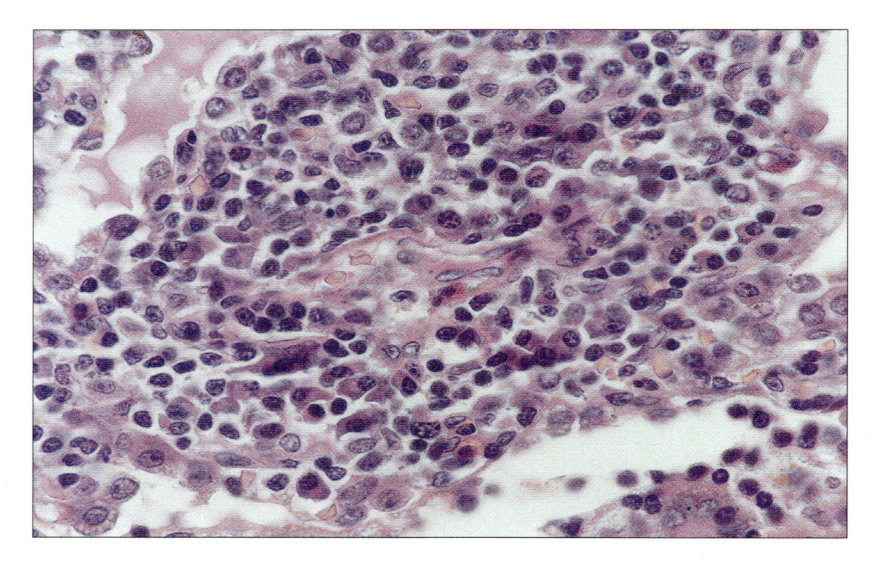

(**e**) In some areas, the interstitial infiltrate is composed of a mixture of small lymphoid cells and plasma cells. (H&E stain)

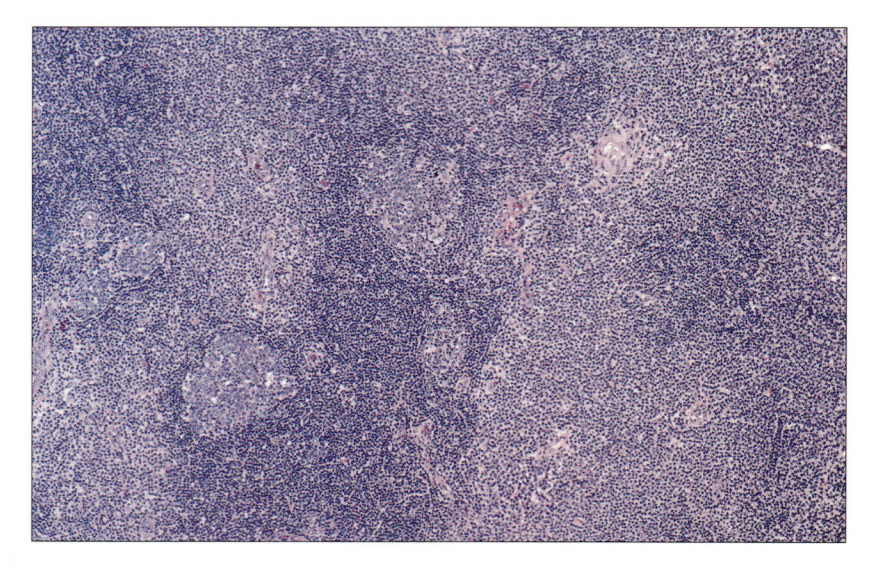

Figure 7.2

MALT lymphoma – Orbit:

(**a**) The lymphoma consists of bands of pale cells surrounding reactive lymphoid follicles. (H&E stain)

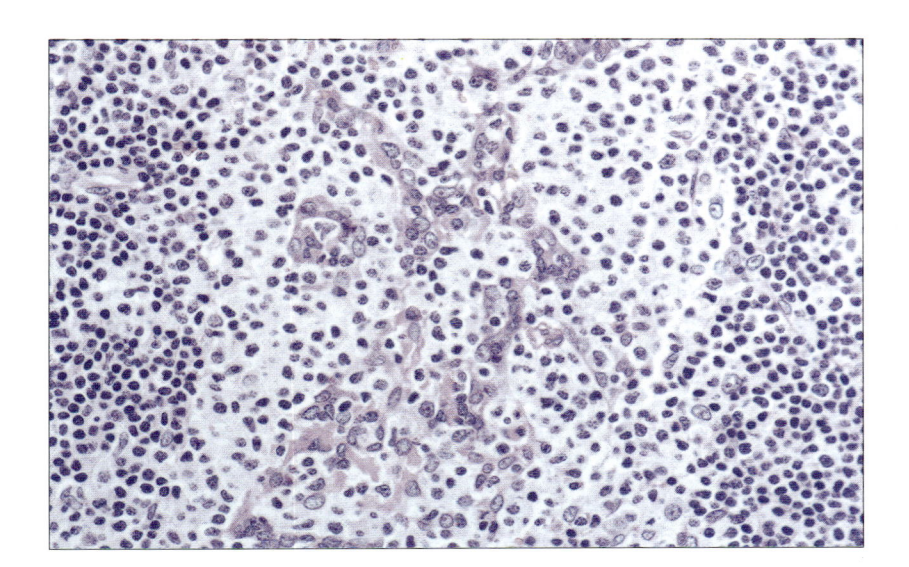

Figure 7.2 *continued*

(b) Monocytoid B cells with abundant pale cytoplasm surround and infiltrate lacrimal gland epithelium. (H&E stain)

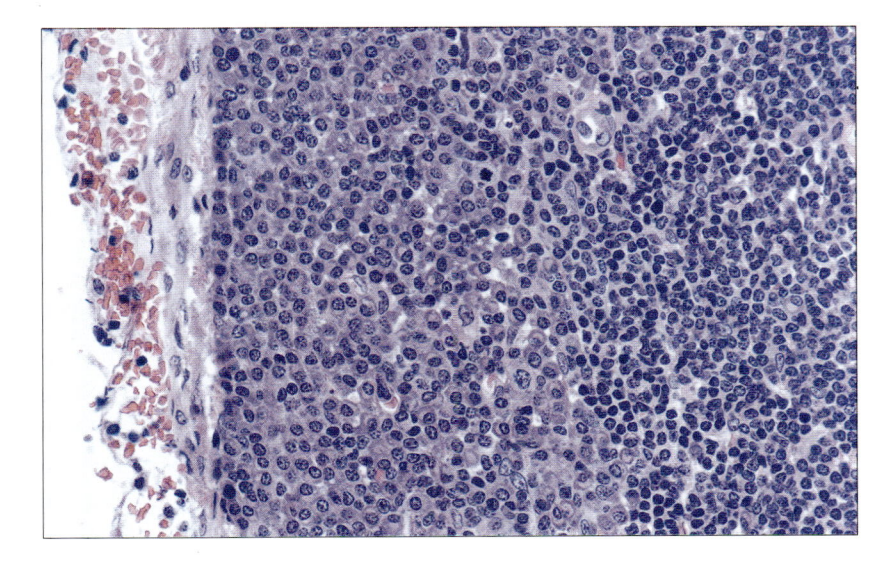

(c) A broad zone of plasma cells with abundant pink cytoplasm is adjacent to a band of small lymphocytes with scant cytoplasm. (H&E stain)

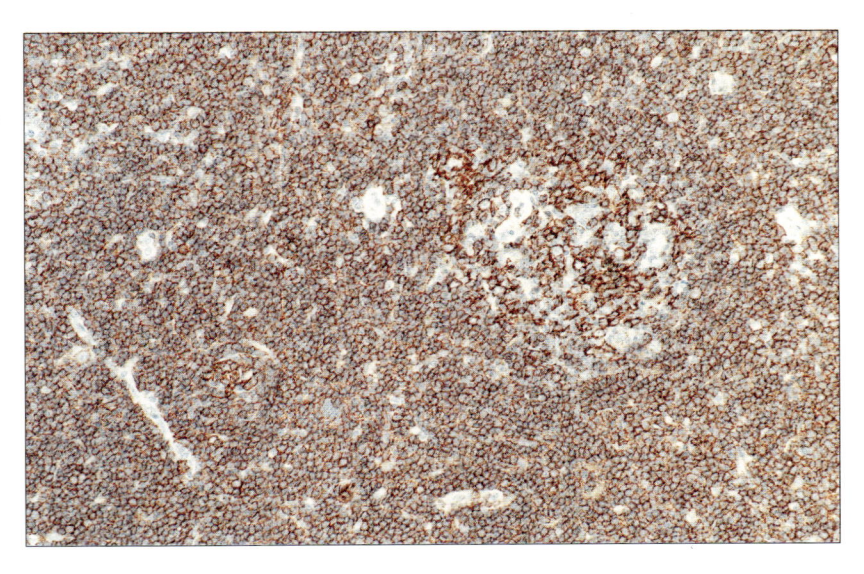

(d) With antibody to B cells (L26), most lymphoid cells are stained. A small reactive follicle is present. (Immunoperoxidase technique on paraffin sections)

Contd

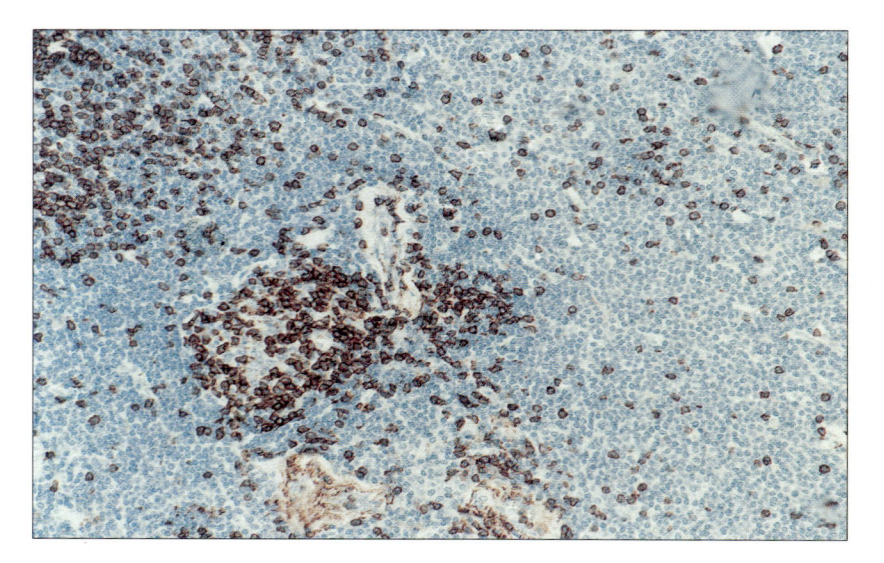

Figure 7.2 *continued*

(e) With antibody to T-cell-associated antigen (CD45RO), scattered cells are stained. T cells are more numerous in the reactive follicle than in the surrounding lymphoma. (Immunoperoxidase technique on paraffin sections)

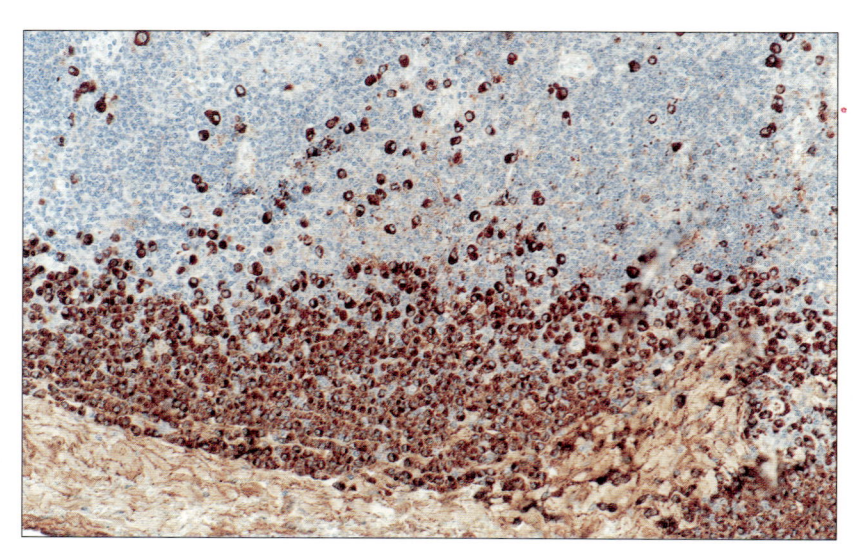

The plasma cells forming a band express monotypic cytoplasmic immunoglobulin (**f,g**), with nearly all plasma cells expressing κ (**f**), and only rare λ^+ (**g**) plasma cells. (Immunoperoxidase technique on paraffin sections)

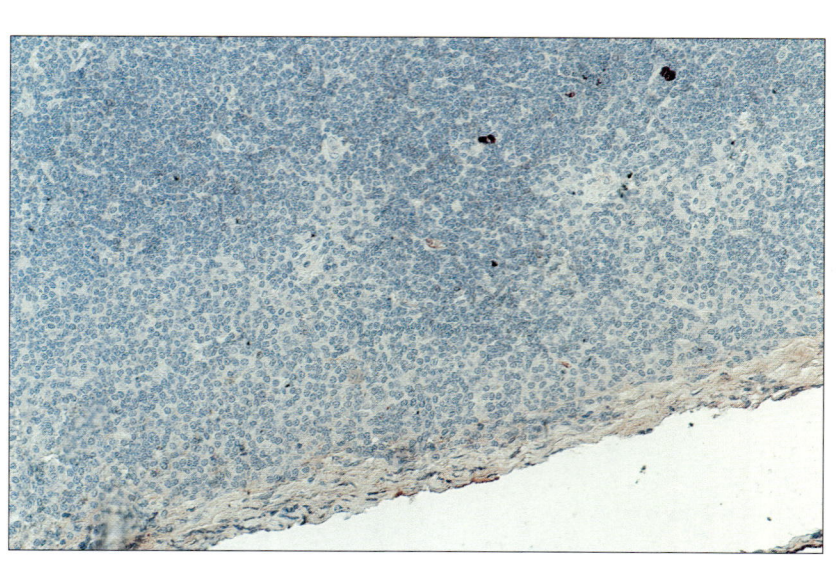

(f)

(g)

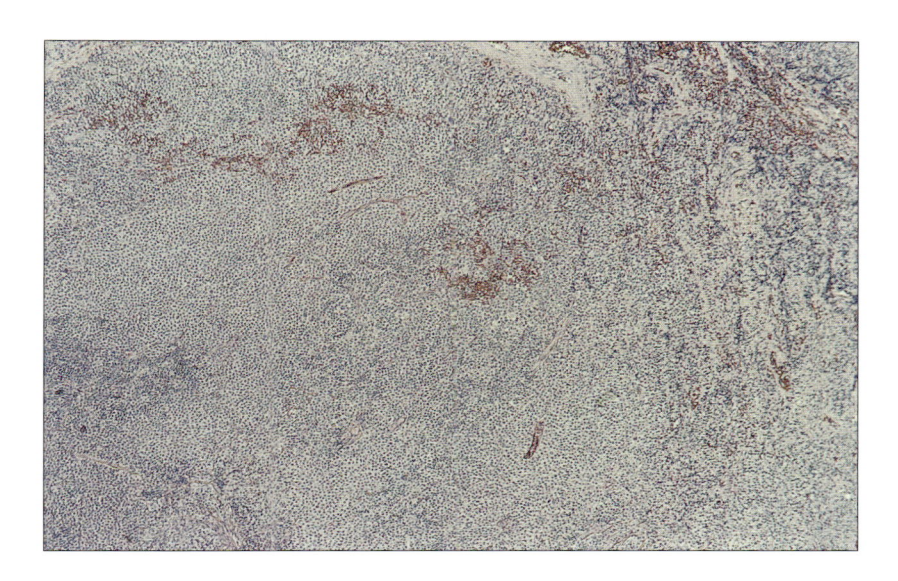

Figure 7.3

MALT lymphoma – Parotid:

Low-power examination shows obliteration of the normal parenchyma by sheets of monocytoid B cells (**a**), in some areas with an admixture of aggregates of darker small lymphocytes (**b**). (H&E stain)

(a)

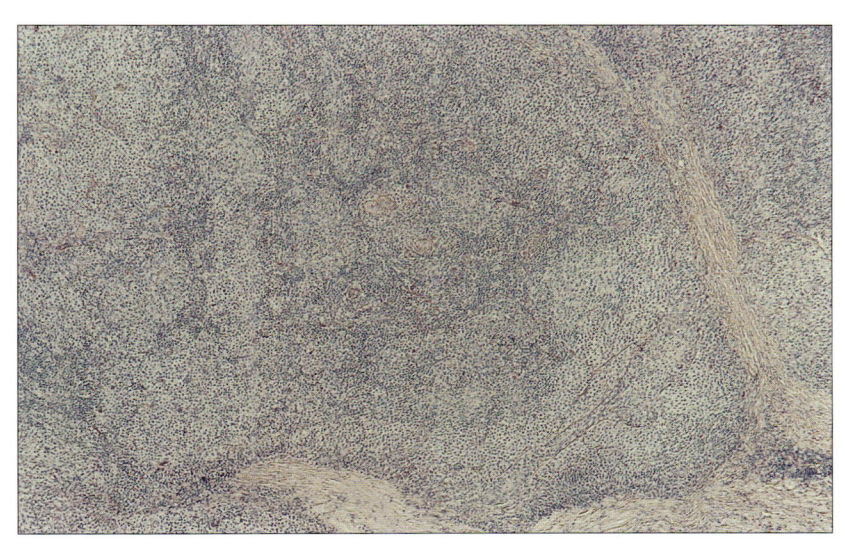

(b)

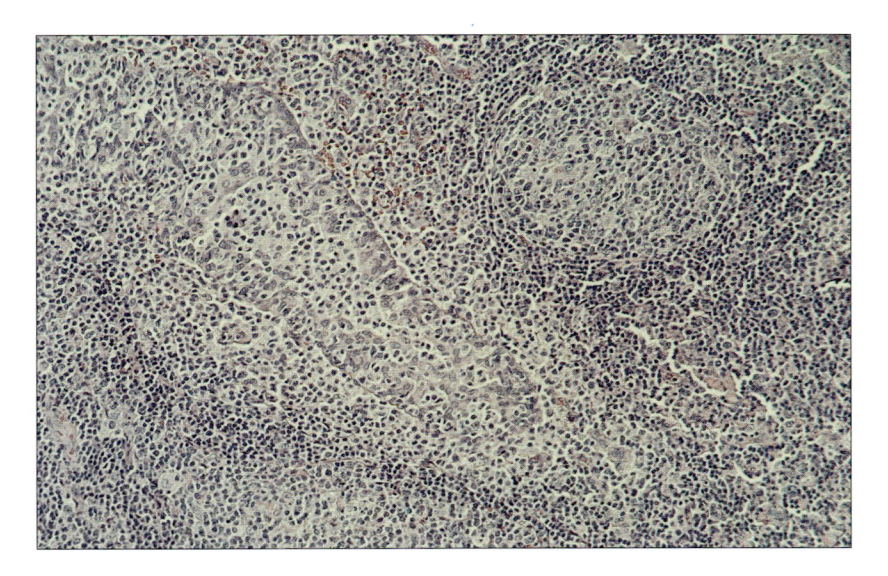

(c) A reactive lymphoid follicle and a large prominent lymphoepithelial lesion are present. (H&E stain)

Contd

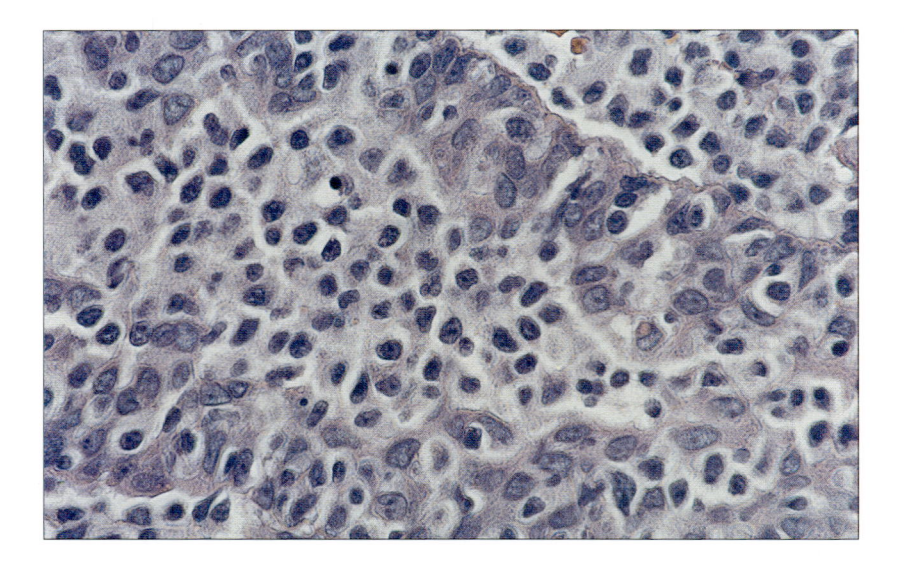

Figure 7.3 *continued*

(d) Higher power of the lymphoepithelial lesion shows monocytoid B cells with abundant pale cytoplasm in association with an expanded island of epithelial cells. (H&E stain)

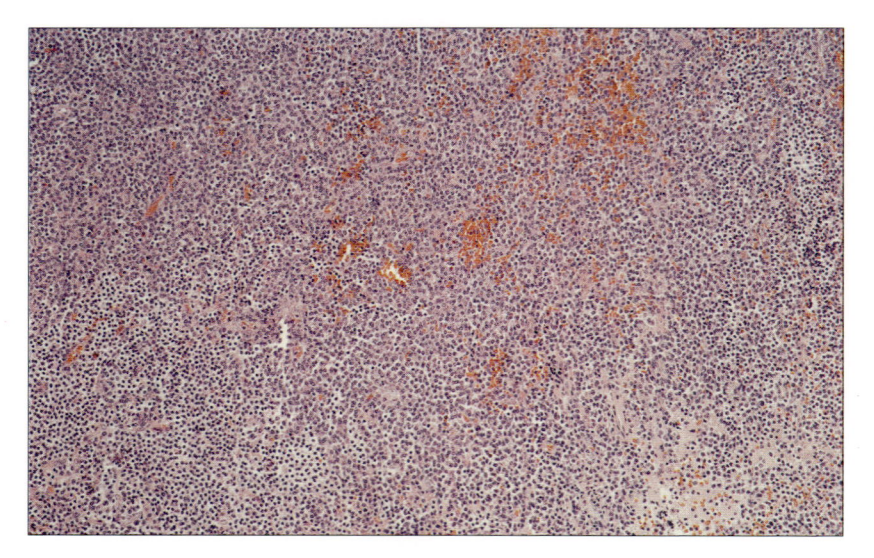

Figure 7.4

MALT lymphoma – nasolacrimal duct region:

(a) Sheets of cells occupy soft tissue around the nasolacrimal duct. (H&E stain)

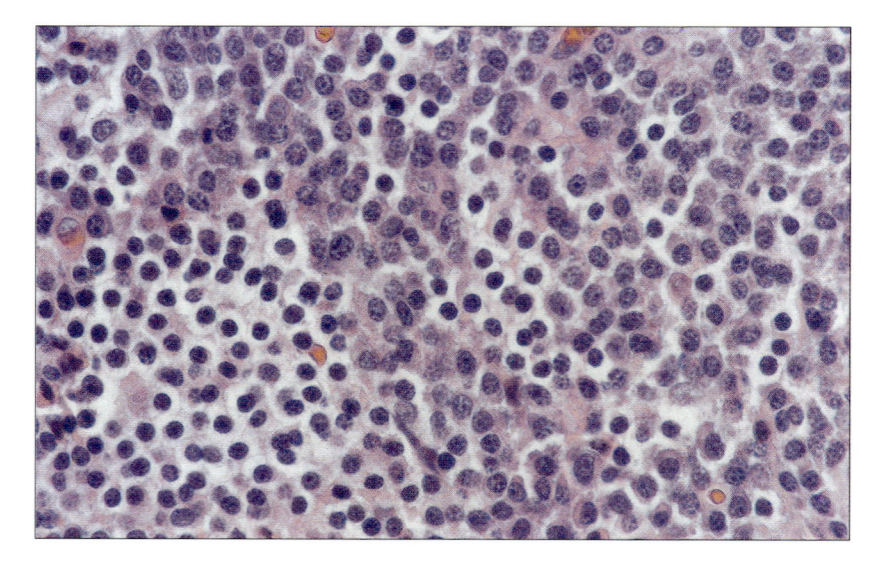

(b) Higher power reveals two populations: marginal-zone cells with clear cytoplasm and plasma cells with amphophilic cytoplasm. (H&E stain)

MALT lymphoma

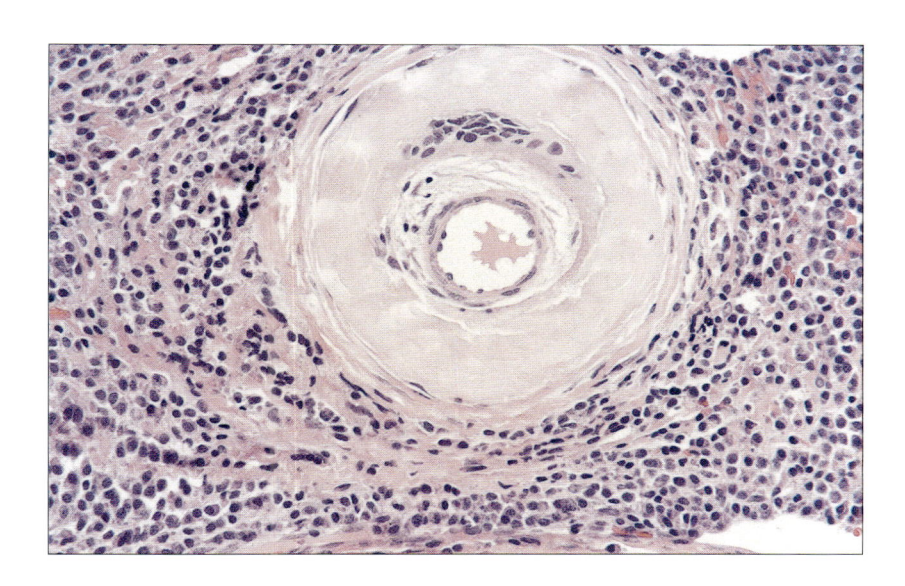

(c) This lymphoma is associated with amyloid deposition in blood vessels. (H&E stain)

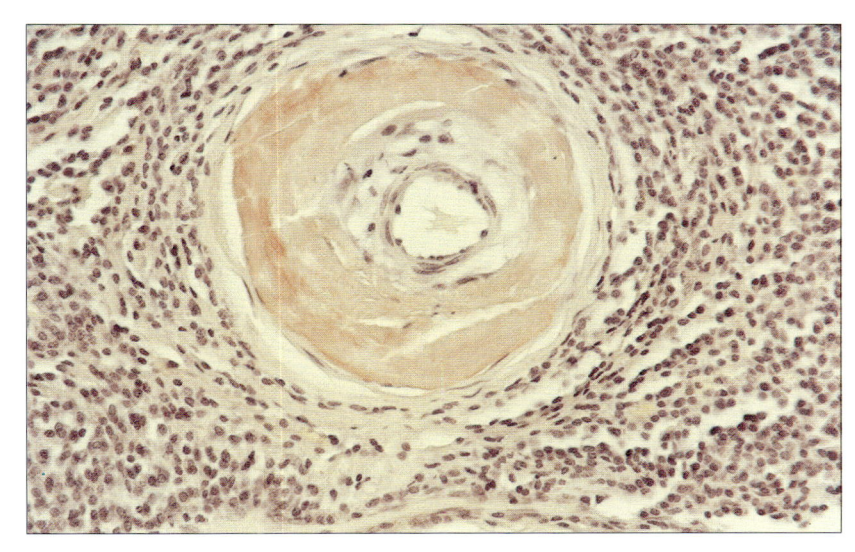

(d) The amyloid stains orange with a Congo red stain.

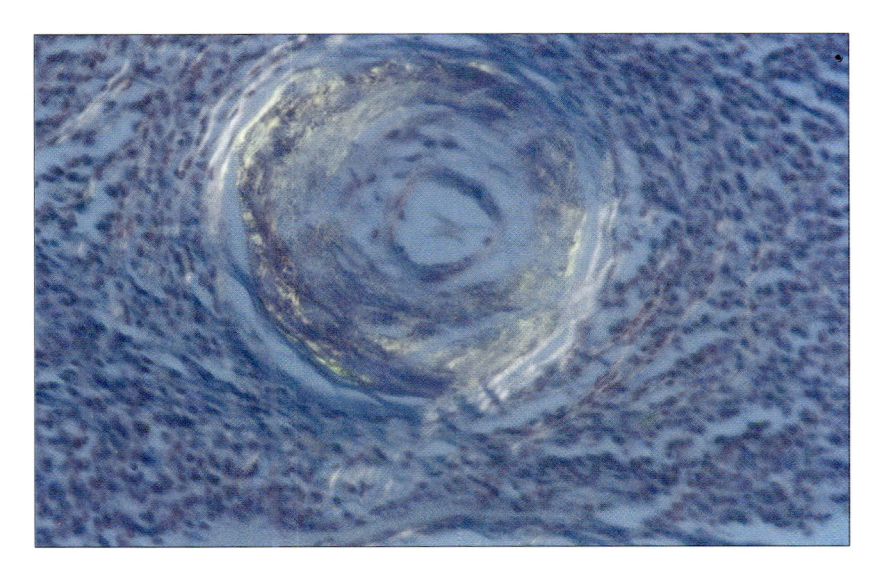

(e) The amyloid shows apple-green birefringence with polarized light. (Congo red stain)

Contd

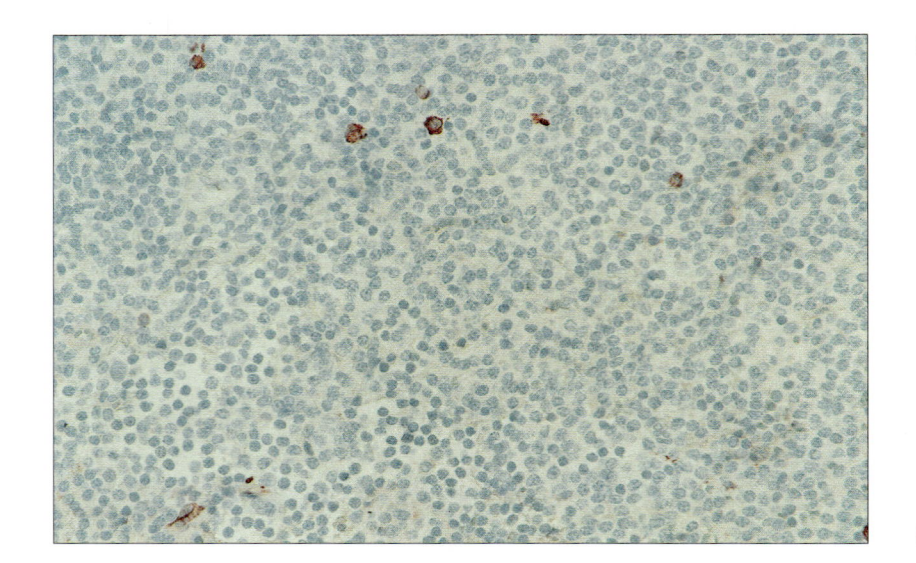

Figure 7.4 *continued*

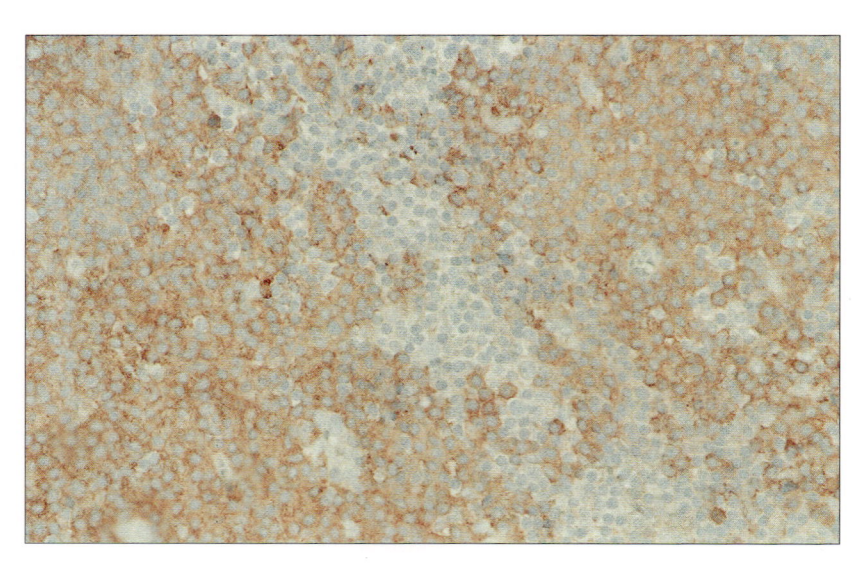

With antibodies to immunoglobulin light chains, only rare cells are κ⁺ (**f**), while numerous cells are λ⁺ (**g**), consistent with prominent plasmacytic differentiation of the lymphoma. (Immunoperoxidase technique on paraffin sections)

(f)

(g)

8 Burkitt's lymphoma/leukemia

Definition and classification

Burkitt's lymphoma was first described by Dennis Burkitt in African children who presented with large tumors of the facial bones, particularly the jaw. Subsequently tumors of similar morphology but affecting different anatomic sites were noted at a lower frequency in Europe and the USA. The Rappaport classification called Burkitt's lymphoma by the name 'diffuse undifferentiated lymphoma'. The Working Formulation adopted the Lukes and Collins terminology: 'diffuse small non-cleaved cell lymphoma, Burkitt's type'.

A type of lymphoma that occurs more commonly in adults was observed to be similar in histologic appearance to Burkitt's lymphoma, but showed much more heterogeneity in the size and shape of the nucleus than was typical of the monotonous Burkitt's lymphoma. This tumor was called 'diffuse small non-cleaved cell lymphoma, non-Burkitt's type'.

In the REAL classification, Burkitt's lymphoma is called 'Burkitt's lymphoma'. The entity that was called non-Burkitt's type was designated a provisional entity in the new classification and called 'high-grade B-cell lymphoma, Burkitt-like'. The pathologists of the Non-Hodgkin's Lymphoma Classification Project found that reproducibly distinguishing Burkitt's from Burkitt-like lymphoma was difficult on the basis of light microscopy alone. Furthermore, more careful molecular analysis of Burkitt-like lymphoma cases suggested that this was not a discrete clinicopathologic entity, and, in particular, these cases uniformly lacked expression of c-MYC, a nearly universal feature of Burkitt's lymphoma. In light of the difficulty in making the diagnosis and the apparent heterogeneity of molecular features, Burkitt-like lymphoma is not a named entity in the new WHO classification. Cases that look similar to Burkitt's lymphoma but have more cellular heterogeneity and are not associated with c-MYC activation will be classified as diffuse large B-cell lymphomas.

Frequency

The endemic regions of Burkitt's lymphoma are Equatorial Africa and New Guinea, and in these areas the annual incidence of the disease is 2.2–3.8/100 000. The peak incidence is at age 5–8 years. In epidemic regions, Burkitt's lymphoma accounts for about 50% of all childhood cancers. In non-endemic regions, the annual incidence in children under the age of 16 years is 0.1–0.3/100 000: 20–40 times lower than in endemic areas. Even though Burkitt's lymphoma is rarer in Western countries, it represents the most common form of childhood lymphoma, accounting for 35–45% of cases. Among the 1400 cases in the Non-Hodgkin's Lymphoma Classification Project, 10 were Burkitt's lymphomas. The only African country represented in this study was South Africa, where the incidence is similar to that in Western countries.

Burkitt's lymphoma is also one of the more common lymphomas complicating the clinical course of HIV infection; about one-third of lymphomas in AIDS patients are Burkitt's lymphomas. Like non-epidemic Burkitt's lymphoma, AIDS-associated Burkitt's lymphoma is much more common in men than women and in Whites than in African–Americans.

Pathology

Histology

The tumor grows in a diffuse pattern, and is composed of sheets of monomorphic cells with little perceptible variation from cell to cell. The cells are medium-sized (larger than small lymphocytes, smaller than large cell lymphoma cells), with round nuclei, clumped chromatin, several (two to five) darkly staining nucleoli, and moderately abundant basophilic cytoplasm. Interspersed between tumor cells are occasional macrophages ingesting apoptotic tumor cells; these cells are described as giving the tumor a 'starry sky' appearance.

Immunophenotype

The cells are mature B lymphocytes with surface immunoglobulin (usually IgM), and they express CD19, CD20, CD22, CD79a and usually CD10. They are terminal deoxynucleotide transferase (TdT)-negative, CD5$^-$ and CD23$^-$, and express no T-cell markers. All the tumor cells are in cycle, giving this tumor a 100% growth fraction, and thus the cells all stain with Ki-67, an antibody against a DNA polymerase only expressed in dividing cells. The normal counterpart of the Burkitt's lymphoma cell is not fully defined. The cells demonstrate immunoglobulin gene mutations that commonly occur in germinal centers; however, they are not follicular center cells. It is possible that they originate in Peyer's patches or other extranodal sites of antibody affinity maturation.

Genetics

The molecular hallmark of Burkitt's lymphoma is activation of the c-*MYC* gene. Typically, this activation occurs as a consequence of chromosomal rearrangement that brings the c-*MYC* gene on chromosome 8q24 into proximity to the transcriptionally active immunoglobulin genes. Chromosome breaks at 8q24 are present in all Burkitt's lymphomas, and are almost non-existent in any other lymphoma. In 80% of cases, the translocation involves the immunoglobulin heavy-chain gene on chromosome 14q32; in 15% of cases, 8q24 translocates to the immunoglobulin κ light chain on chromosome 2p11; and in 5% of cases, the c-*MYC* gene translocates to the immunoglobulin λ light-chain gene on chromosome 22q11.

The common t(8;14)(q24;q32) translocation is the exclusive lesion found in epidemic Burkitt's lymphoma, and it differs from the t(8;14) translocation in sporadic (non-epidemic) Burkitt's lymphoma. In epidemic Burkitt's lymphoma, the breakpoint on chromosome 8 is more than 1000 kb 5' to the c-*MYC* gene, and the chromosome 14 breakpoint is within the J_H region of the heavy-chain gene. When the translocation takes place, mutations are introduced into the 5' non-coding regions of the gene that contribute to the overexpression of the gene. In the t(8;14) in sporadic Burkitt's lymphoma, the chromosome 8 breakpoint decapitates the first exon of c-*MYC*, and the chromosome 14 breakpoint is within the immunoglobulin switch region. The nature of these translocations suggests that they occur at the pro-B-cell stage of differentiation when the immunoglobulin genes are rearranging. All of the translocations result in the overexpression of c-MYC and the proliferation of the overexpressing cell. Why the cell does not become overtly neoplastic until it differentiates into a mature B cell is unknown.

In addition to the translocations, in about 50% of Burkitt's lymphomas, the c-MYC protein bears point mutations in exon 2 that are similar to those present in the transforming v-MYC analogue of c-MYC. These mutations further augment the transforming power of c-MYC because the mutated proteins cannot bind to the retinoblastoma (RB)-related p107 protein that acts as an inhibitor of c-MYC activity.

About 95% of endemic Burkitt's lymphomas and 20% of sporadic Burkitt's lymphomas are infected with monoclonal Epstein–Barr virus (EBV). The monoclonality of the virus suggests that it was present in the cell at the time of neoplastic transformation. The role of the virus in lymphomagenesis is unclear, especially in view of the fact that the virus is latent in the tumor cells. Only a noncoding RNA molecule (EBER) and a single viral protein (EBNA1) are expressed, and these viral components are not sufficient to cause malignant transformation.

Inactivation of *p53* is noted in 30–40% of Burkitt's lymphomas, and in many cases there are also deletions of chromosome 6q. The additional genetic lesions probably contribute to the pathogenesis of the disease. Activation of c-*MYC* has not been noted in Burkitt-like lymphoma – a finding that fosters the idea that Burkitt-like lymphoma is not a discrete entity and should be considered a form of diffuse large B-cell lymphoma.

Clinical characteristics

Burkitt's lymphoma has a male-to-female ratio of 2–4:1. Endemic Burkitt's lymphoma most commonly affects the jaw (70%), and involves, in descending order, the gastrointestinal tract (60%), central nervous system (20%) and orbit (10%). The pattern of distribution of sporadic Burkitt's lymphoma is different: 80% of cases involve the gastrointestinal tract, 40% involve the lymph nodes and 25% involve the bones and bone marrow; a small number of cases involve unusual sites like the testis and breast, but lymphomas involving the testis and breast are usually Burkitt's lymphomas. Leptomeningeal spread to the central nervous system (CNS) can occur in patients with bone, bone marrow or testicular involvement. An important subset of patients present with dominant bone marrow involvement and a clinical picture of acute leukemia without tumor masses outside the marrow. In the FAB classification system, Burkitt's leukemia is called L3 or 'B-cell acute lymphoblastic leukemia'. The total fraction of Burkitt's lymphoma that is leukemia is somewhat difficult to estimate, because these entities were approached as separate diseases for many years. However, the incidence of acute lymphoid leukemia is about 15–20-fold higher than the incidence of Burkitt's lymphoma. Given that Burkitt's leukemia represents about 2% of acute leukemias, Burkitt's leukemia may represent 30% of all cases of Burkitt's lymphoma.

The median age of onset is related to the frequency of the disease, and varies in different geographic sites: in endemic regions where the disease prevalence is high, the median age is lower (age 5–8 years); in non-endemic regions where the disease prevalence is lower, the median age is 14 years. In the USA and Europe, most patients are children or adolescents; the disease is rare in people over age 40 years.

Because of the high growth fraction of the tumor, clinical progression of disease is rapid, and

Table 8.1
Staging of Burkitt's lymphoma

St Jude staging system
Stage I	Single tumor (extranodal)
	Single anatomic area (nodal)
	Excluding mediastinum or abdomen
Stage II	Single tumor (extranodal) with regional node involvement
	Primary gastrointestinal tumor with or without mesenteric nodes, resected
	Two or more nodal areas or two single extranodal tumors on same side of diaphragm
Stage III	Two or more nodal areas or two single extranodal tumors on both sides of diaphragm
	All primary intrathoracic tumors
	All extensive primary intraabdominal disease
	All primary paraspinal or epidural tumors, regardless of other sites
Stage IV	Any of the above with initial CNS or bone marrow (>25%) involvement

Uganda Cancer Institute staging system
Stage A	Single or multiple jaw tumors; no other site of involvement
Stage AR	Abdominal tumor more than 90% resected
Stage B	Multiple sites of disease outside the abdomen
Stage C	Tumor confined to the abdomen
Stage D	Abdominal tumor and extraabdominal tumor (except single jaw tumor)

little time should elapse between diagnosis and treatment. Thus staging needs to be accomplished in hours rather than days. Two staging systems have been employed for Burkitt's lymphoma (Table 8.1). An argument could be made to perform exploratory laparotomy on patients with large abdominal masses and to resect as much disease as possible; data from uncontrolled studies suggest that patients whose tumors are surgically debulked fare better than those treated with combination chemotherapy without surgical debulking. However, definitive chemotherapy cannot be withheld from patients for more than 48 hours postoperatively lest the tumor regrow. This early postoperative intervention is uncommonly associated with wound infections or dehiscence.

A number of disease-related problems may complicate management. Intestinal obstruction, most commonly related to intussusception, perforation or hemorrhage, airway obstruction from pharyngeal tumor growth, respiratory difficulties related to pleural effusions, or cardiac tamponade from pericardial effusions may occur. Massive abdominal disease may slow blood flow in major vessels and produce thrombosis that could lead to fatal pulmonary thromboembolism. Appropriate prophylaxis to prevent a catastrophe is important to consider. Once a diagnosis of Burkitt's lymphoma has been made, and while minimal staging tests are being performed, patients should be hydrated vigorously, have their urine made alkaline, and begin allopurinol to prevent the consequences of rapid tumor lysis upon initiation of chemotherapy. The massive discharge of intracellular contents from dying tumor cells can produce sudden death from hyperkalemia or can induce acute renal failure from urate nephropathy. The risk of acute tumor lysis syndrome is related to the tumor burden. If renal failure occurs despite prophylaxis, treatment should continue with hemodialysis support.

Treatment

It was once thought that adults with Burkitt's lymphoma had a poorer prognosis than children and that patients with Burkitt's leukemia had a poorer prognosis than patients with other forms of lymphoblastic leukemia. However, with the application of treatment principles derived from management of acute leukemia (intensive induction, consolidation, maintenance, CNS prophylaxis), the prognoses for adults and children with Burkitt's lymphoma have become similar, and Burkitt's leukemia is curable in the majority of cases.

Patients with limited or localized disease (St Jude stages I and II, Uganda stages A and AR) are cured in 90–100% of cases with combination chemotherapy regimens that employ intensive therapy for only two to three months. The German Berlin–Frankfurt–Münster BFM 86 protocol (see Chapter 11), the French Society of Pediatric Oncology LMB 86 protocol (see Figure 8.1) and the National Cancer Institute's CODOX-M regimen all report extremely high long-term survival rates without life-threatening toxicity. Radiation therapy does not improve the results.

For patients with advanced disease (stage III and stage IV), BFM 86, LMB 89, and the NCI protocol alternating CODOX-M and IVAC produce similar results: long-term survival in 75–92% of stage III patients and 75–87% of stage IV patients (see Table

Table 8.2
Outcome of treatment in advanced Burkitt's lymphoma

Treatment protocol	No. of patients	Event-free survival	
		Stage III	Stage IV
Total B	29	81%	37% (17% for leukemia)
POG 9317	68	87%	63% (83% for leukemia)
HiC-COM	20	92%	50%
BFM 86	150	73%	75%
SFOP 89	181	87%	85% (87% for leukemia)
CODOX-M/IVAC	38	92%	81%
SFOP LMB 86 adults	53	76%	57%

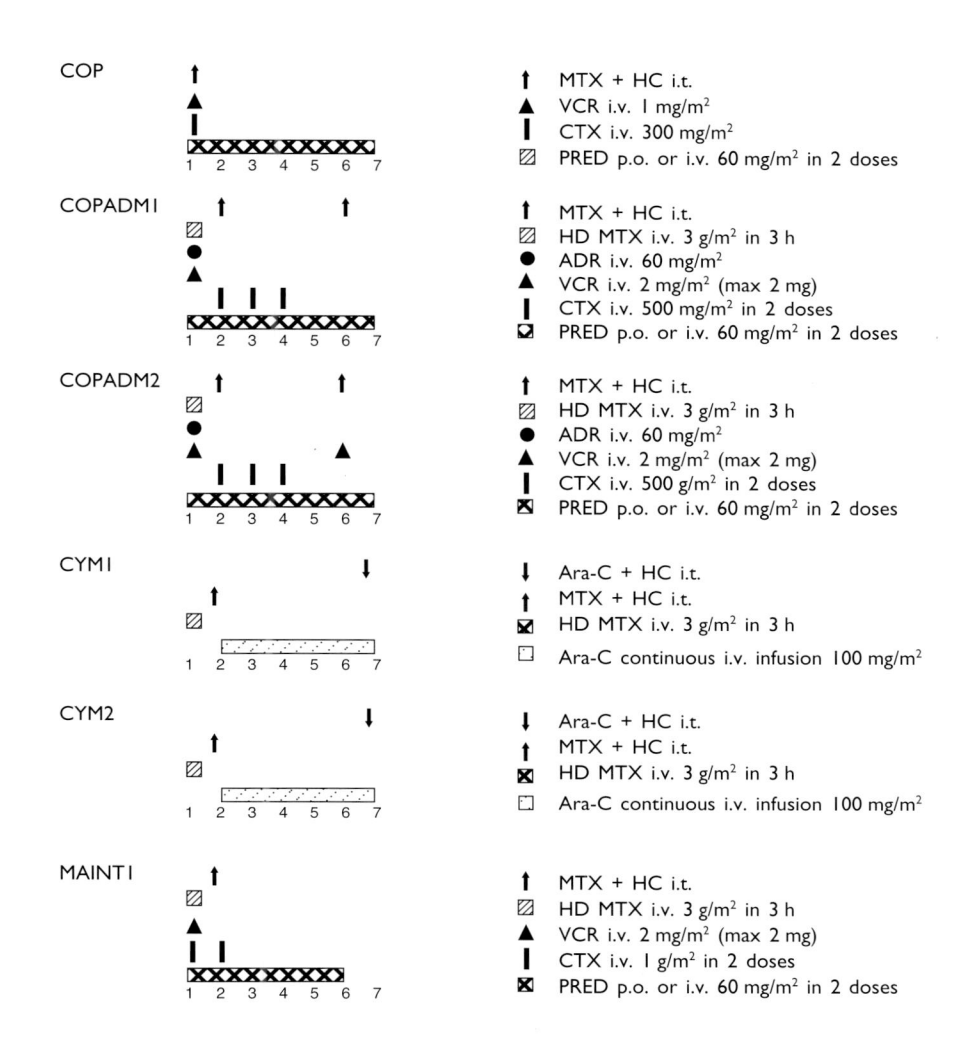

Figure 8.1
The LMB 86 protocol of the Société Française d'Oncologie Pédiatrique (SFOP) for B-cell lymphoma/leukemia. Therapy is tailored to the patient's tumor burden. Those with disease completely resected (low risk) receive induction chemotherapy without high-dose methotrexate. Those with residual disease but with less than 70% tumor cells in the bone marrow (intermediate risk) receive 3 gm/m² doses of high-dose methotrexate. Those with greater than 70% tumor cells in the bone marrow (high risk) receive 8 gm/m² doses of high-dose methotrexate. In addition, high-risk patients receive more aggressive consolidation and a second type of maintenance therapy for four monthly cycles, rather than the single cycle that intermediate-risk patients get. High-risk patients also receive cranial radiation (2400 cGy) during maintenance therapy. MTX, methotrexate (HD, high-dose); HC, hydrocortisone; VCR, vincristine; CTX, cyclophosphamide; PRED, prednisone; ADR, Adriamycin (doxorubicin); Ara-C, cytosine arabinoside. (Reproduced from Canellos GP et al, *The Lymphomas*, 1997, based on data provided by Dr C Patte, and with permission from WB Saunders.)

8.2). Patients who relapse typically have marrow progression. The use of high-dose therapy and bone marrow transplantation has not been shown to cure a larger fraction of patients when it is a component of primary treatment. However, 33–49% of relapsed patients may be rescued with high-dose therapy and autologous stem cell transplantation.

Relapse of disease occurs within eight months of starting treatment or it does not occur at all. The rapid proliferation of the tumor cells makes a relapse apparent quickly; even if a single cell remained alive after treatment, it would produce clinically apparent disease within four or five months. Rare late relapses have been seen in endemic Burkitt's lymphomas, where treatment approaches are generally less aggressive; however, the development of what appears to be recurrent tumor in HIV-infected patients may actually be the development of an independent neoplasm derived from a different clone of cells.

Patients with Burkitt's lymphoma complicating the course of AIDS have a much poorer prognosis – not because the disease is resistant to treatment but because the treatment has greater toxicity in patients with immunodeficiency. Where aggressive treatment has been given, response rates are similar to those obtained in patients without immunodeficiency. However, the high death rate from complicating serious infections makes aggressive therapy difficult to administer.

Bibliography

Bowman PW, Shuster JJ, Cook B et al, Improved survival for children with B cell acute lymphoblastic leukemia and stage IV small noncleaved cell lymphoma: A Pediatric Oncology Group Study. *J Clin Oncol* 1996; **14:** 1252–61.

Burkitt D, O'Conor GT, Malignant lymphoma in African children. I. A clinical syndrome. *Cancer* 1961; **14:** 258–69.

Haddy TB, Adde M, Magrath I, CNS involvement in small noncleaved-cell lymphoma: Is CNS disease per se a poor prognostic sign? *J Clin Oncol* 1991; **9:** 1973–82.

Hoelzer D, Ludwig WD, Thiel E et al, Improved outcome in adult B-cell acute lymphoblastic leukemia. *Blood* 1996; **87:** 495–508.

Ladenstein R, Pearce R, Hartmann O et al, High-dose chemotherapy with autologous bone marrow rescue in children with poor-risk Burkitt's lymphoma: a report from the European Lymphoma Bone Marrow Transplantation Registry. *Blood* 1997; **90:** 2921–30.

Link MP, Shuster JJ, Donaldson SS et al, Treatment of children and young adults with early-stage non-Hodgkin's lymphoma. *N Engl J Med* 1997; **337:** 1259–66.

Magrath I, Adde M, Shad A et al, Adults and children with small noncleaved cell lymphoma have similar excellent outcome when treated with the same chemotherapy regimen. *J Clin Oncol* 1996; **14:** 925–35.

Patte C, Michon J, Frappaz D et al, Therapy of Burkitt and other B-cell acute lymphoblastic leukaemia and lymphoma: experience with the LMB protocols of the SFOP (French Paediatric Oncology Society) in children and adults. *Baillière's Clin Haematol* 1994; **7:** 339–48.

Patte C, Philip T, Rodary C et al, High survival rate in advanced-stage B-cell lymphomas and leukemias without CNS involvement with a short intensive polychemotherapy: results from the French Pediatric Oncology Society of a randomized trial of 216 children. *J Clin Oncol* 1995; **13:** 359–68.

Preudhomme C, Dervite I, Wattel E et al, Clinical significance of p53 mutations in newly diagnosed Burkitt's lymphoma and acute lymphoblastic leukemia: a report of 48 cases. *J Clin Oncol* 1995; **13:** 812–20.

Soussain C, Patte C, Ostronoff M et al, Small noncleaved cell lymphoma and leukemia in adults. A retrospective study of 65 adults treated with the LMB pediatric protocols. *Blood* 1995; **85:** 664–74.

Spina M, Tirelli U, Zagonel V et al, Burkitt's lymphoma in adults with and without human immunodeficiency virus infection: a single-institution clinicopathologic study of 75 patients. *Cancer* 1998; **82:** 766–74.

Sweetenham JW, Pearce R, Taghipour G et al, Adult Burkitt's and Burkitt-like non-Hodgkin's lymphoma – outcome for patients treated with high-dose therapy and autologous stem-cell transplantation in first remission or at relapse: results from the European Group for Blood and Marrow Transplantation. *J Clin Oncol* 1996; **14:** 2465–72.

Todeschini G, Tecchio C, Degani D et al, Eighty-one percent event-free survival in advanced Burkitt's lymphoma/leukemia: no differences in outcome between pediatric and adult patients treated with the same intensive pediatric protocol. *Ann Oncol* 1997; **8**(Suppl 1): 77–81.

Yano T, Van Krieken JJ, Magrath I et al, Histogenetic correlations between subcategories of small noncleaved cell lymphomas. *Blood* 1992; **79:** 1282–90.

Burkitt's lymphoma

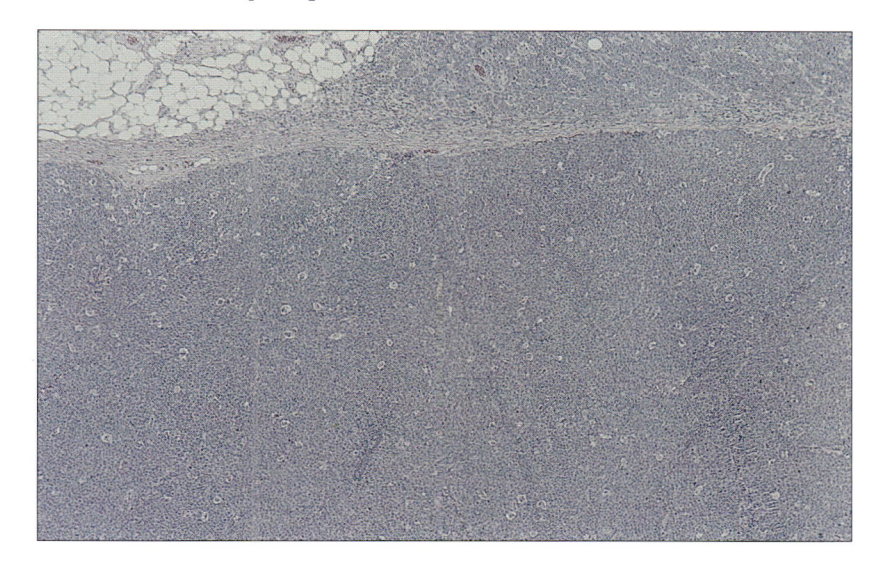

Figure 8.2

Burkitt's lymphoma:

(a) There is obliteration of the normal lymph node architecture and extension into perinodal fat. (H&E stain)

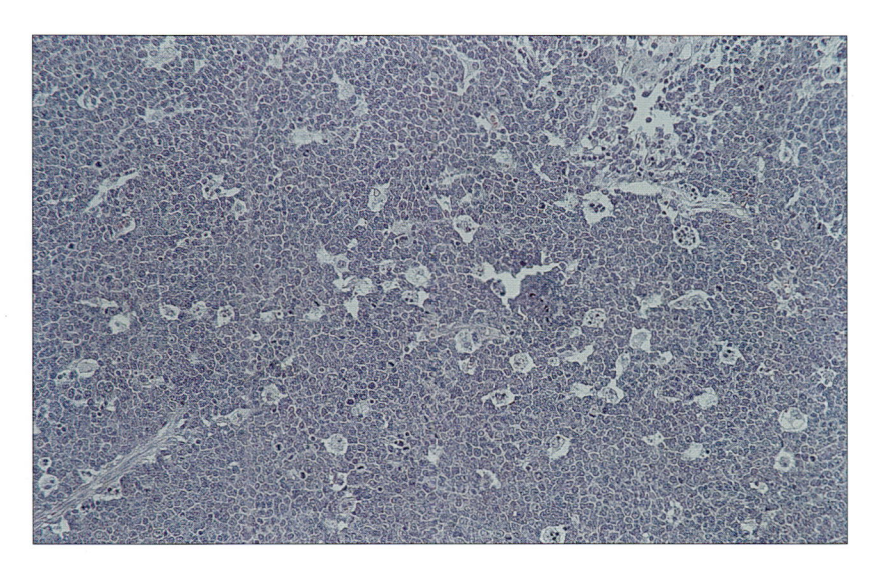

(b) A 'starry sky' pattern is prominent, owing to the presence of many tingible body macrophages. (H&E stain)

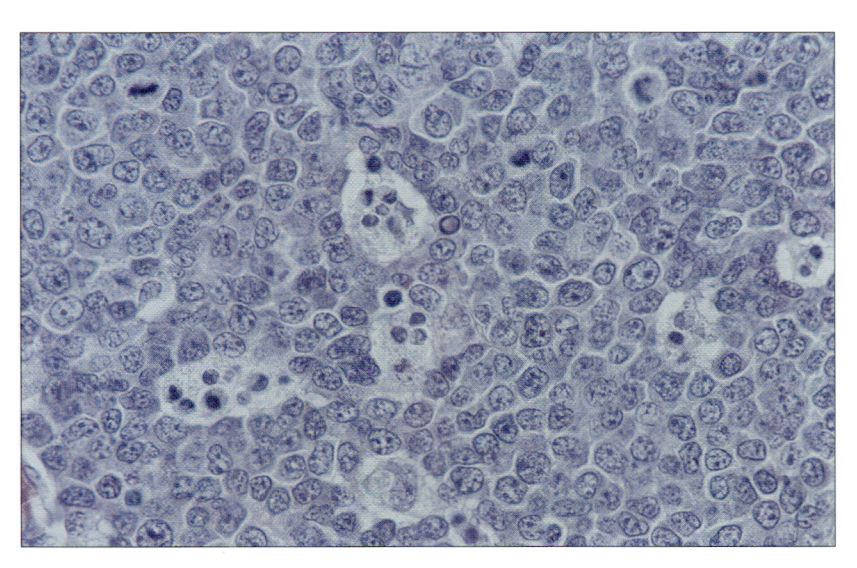

(c) The neoplastic cells are intermediate-sized cells with round nuclei, granular chromatin and a high mitotic rate; several tingible body macrophages are also seen. (H&E stain)

High-grade B-cell lymphoma, Burkitt-like

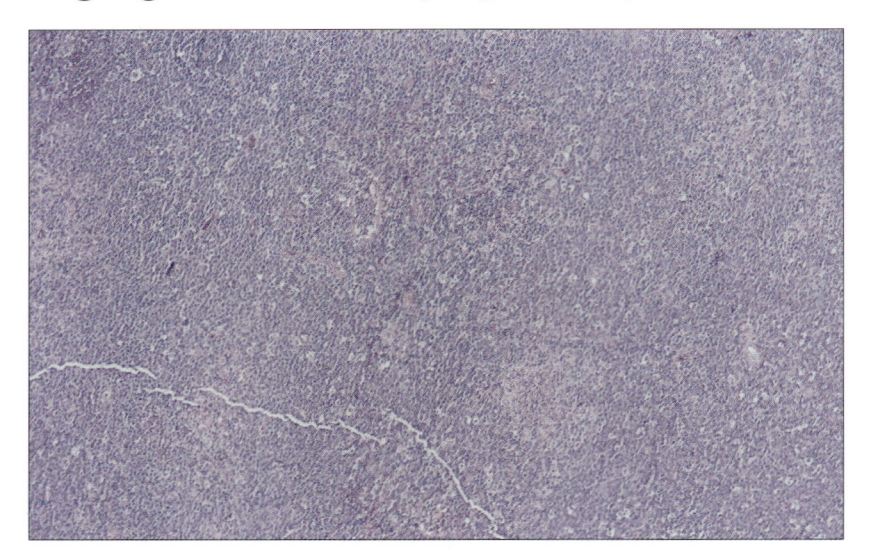

Figure 8.3

High-grade B-cell lymphoma, Burkitt-like:

(a) Low power shows a diffuse cellular infiltrate. (H&E stain)

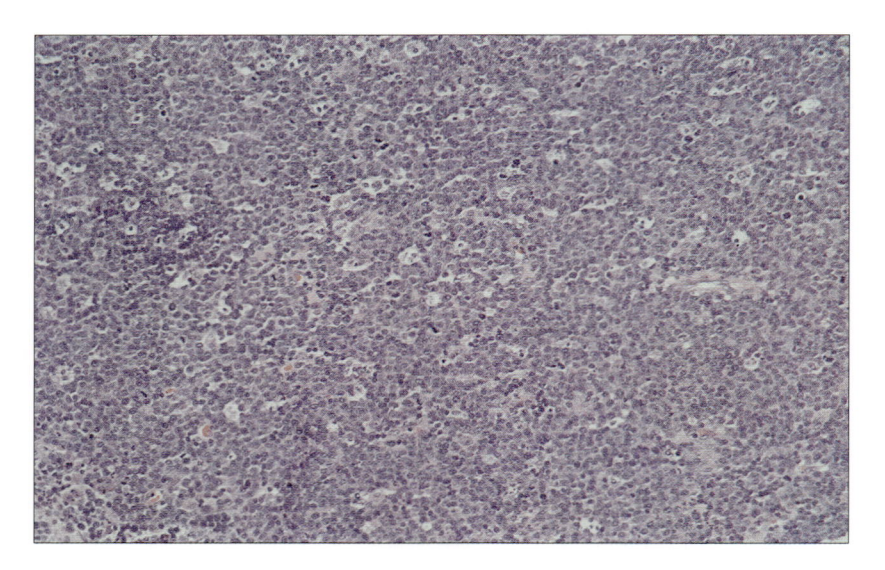

(b) A 'starry sky' pattern is seen. (H&E stain)

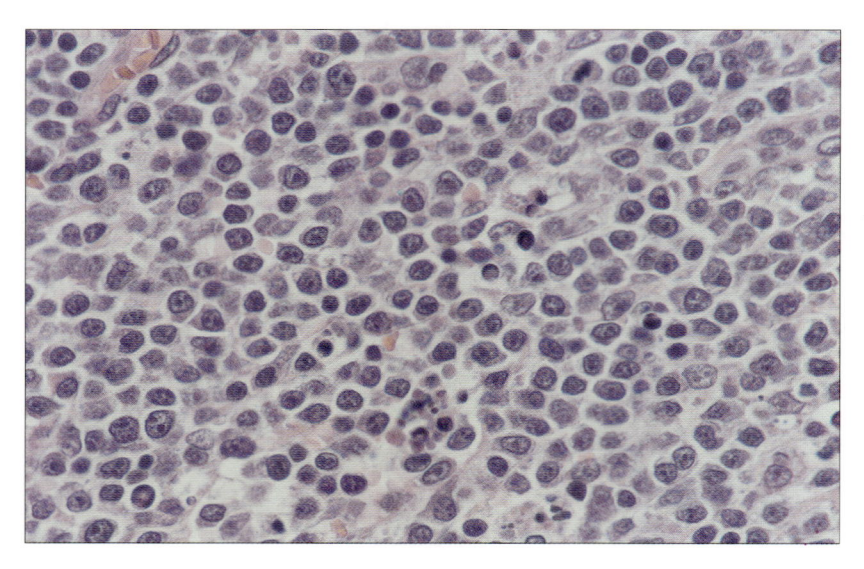

(c) The neoplastic cells are, on average, intermediate in size, although they vary somewhat more in size than classic Burkitt's cells, and some of them appear slightly plasmacytoid. (H&E stain)

9 Anaplastic large T/null cell lymphoma

Definition and classification

Anaplastic large T/null cell lymphoma is one of the recently recognized subtypes of non-Hodgkin's lymphoma. In the past, it was frequently confused with other neoplasms. It was often diagnosed as anaplastic carcinoma, undifferentiated malignant neoplasm, or malignant histiocytosis. Discovery of the CD30 or Ki-1 antigen allowed recognition of this particular subtype of lymphoma, since it essentially always displayed the CD30 antigen. Subsequent recognition of a specific genetic abnormality guaranteed the acceptance of anaplastic large cell lymphoma as a specific subtype.

The anaplastic appearance in a diffuse large cell lymphoma can also be seen with B-cell lymphomas. However, in the REAL classification, only the T/null cell lymphomas are separately recognized. This is related to their unusual clinical characteristics and their surprisingly good clinical outcome. B-cell lymphomas with the same histologic appearance do not appear to have a different clinical course to that of other diffuse large B-cell lymphomas.

Frequency

Anaplastic large T/null cell lymphoma represents approximately 2% of all non-Hodgkin's lymphomas. In the International Lymphoma Classification Study it did not differ significantly by geographic site. However, unless pathologists are aware of the distinctive histological, immunophenotypic and genetic features of the disorder, it will be underdiagnosed. Because of the good prognosis, this would represent a major error.

Pathology

Histology (Table 9.1)

In many cases, anaplastic large T/null cell lymphoma has the appearance of a carcinoma. The tumor cells are large, and have pleomorphic, horseshoe-shaped or multiple nuclei. They may occasionally resemble Reed–Sternberg cells. They usually have multiple, prominent nucleoli.

Table 9.1
Histologic features of anaplastic large T/null cell lymphoma

- Large blastic cells
- Pleomorphic, horseshoe-shaped or multiple nuclei
- Usually multiple, prominent nucleoli
- May resemble Reed–Sternberg cells
- Tumor cells larger and with more abundant cytoplasm than usually seen in lymphoma
- Cohesive growth pattern often involving lymph node sinuses

The tumor cells tend to be larger and have more abundant cytoplasm than is seen in other types of non-Hodgkin's lymphoma. These findings, when combined with a cohesive growth pattern and involvement of lymph node sinuses, lead to confusion with carcinomas. Some anaplastic large T/null cell lymphomas can present with a lymphohistiocytic appearance in which reactive histiocytes predominate and the neoplastic cells are often smaller than those usually seen in this histologic subtype. A small cell variant has also been described.

The occurrence of anaplastic large T/null cell lymphoma with features like those of Hodgkin's disease has led to proposals for an intermediate lymphoma between anaplastic large T/null cell lymphoma and Hodgkin's disease. However, at the present time, it is suggested that these patients should be diagnosed as having either anaplastic large T/null cell lymphoma or Hodgkin's disease.

Immunophenotype (Table 9.2)

The characteristic immunophenotype in patients with anaplastic large T/null cell lymphoma includes features that demonstrate the tumors to be of T-cell origin and display the Ki-1 or CD30 antigen. Thus the tumor cells are usually $CD3^+$ and $CD30^+$. However, some will not display either T- or B-cell markers (i.e. null cells). Tumor cells also often display epithelial membrane antigen (EMA). Because of the characteristic genetic abnormalities noted below, the tumor cells will often stain positive for anaplastic lymphoma kinase (ALK) protein. The tumor cells will be $CD20^-$ and $CD15^-$.

Genetics (Table 9.2)

The acceptance of anaplastic large T/null cell lymphoma as a specific subtype of lymphoma was confirmed by the recognition of a characteristic cytogenetic abnormality and accompanying oncogene expression. The cytogenetic abnormality is the t(2;5)(p23;q35) translocation. This leads to overexpression of the *ALK* gene and results in overproduction of the ALK protein. It appears that this protein is key to the malignant expression of these cells.

Table 9.2
Immunophenotype and genetics of anaplastic large T/null cell lymphoma

Characteristic	Results
Immunophenotype	$CD3^+$, $CD30^+$, EMA^+, ALK^+ $CD20^-$, $CD15^-$
Cytogenetics	t(2;5)(p23;q35)
Oncogenes	*ALK*

Clinical characteristics (Table 9.3)

Anaplastic large T/null cell lymphoma is one of the most distinctive subtypes of non-Hodgkin's lymphoma. It occurs at a much lower average age than other large cell lymphomas, with a median age in the mid 30s. There is a striking male predominance, with only approximately 30% of patients being female.

As with other large cell lymphomas, approximately 50% of patients have disease confined to one side of the diaphragm and 50% of patients have more extensive disease. Stage I disease is seen in approximately 20% of patients and stage IV disease in approximately 40%. Approximately 50% of patients will complain of fevers, night sweats or weight loss. An elevated level of serum lactate dehydrogenase (LDH) is seen in approximately 45% of patients. In the International Lymphoma Classification Study, 74% of patients were fully active, and tumor masses as large as 10 cm were only seen in 17% of patients. Extranodal sites of involvement are seen in approximately 60% of patients. However, bone marrow and gastrointestinal-tract involvement are unusual. While skin involvement is seen frequently in this lymphoma, disease confined to the skin needs to be approached cautiously. Lymphomatoid papulosis and similar disorders have the histologic characteristics of anaplastic large T/null cell lymphoma, and also display the CD30 antigen. However, they follow a much more indolent clinical course. Patients whose tumors have the histologic appearance of anaplastic large T/null cell lymphoma but

Table 9.3	
Clinical characteristics of anaplastic large T/null cell lymphoma	
Characteristic	**Result**
Median age	34 years
Percent male	69%
Stage I	16%
Stage IE	3%
Stage II	22%
Stage IIE	10%
Stage III	10%
Stage IV	39%
B symptoms	53%
Elevated LDH	45%
Karnofsky $\leq$ 70	26%
Tumor mass $\geq$ 10 cm	17%
Any extranodal site	59%
Bone marrow positive	13%
GI-tract involved	9%
IPI score 0/1	61%
2/3	18%
4/5	21%

are confined to the skin should be approached conservatively. Many of these patients will not have a progressive, aggressive lymphoma, and may have a very different disease.

The comparatively good prognosis seen in anaplastic large T/null cell lymphoma is reflected in the proportion of patients with adverse risk factors in the International Prognostic Index. Approximately 60% of patients will have none or only one adverse risk factor, and only approximately 20% will have four or five adverse risk factors.

Treatment and outcome

Anaplastic large T/null cell lymphoma has one of the best prognoses of any type of non-Hodgkin's lymphoma. Only MALT lymphomas have a similarly positive clinical outcome. The overall survival and failure-free survival in patients with anaplastic large T/null cell lymphoma are shown in Figure 9.1.

The paradox of a highly aggressive histologic appearance and excellent response to therapy is found in anaplastic large T/null cell lymphoma. The reason for this paradox is not clear. However, confusion of this lymphoma with anaplastic carcinoma, leading to the patient not receiving effective anti-lymphoma therapy, is a clinical tragedy. The optimal therapy for these patients is not clear. However, treatments that have proven effective for diffuse large B-cell lymphoma are usually utilized. Most patients receive an effective combination chemotherapy regimen as the initial treatment. Patients with localized disease might have their total number of chemotherapy cycles reduced and

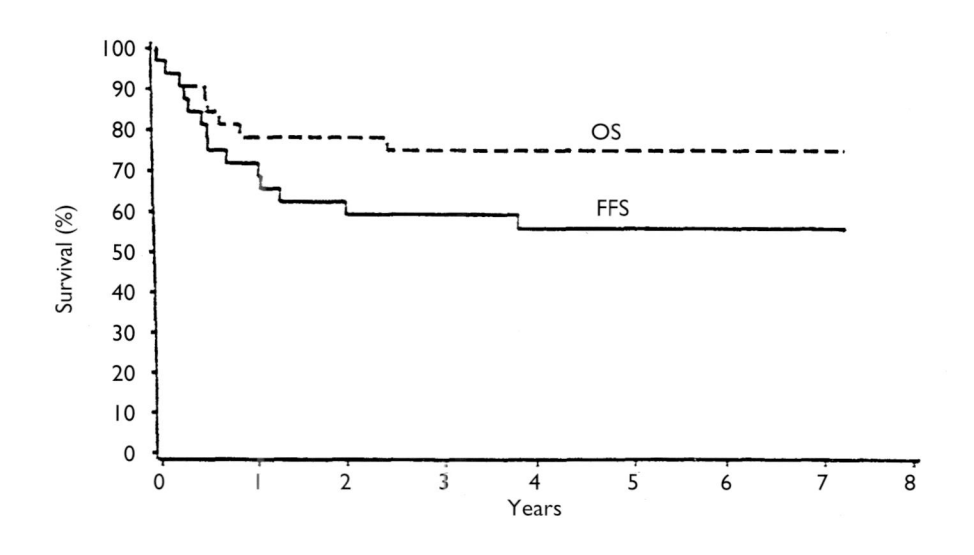

Figure 9.1
Overall survival (OS) and failure-free survival (FFS) for patients with anaplastic large T/null cell lymphoma.

involved-field radiotherapy substituted. These patients appear to respond to high-dose therapy and autologous transplantation after relapse as well as other patients with diffuse large cell lymphomas.

Bibliography

Cabanillas F, Armitage J, Pugh WC et al, Lymphomatoid papulosis: a T-cell dyscrasia with a propensity to transform into malignant lymphoma. *Ann Intern Med* 1995; **122:** 210–17.

De Bruin PC, Beljaards RC, van Heerde P et al, Differences in clinical behavior and immunophenotype between primary cutaneous and primary nodal anaplastic large cell lymphoma of T-cell or null cell phenotype. *Histopathology* 1993; **23:** 127–35.

Greer J, Kinney M, Collins R et al, Clinical features of 31 patients with Ki-1 anaplastic large-cell lymphoma. *J Clin Oncol* 1991; **9:** 539–47.

Harris NL, Jaffe ES, Stein H et al, A revised European–American classification of lymphoid neoplasms: a proposal from the International Lymphoma Study Group. *Blood* 1994; **84:** 1361–92.

Kinney MC, Collins RD, Greer JP et al, A small-cell-predominant variant of primary Ki-1 (CD30)+ T-cell lymphoma. *Am J Surg Pathol* 1993; **17:** 859–68.

Mason D, Bastard C, Rimokh R et al, CD30-positive large cell lymphomas ('Ki-1 lymphoma') are associated with a chromosomal translocation involving 5q35. *Br J Haematol* 1990; **74:** 161–8.

Non-Hodgkin's Lymphoma Classification Project, A clinical evaluation of the International Lymphoma Study Group classification of non-Hodgkin's lymphoma. *Blood* 1997; **89:** 3909–18.

Pileri S, Bocchia M, Baroni C et al, Anaplastic large cell lymphoma (CD30+/Ki-1+). Results of a prospective clinicopathologic study of 69 cases. *Br J Haematol* 1994; **86:** 513–23.

Pileri S, Falini B, Delsol G et al, Lymphohistiocytic T-cell lymphoma (anaplastic large cell lymphoma CD30+/Ki-1+ with a high content of reactive histiocytes). *Histopathology* 1990; **16:** 383–91.

Pileri SA, Pulford K, Mori S et al, Frequent expression of the NPM–ALK chimeric fusion protein in anaplastic large-cell lymphoma, lympho-histiocytic type. *Am J Pathol* 1997; **150:** 1207–11.

Pulford K, Lamant L, Morris SW et al, Detection of anaplastic lymphoma kinase (ALK) and nucleolar protein nucleophosmin (NPM)–ALK proteins in normal and neoplastic cells with the monoclonal antibody ALK1. *Blood* 1997; **89:** 1394–404.

Shiota M, Nakamura S, Ichinohasama R et al, Anaplastic large cell lymphomas expressing the novel chimeric protein p80NPM/ALK: a distinct clinicopathologic entity. *Blood* 1995; **86:** 1954–60.

Shulman LN, Frisard B, Antin JH et al, Primary Ki-1 anaplastic large cell lymphoma in adults: clinical characteristics and therapeutic outcome. *J Clin Oncol* 1993; **11:** 937–42.

Stein H, Mason DY, Gerdes J et al, The expression of Hodgkin's disease associated antigen Ki-1 in reactive and neoplastic lymphoid tissue: evidence that Reed–Sternberg cells and histiocytic malignancies are derived from activated lymphoid cells. *Blood* 1985; **66:** 848–58.

Anaplastic large T/null cell lymphoma

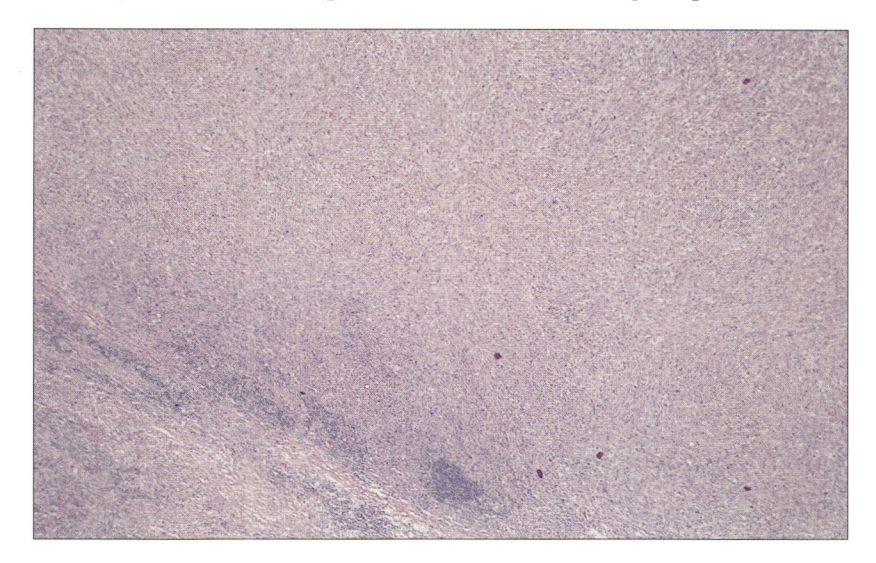

Figure 9.2

Anaplastic large T/null cell lymphoma:

(a) Lymphoma diffusely involves the lymph node. (H&E stain)

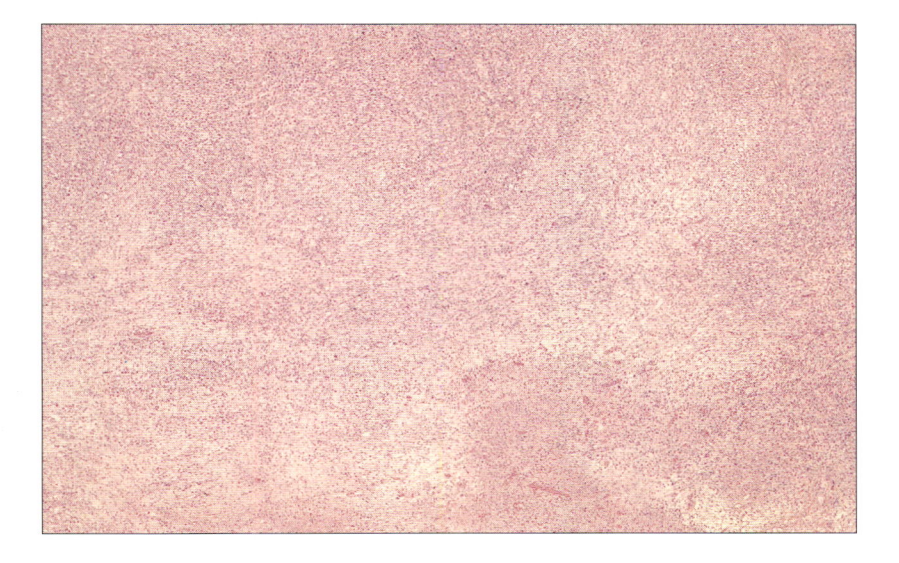

(b) There are irregular eosinophilic areas of necrosis within the lymphoma. (H&E stain)

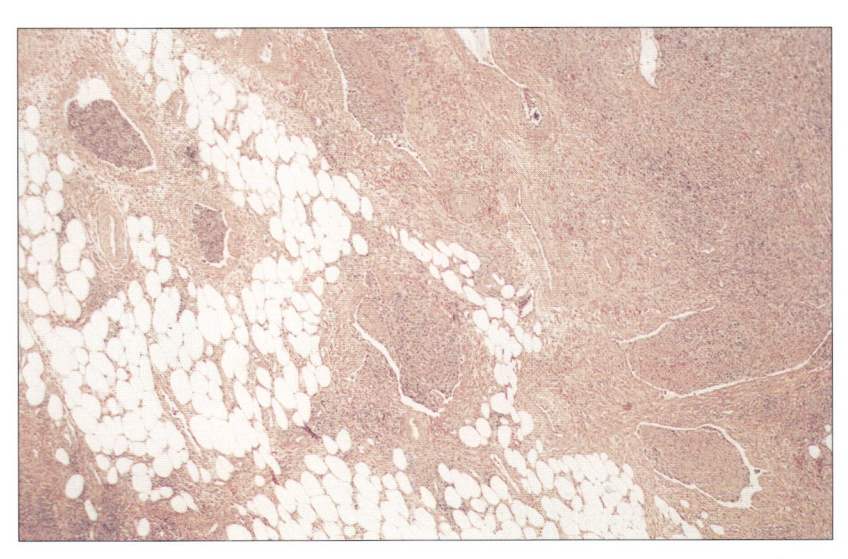

(c) Aggregates of tumor cells fill large lymphatics outside the lymph node. (H&E stain)

Contd

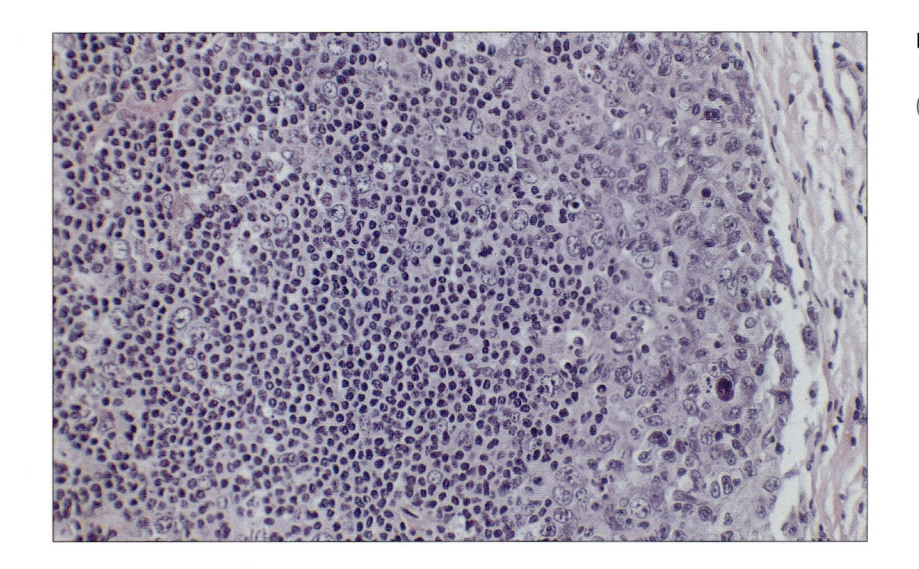

Figure 9.2 *continued*

(d) Neoplastic cells fill the subcapsular sinus. (H&E stain)

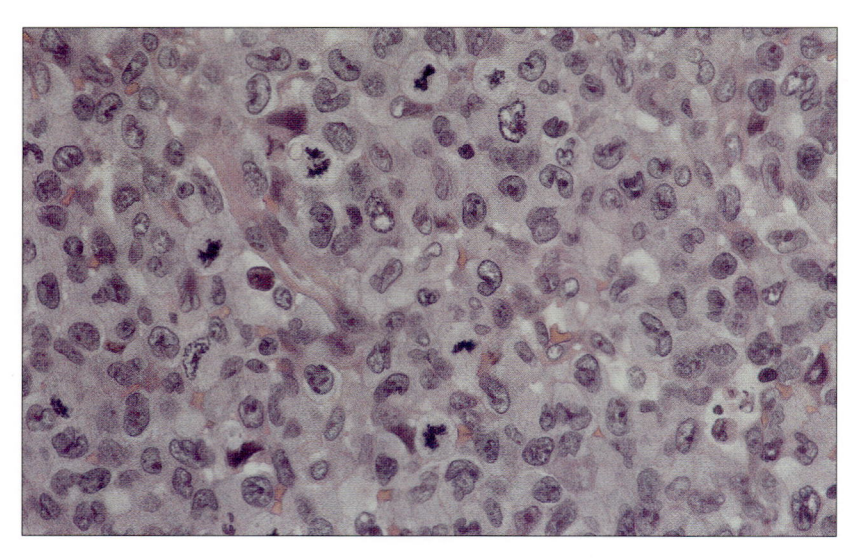

(e) High-power examination shows large cells with oval to indented nuclei, abundant pale cytoplasm and a high mitotic rate. (H&E stain)

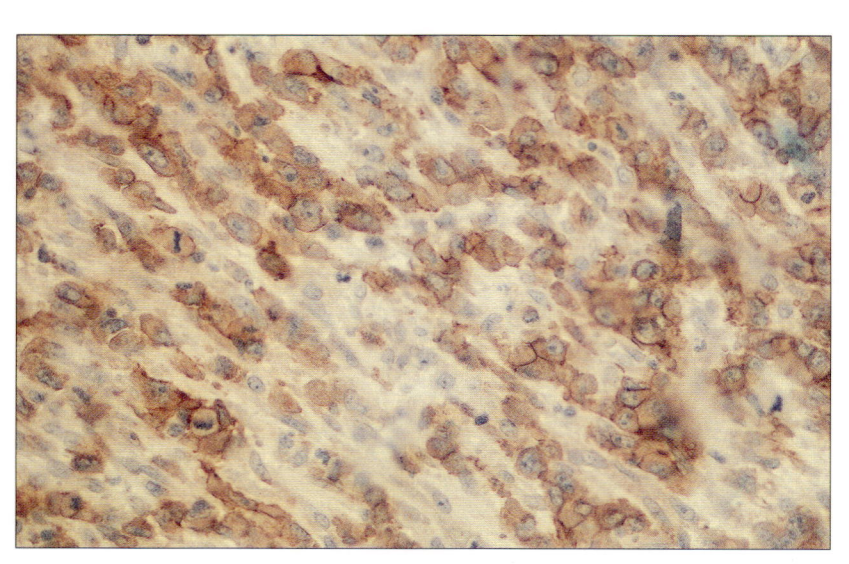

(f) There is diffuse strong staining for CD30. (Immunoperoxidase technique on paraffin sections)

Anaplastic large T/null cell lymphoma, Hodgkin-like/related

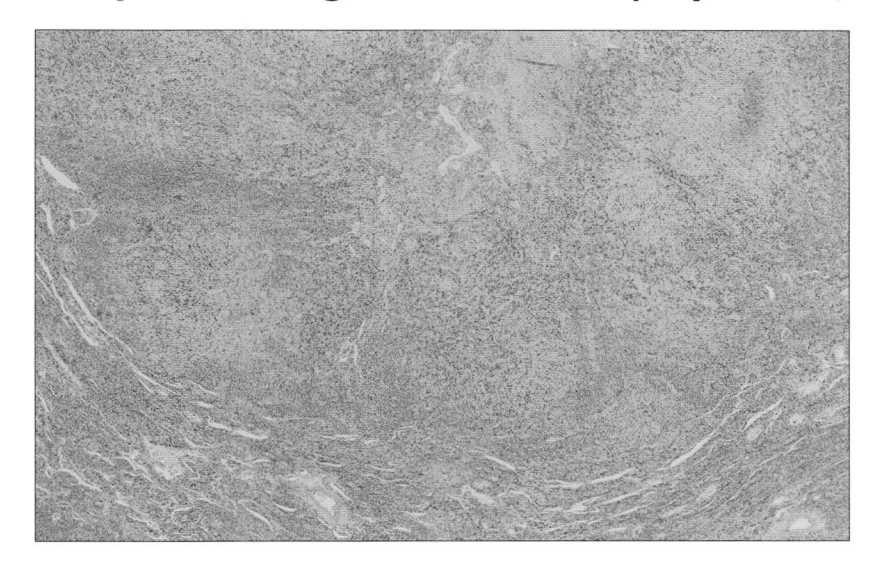

Figure 9.3

Anaplastic large T/null cell lymphoma, Hodgkin-like or Hodgkin-related:

(a) The lymph node is partially replaced by a multinodular lesion of mottled blue and pink color. (H&E stain)

(b) Individual nodules are centrally necrotic, and contain a mixture of lymphocytes, histiocytes, eosinophils and large atypical cells. (H&E stain)

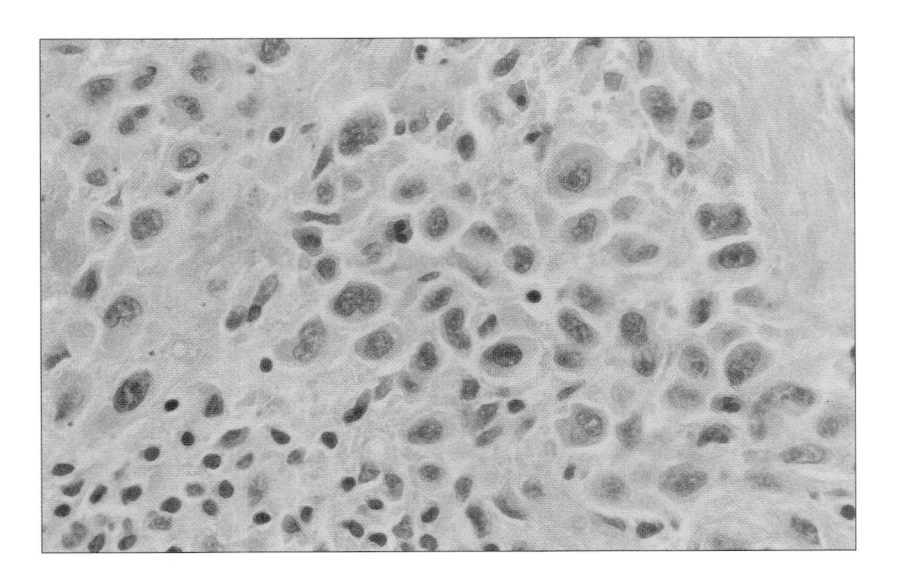

(c) Adjacent to the necrosis, large cells, with vesicular nuclei, very prominent nucleoli and abundant eosinophilic cytoplasm are present in large numbers. (H&E stain)

Contd

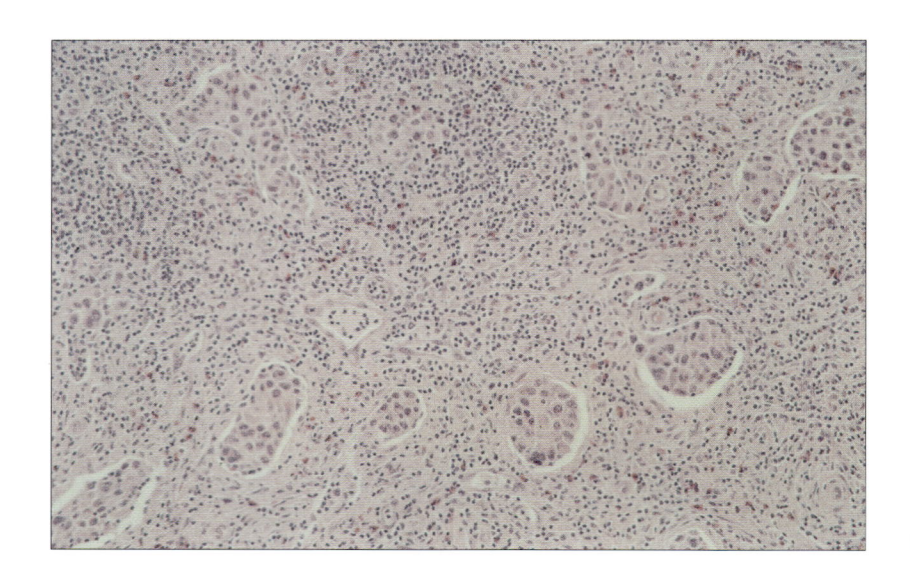

Figure 9.3 *continued*

Many sinuses contain large atypical tumor cells (**d**); seen at higher power in (**e**). (H&E stain)

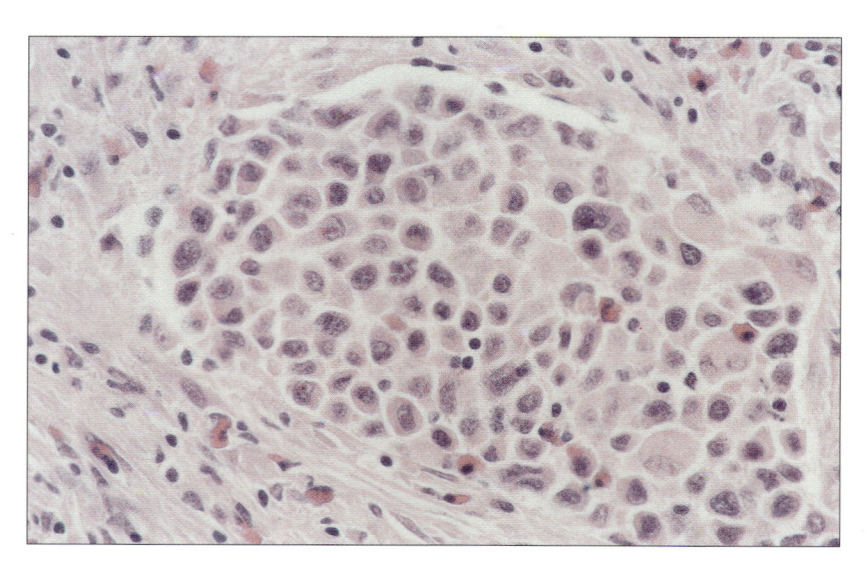

(d)

(e)

10 Primary mediastinal large B-cell lymphoma

Definition and classification

Primary mediastinal large B-cell lymphoma was first described as a distinct clinicopathologic entity in the 1980s. It is recognized in both the REAL and WHO classifications. The disease originates in the thymus, and produces a large anterior mediastinal mass that can lead to airway compromise and superior vena cava syndrome. Although it resembles nodal large cell lymphomas, it has discrete morphologic, phenotypic and genetic features. It is derived from thymic B cells and is considered a peripheral B-cell neoplasm.

Frequency

The disease is rare, and its precise frequency is difficult to discern with accuracy because of its relatively recent identification. The best estimate derives from a retrospective analysis of the large cell lymphoma studies of the French Groupe d'Etude des Lymphomes de l'Adult (GELA). Among 1057 patients with large cell lymphoma, 141 (13%) had primary mediastinal large B-cell lymphoma. Reports describing the same disease process have come from Asia, Japan and the Middle East. In a review of 1400 cases of non-Hodgkin's lymphoma from nine centers all over the world, primary mediastinal large B-cell lymphoma was found to account for 2% of the cases.

Pathology (Table 10.1)

Histology

The cytology resembles that of other diffuse large cell lymphomas; the nuclei of the tumor cells can mimic large non-cleaved cells (centroblastic), large cleaved cells (centrocytic), multilobated cells

Table 10.1
Comparison of diffuse large B-cell lymphoma and mediastinal large B-cell lymphoma

	Diffuse large B-cell lymphoma	Mediastinal large B-cell lymphoma
Median age	55 years	35 years
Sex distribution (M:F)	55:45	30–40:70–60
Nodal/extranodal presentation	65%/35%	0%/100%
Bulky disease	30%	60–75%
Histology	Standard	Similar, but pale cytoplasm and sclerosis
Clonal B cell	Yes	Yes
Surface immunoglobulin	Yes	No
CD20, CD79a	Yes	Yes
BCL6 translocation	Common	Rare
Extra chromosome fragments	Occasional	Common, 9p, Xq

(Reed–Sternberg-like), and occasionally even immunoblasts. The cells have abundant pale cytoplasm, sometimes called 'clear', and bands of sclerosis are a frequent feature, though it may be patchy. The tumor has a diffuse pattern of growth; compartmentalization of the tumor by sclerosis is not a nodular growth pattern. Residual thymus may be present in the tumor.

Immunophenotype/immunohistology

The cells are B cells with an unusual phenotype. They express CD20, CD22 and CD79a, which are typical of B cells; however, they do not express either surface or cytoplasmic immunoglobulin in most cases. Immunoglobulin genes are clonally rearranged, but T-cell receptor genes are not. Often the tumor cells are CD23$^+$, and light staining with anti-CD30 can sometimes be seen. This phenotype is characteristic of the rare B cells found in the thymic medulla. Therefore it is felt that the tumor arises from a thymic medullary B cell.

Genetics

No characteristic chromosome translocation has been identified. However, a variety of genetic alterations have been described. Interestingly, the abnormalities are largely non-overlapping with the genetic lesions found in diffuse large cell lymphomas. In particular, *BCL6* translocations are very rare in primary mediastinal large B-cell lymphoma. Mutations involving c-*MYC* and *p53*, amplification of *REL*, activation of *NFκB*, and gain of chromosomes 9p, 12q and Xq have been described. Gain of Xq coincided with gain of 9p, but the other lesions rarely coexist in the same tumor. Thus it is unclear that there is a single molecular pathogenesis for this tumor.

Clinical characteristics/natural history (Table 10.1)

Primary mediastinal large B-cell lymphoma affects younger patients than do other adult lymphomas. The median age is the mid-30s; children and older adults may be affected as well, but the disease is rare in people over age 65 years. About 60–70% of affected individuals are women. Over 90% of patients present with symptoms of cough, dyspnea and/or chest pain. About one-third have B symptoms. One-third to one-half of patients will have signs and symptoms of superior vena cava syndrome, thoracic and neck vein distension, facial edema, conjunctival swelling, and occasionally arm edema. Radiographic examination identifies a massive anterior mediastinal mass in 60–75% of patients and pleural effusion in about 33%, and when patients are staged with CT scan, 30% have pericardial effusions and the tumor shows areas of attenuated signal, suggesting the presence of necrosis in about half. Contiguous infiltration of the lung is seen in about half of the patients.

The disease must be distinguished from other causes of anterior mediastinal masses, including thymoma, Hodgkin's disease, lymphoblastic lymphoma, thymic MALT lymphoma, epithelial cancers, and, in males, mediastinal germ cell tumors. This requires an open excisional biopsy with sufficient tissue obtained for formalin fixation (hematoxylin and eosin-stained histology) and saline (fresh freezing for immunophenotyping and immunohistology).

The tumor almost never involves lymph nodes. When it spreads beyond the mediastinum and the pleural cavity, it involves sites not commonly involved with lymphoma, such as the kidneys, adrenals, liver and ovaries. Bone marrow involvement is rare. High lactate dehydrogenase (LDH) levels and pleural effusions have been said to be poor prognostic indicators, as have poor performance status and the presence of a pericardial effusion. The GELA group found that their 141 patients stratified on the basis of the International Prognostic Index (IPI) were comparable in their survival to similarly treated patients with diffuse large cell lymphoma. However, the MD Anderson Cancer Center group found the IPI to be less useful in their 37 patients. They noted that serum β_2-microglobulin levels were unusually low in patients with primary mediastinal large B-cell lymphoma based on what was expected given the tumor bulk. However, when they adjusted the threshold for poor risk to the disease (that is, used a lower level as the discriminator between good and bad prognosis), they were able to use their tumor score model to separate two groups of patients: a good group with overall survival of 80% and a poorer group with overall survival of 55%.

Treatment

There have been no randomized treatment trials focusing on patients with primary mediastinal large B-cell lymphoma. However, series enrolling 16–141 patients have been reported, and permit some conclusions to be drawn. First, radiation therapy alone is ineffective in this disease. Second, the use of CHOP chemotherapy led to the early impression that the prognosis of patients with primary mediastinal large B-cell lymphoma was worse than that for the more common diffuse large cell lymphoma. However, with the application of more aggressive combination chemotherapy programs, it appears that the complete response rate, disease-free survival and overall survival of patients with primary mediastinal large B-cell lymphoma are at least as good and probably better than those for diffuse large cell lymphoma.

The GELA group used LNH84 and LNH87 in both primary mediastinal large B-cell lymphoma and diffuse large cell lymphoma, and found a superior complete response rate (79% versus 68%) and superior three-year overall survival rate (66% versus 61%) for patients with mediastinal large B-cell lymphoma. However, this difference was due to the distribution of poor prognostic factors in the IPI index; when the same risk groups were compared with each other, the outcome was the same. No radiation therapy was used in this study.

Many groups have empirically delivered radiation therapy to responding patients. It is difficult to assess whether this has improved treatment outcome.

In centers that have used CHOP and other more aggressive multidrug regimens, the results have clearly favored the more aggressive regimens. Todeschini and colleagues from Verona used CHOP in their first six patients without achieving a single complete response; in the 15 patients treated with more aggressive regimens (MACOP-B and F-MACHOP), 13 (87%) achieved a complete response, and only one of the complete responders relapsed. Lazzarino and colleagues at the University of Pavia treated 30 patients; the complete response rate to CHOP was 36%, while that to MACOP-B or VACOP-B was 73% ($p = 0.047$). Zinzani and colleagues at Bologna used MACOP-B or F-MACHOP in 22 patients; 21 (95%) achieved a complete response, and overall survival at two years was 87%. The two relapses occurred at 7 and 10 months after treatment.

In general, when relapses occur, they do so in the mediastinum and within the first 6–12 months after treatment; late relapses are rare. It was initially thought that relapsed disease was refractory to further treatment. However, a recent analysis of the efficacy of high-dose therapy and autologous stem cell transplantation in relapsed and refractory diffuse large cell lymphoma has called that conclusion into question. Among 90 patients treated at the MD Anderson Cancer Center, 31 (34%) had primary mediastinal large B-cell lymphoma. Overall survival for the entire group was 42%, and an analysis of prognostic factors identified LDH level, Ann Arbor stage and primary mediastinal localization as independent favorable prognostic factors for both disease-free and overall survival.

Thus the accumulated treatment experience with primary mediastinal large B-cell lymphoma would suggest that MACOP-B, VACOP-B or F-MACHOP should be the first regimen employed. The use of radiation therapy is not completely defined. The excellent results obtained in the GELA studies without radiation therapy raise a question about its necessity. The choices appear to be to use it in everyone or to use it selectively in patients whose mediastinal mass remains gallium-positive at the end of six cycles of chemotherapy. Primary mediastinal large B-cell lymphoma is always gallium-positive at diagnosis, and persistent positivity after therapy is a harbinger of relapse. Over 40% of patients have residual radiographic abnormalities in the mediastinum even after successful treatment, so chest radiographs and CT scans are not useful in making therapeutic decisions. Whether radiation therapy benefits all patients or just those with residual mediastinal gallium uptake needs to be ascertained in a clinical trial. If patients fail to achieve a complete response and cannot be converted to one by radiation therapy, or if they relapse from complete response, the use of high-dose therapy and stem cell support may rescue more than half of them. With the appropriate application of currently available tools, the long-term survival of patients with primary mediastinal large B-cell lymphoma may be 70–75%.

Bibliography

Addis B, Isaacson P, Large cell lymphoma of the mediastinum: a B cell tumor of probably thymic origin. *Histopathology* 1986; **10:** 379–90.

Cazals-Hatem D, Lepage E, Brice P et al, Primary mediastinal large B-cell lymphoma. A clinicopathologic study of 141 cases compared with 916 nonmediastinal large B-cell lymphomas, a GELA (Groupe d'Etude des Lymphomes de l'Adulte) study. *Am J Surg Pathol* 1996; **20:** 877–88.

Chim CS, Liang R, Chan AC et al, Primary B cell lymphoma of the mediastinum. *Hematol Oncol* 1996; **14:** 173–9.

Joos S, Otano-Joos MI, Ziegler S et al, Primary mediastinal (thymic) B-cell lymphoma is characterized by gains of chromosomal material including 9p and amplification of the REL gene. *Blood* 1996; **87:** 571–8.

Kanaveros P, Gaulard P, Charlotte F et al, Discordant expression of immunoglobulin and its associated molecule mb-1/CD79a is frequently found in mediastinal large B cell lymphomas. *Am J Pathol* 1995; **146:** 735–41.

Lamarre L, Jacobson JO, Aisenberg AC, Harris NL, Primary large cell lymphoma of the mediastinum. A histologic and immunophenotypic study of 29 cases. *Am J Surg Pathol* 1989; **13:** 730–9.

Lazzarino M, Orlandi E, Paulli M et al, Primary mediastinal B-cell lymphoma with sclerosis: an aggressive tumor with distinctive clinical and pathologic features. *J Clin Oncol* 1993; **11:** 2306–13.

Lazzarino M, Orlandi E, Paulli M et al, Treatment outcome and prognostic factors for primary mediastinal (thymic) B-cell lymphoma: a multicenter study of 106 patients. *J Clin Oncol* 1997; **15:** 1646–53.

Moller P, Moldenhauer G, Momburg F et al, Mediastinal lymphoma of clear cell type is a tumor corresponding to terminal steps of B-cell differentiation. *Blood* 1987; **69:** 1087–95.

Popat U, Przepiorka D, Champlin R et al, High-dose chemotherapy for relapsed and refractory diffuse large B-cell lymphoma: mediastinal localization predicts for a favorable outcome. *J Clin Oncol* 1998; **16:** 63–9.

Romaguera JE, Rodriguez Diaz-Pavon J, Carias L et al, Use of the International Prognostic Index and the tumor score to detect poor-risk patients with primary mediastinal large B-cell lymphoma: a study of 37 previously untreated patients. *Leuk Lymphoma* 1998; **28:**; 295–306.

Shaffer K, Smith D, Kirn D et al, Primary mediastinal large B-cell lymphoma: radiologic findings at presentation. *Am J Roentgenol* 1996; **167:** 425–30.

Todeschini G, Ambrosetti A, Meneghini V et al, Mediastinal large B-cell lymphoma with sclerosis: a clinical study of 21 patients. *J Clin Oncol* 1990; **8:** 804–8.

Tsang P, Cesarman E, Chadburn A et al, Molecular characterization of primary mediastinal B cell lymphoma. *Am J Pathol* 1996; **148:** 2017–25.

Zinzani PL, Bendandi M, Frezza G et al, Primary mediastinal B-cell lymphoma with sclerosis: clinical and therapeutic evaluation of 22 patients. *Leuk Lymphoma* 1996; **21:** 311–16.

Primary mediastinal large B-cell lymphoma

Figure 10.1

Primary mediastinal large B-cell lymphoma:

(a) The specimen shows a diffuse cellular infiltrate. (H&E stain)

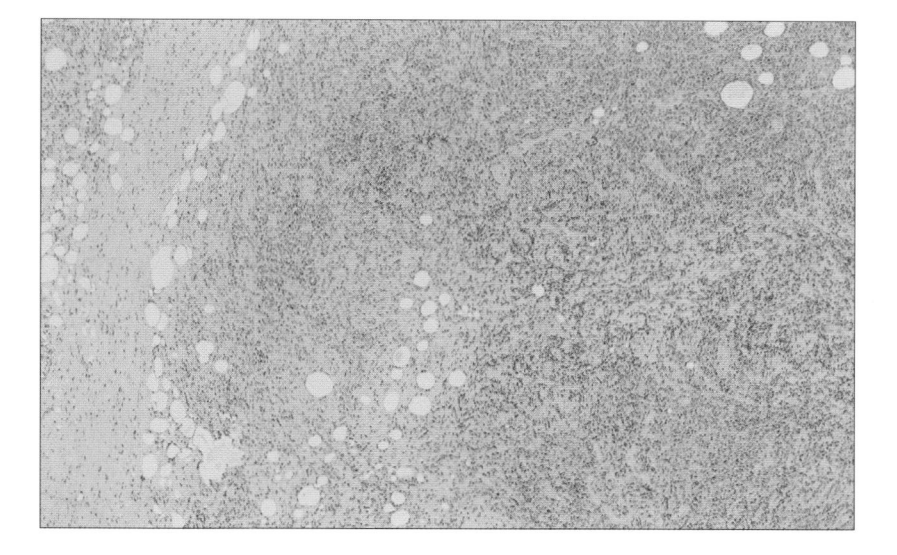

(b) In areas, there is band-like fibrosis and involvement of mediastinal fat. (H&E stain)

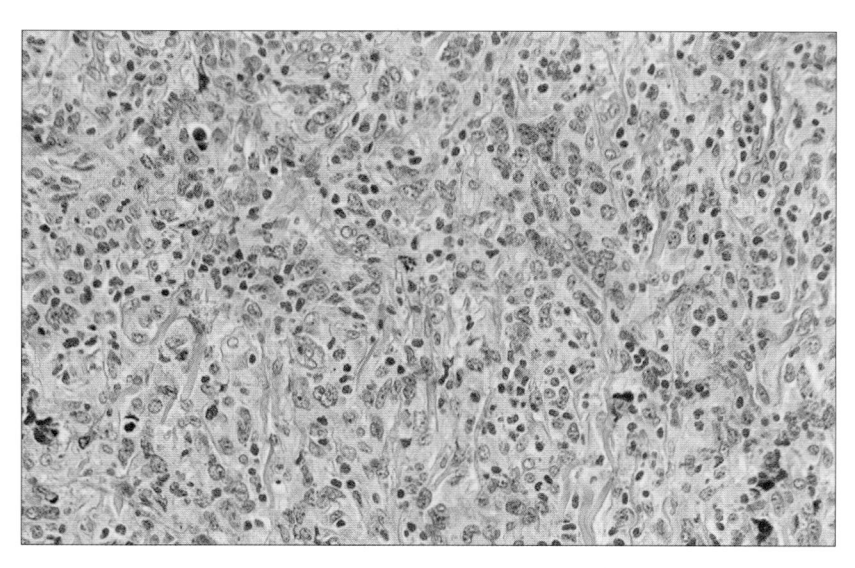

(c) The tumor is associated with deposition of fine collagen fibers, sometimes imparting a nesting pattern to the neoplastic cells. (H&E stain)

Contd

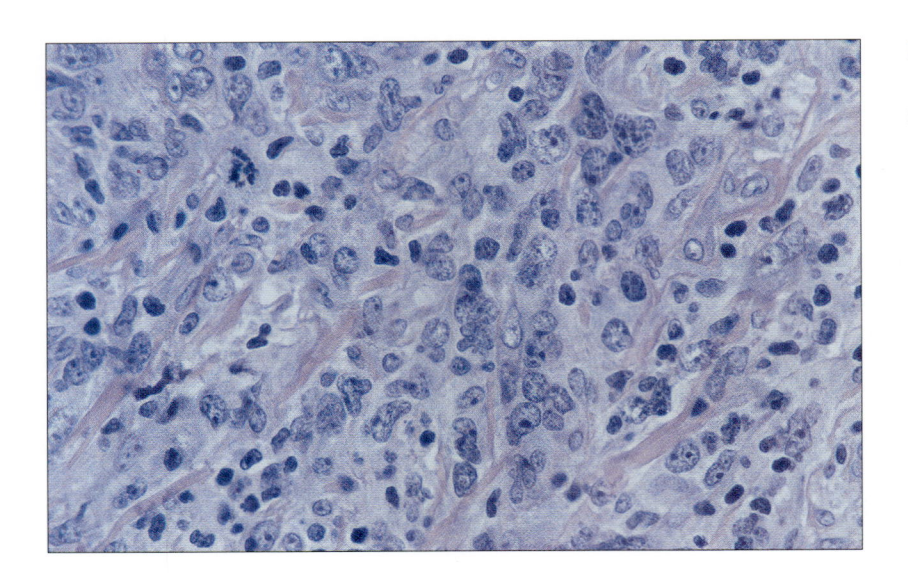

Figure 10.1 *continued*

(d) The tumor cells are large lymphoid cells with a moderate amount of pale cytoplasm. (H&E stain)

11 Lymphoblastic leukemia/lymphoma

Definition and classification

Lymphoblastic lymphoma is a neoplasm of precursors of T cells and B cells that is morphologically indistinguishable from acute lymphoid leukemias. Lymphoblastic lymphoma and acute lymphoid leukemias also share phenotypes and genetic lesions. The distinctions between lymphomas and leukemias derived from the same precursors are clinical differences that are usually arbitrary and often subtle. A particular patient is said to have acute leukemia based upon the percentage of bone marrow involvement (>25% in children, >30% in adults). Patients with lymphoblastic lymphoma often are young, male and present with an anterior mediastinal mass, and the bone marrow, when involved, is less than 30% replaced by tumor. Late in the course of the disease, patients may have greater than 30% marrow involvement. Generally, patients who were originally considered to have lymphoblastic lymphoma do not have the diagnosis changed to leukemia when marrow involvement passes the diagnostic threshold.

In the Rappaport classification, lymphoblastic lymphoma was called 'diffuse small cleaved cell lymphoma' because of the diffuse pattern of growth and the convoluted nuclear contour of the tumor cells. The clinicopathologic entity was first recognized in 1975 and lymphoblastic lymphoma became an official category in the Working Formulation. About 90% of the cases diagnosed as lymphoblastic lymphoma are tumors of T-cell precursors, often with common thymocyte cell surface phenotype; 10% of cases are derived from B-cell precursors. By contrast, about 75% of acute lymphoid leukemias are derived from B-cell precursors, 15% are tumors of T-cell precursors and 10% are cells with lymphoid morphology with some myeloid cell markers. These differences in disease distribution between neoplasms derived from T-cell precursors and B-cell precursors reflect the pattern of normal lymphopoiesis of T and B cells. Nearly all of B-cell development takes place – and thus the largest fraction of B-cell precursors reside – in the bone marrow, and neoplasia in these cells arise in the marrow. By contrast, only a small number of the precursor T cells are in the marrow. Pre-thymocytes then migrate from the marrow to the thymus, where most of the stages of T-cell development take place. Thus most tumors of precursor T cells arise in the thymus and relatively few arise in the bone marrow.

In recent years, it has become clear that lymphoblastic lymphoma and acute lymphoid leukemia are related and are best treated as though they were the same disease. The discussion here will, however, focus on lymphoblastic lymphoma.

Frequency

Lymphoblastic lymphoma is rare. It accounted for 1.7% of a series of 1400 cases of lymphoma collected in nine centers worldwide as part of the Non-Hodgkin's Lymphoma Classification Project. There are around 1000 cases per year in the USA.

Pathology

Histology

Thymic tumors in patients with lymphoblastic lymphoma generally show sheets of neoplastic cells that are larger than normal lymphocytes (but smaller than the cells of diffuse large cell lymphoma), with large nuclei, most often with convoluted borders (but occasionally non-convoluted), finely stipled chromatin, poorly defined nucleoli, and sparse, pale cytoplasm, sometimes with vacuoles present. Mitoses are frequent. Involved lymph nodes are usually totally effaced, but some may show preservation of occasional lymphoid follicles, reflecting the predilection of the tumor for the paracortical, interfollicular and medullary cord areas of the node. When the FAB classification of acute leukemia is applied to these lymphoblasts, the cells generally fall into the L1 or L2 groups.

The differential diagnosis of lymphoblastic lymphoma includes the blastic variant of mantle-cell lymphoma (MCL). Usually, blastic MCL cells have more cytoplasm than lymphoblastic lymphoma cells, but the most effective way to distinguish these tumors is by immunophenotype. Lymphoblastic lymphoma cells always express terminal deoxynucleotide transferase (TdT). Blastic MCL cells express surface immunoglobulin and are TdT$^-$. The distinction is most relevant in adults, because blastic MCL is exceedingly rare in children.

Immunophenotype

The vast majority of lymphoblastic lymphomas are derived from T-cell precursors. They express CD7 and cytoplasmic CD3, but there is no CD3 at the cell surface. CD5 and CD2 are usually expressed (see Figure 11.1). T-cell lymphoblastic lymphomas most often express the phenotype of cortical thymocytes. The 10% of cases that are derived from B-cell precursors are often CD19$^+$ and CD10$^+$. CD20 is present in about half of the cases. Cytoplasmic CD79a (part of the surface immunoglobulin signalling complex) is a reliable marker. B-cell lymphoblastic lymphoma is usually HLA-DR$^+$ and shares features of either pre-B-cell (cytoplasmic μ-chain) or common ALL. In difficult cases, the two most useful markers to assign lineage are CD3 and CD79a. Antibodies to both molecules work in paraffin-fixed tissue; CD3 is present in tumors of T-cell lineage and CD79a is present in tumors of B-cell lineage. Lymphoblastic lymphomas of both lineages are TdT$^+$.

Genetics

No single chromosome translocation or genetic lesion characterizes lymphoblastic lymphomas. A large number of lesions have been defined (see Table 11.1). No obvious correlations between genetic lesions and clinical course have been discerned. In general, B-cell tumors fare a bit better than T-cell tumors given the same therapy, but none of the genetic lesions found in a particular lineage has prognostic significance. The genetic abnormalities seen in lymphoblastic lymphoma mimic the lesions seen in acute lymphoid leukemia. As in B-cell neoplasia, many of the genetic abnormalities in T-cell tumors appear to relate to errors that occur during the rearrangement of the T-cell antigen receptor (*TCR*) genes on chromosomes 14q11 (*TCRα/δ* genes), 7q34–q36 (*TCRβ* genes) and 7p15 (*TCRγ* genes). The rearrangements lead to the activation of a variety of genes, most of which are transcription factors that activate genes that are normally not expressed or repress genes that are normally expressed. Such activating rearrangements are likely to be involved in the transformation process.

In addition to the gene-activating translocations, mutations in three tumor suppressor genes are noted in precursor T-cell neoplasms, namely the retinoblastoma gene *RB*, *p53* and *p16*. Homozygous deletions of *p16* on chromosome 9p21 occur most frequently, being detected in up to 80% of patients.

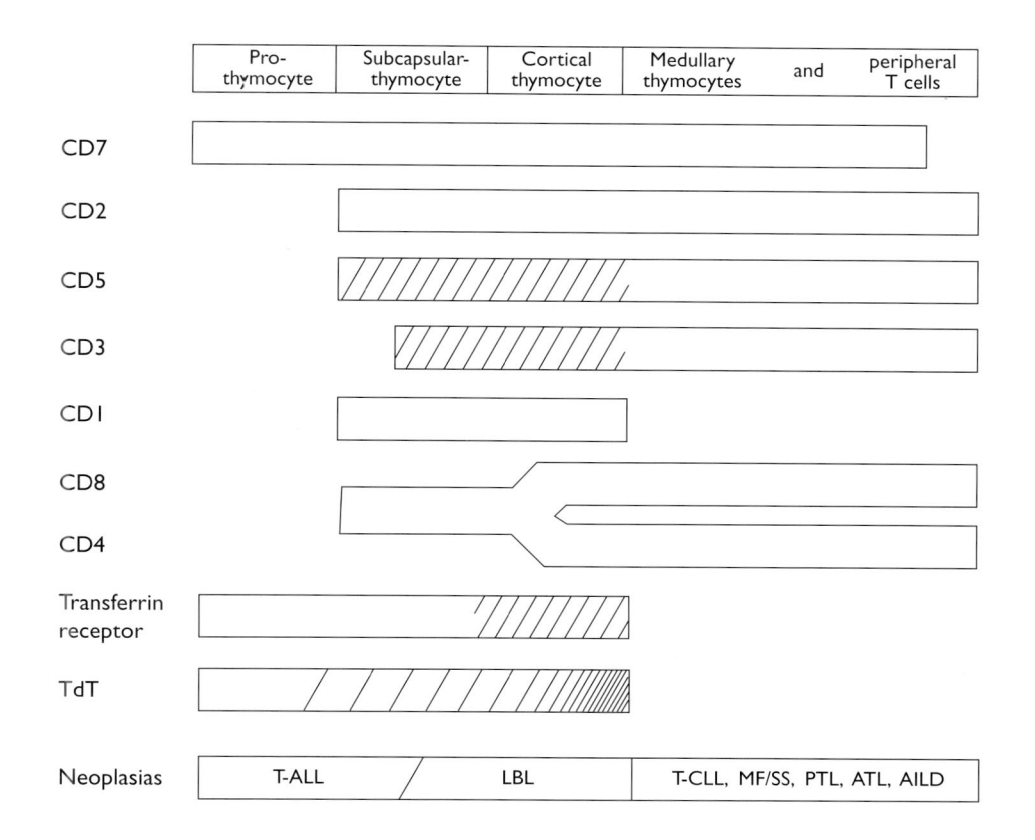

Figure 11.1
Schematic representation of stages of T-cell differentiation and the pattern of marker expression at each stage. Prothymocytes are the earliest recognizable T-cell precursors, and they exist in the bone marrow. These cells migrate to the thymus, enter the subcapsular region, and progressively mature as they migrate through the cortex and into the medulla. The cells of the thymic medulla have a mature peripheral T-cell phenotype. About 85% of the lymphocytes in the thymus are cortical thymocytes, and it is these cells that become malignant in lymphoblastic lymphoma. Hatched bars illustrate stages of development where expression is usually present but may not be in every cell. TdT is terminal deoxynucleotide transferase, an enzyme involved in the generation of the T-cell antigen receptor repertoire. It is an excellent marker for early T-cell and early B-cell development. T-ALL, T-cell acute lymphoblastic leukemia; LBL, lymphoblastic lymphoma; T-CLL, T-cell chronic lymphocytic leukemia; MF/SS, mycosis fungoides/Sézary syndrome; PTL, peripheral T-cell lymphoma; ATL, adult T-cell leukemia/lymphoma; AILD, angioimmunoblastic T-cell lymphoma. (Reproduced from Magrath IT (ed) *The Non-Hodgkin's Lymphomas*, 2nd Ed, 1997, with permission from Edward Arnold.)

Clinical characteristics

T-cell lymphoblastic lymphoma is most common in adolescents and young adults (median age 16 years), but the disease may occur in older people (there is a second smaller peak in the 40s). Males are affected more commonly than females. Patients most commonly present with a mediastinal mass (70%), and may have pleural and/or pericardial effusions. Medical emergencies such as superior vena caval obstruction or pericardial tamponade may be the initial presentations. Patients may have shortness of breath, chest pain, dysphagia, or swelling of the neck, face and upper extremities. Patients have adenopathy involving the neck, axilla and/or supraclavicular regions in 50–80% of cases. Abdominal organs (liver, kidneys, spleen) may be involved late in the disease, but isolated abdominal involvement is very rare. Patients commonly have bone or bone marrow involvement.

Table 11.1
Chromosomal rearrangements in precursor T-cell neoplasms

Gene-activation rearrangement	Rearranged gene at breakpoint	Activated gene near breakpoint	Encoded protein domain
t(8;14)(q24;q11)	TCRα (14q11)	c-MYC (8q24)	bHLH
t(1;14)(p33;q11)	TCRδ (14q11)	SCL/TAL/TCL5 (1p33)	bHLH
t(1;7)(p33;q35)	TCRβ (7q35)	SCL/TAL/TCL5 (1p33)	bHLH
t(1;3)(p33;p21)	TCTA (3p21)	SCL/TAL/TCL5 (1p33)	bHLH
t(7;9)(q35;q34)	TCRβ (7q35)	TAL2 (9q34)	bHLH
t(7;19)(q35;p13)	TCRβ (7q35)	LYL1 (19p13)	bHLH
t(11;14)(p15;q11)	TCRδ (14q11)	RBTN1/TTG1 (11p15)	LIM
t(11;14)(p13;q11)	TCRα/δ (14q11)	RBTN2/TTG1 (11p13)	LIM
t(7;11)(q35;p13)	TCRβ (7q35)	RBTN2/TTG1 (11p13)	LIM
t(10;14)(q24;q11)	TCRα (14q11)	HOX11 (10q24)	Homeobox
t(7;10)(q35;p13)	TCRβ (7q35)	HOX11	Homeobox
t(7;9)(q34;q34)	TCRβ	TAN1 (9q34.3)	Notch
t(1;7)(p34;q34)	TCRβ (7q34)	LCK (1p34)	Receptor tyrosine kinase

Gene fusion rearrangement	Fusion gene	Genes involved in fusion	Encoded protein domains
t(11;19)(p23;p13.3)	ALL1/ENL	ALL1/MLL/HRX (11q23)	Trithorax
		ENL (19p13.3)	Zinc finger
t(X;11)(q13;q23)	ALL1/AFX	ALL1/MLL/HRX (11q23)	Trithorax
		AFX (Xq13)	Zinc finger

bHLH, basic helix–loop–helix

The testes may be involved. Leptomeningeal involvement of the central nervous system is uncommon at diagnosis (10%), but often complicates the late course of the disease, especially in patients with bone and bone marrow involvement. The symptoms of meningeal involvement may be localized pain (nerve root involvement) or cranial nerve symptoms; however, most patients are detected while asymptomatic by the presence of elevated protein levels and malignant cells on spinal tap.

B-cell lymphoblastic lymphoma is rare in adults. Children or adolescents are most commonly affected, and present with peripheral adenopathy, bone lesions, and involvement of the skin, especially in the head and neck region. The vast majority of cases progress to overt leukemia. Mediastinal masses are uncommon.

By Ann Arbor staging, most patients have advanced disease. High lactate dehydrogenase (LDH) level, advanced age and central nervous system involvement are poor prognostic factors.

Treatment

Results of treatment have improved dramatically with the application to lymphoblastic lymphoma of leukemia treatment approaches. The first successful regimen was the LSA_2-L_2 regimen, which includes 10 drugs administered in induction, consolidation and maintenance phases, and incorporates central nervous system prophylaxis in the treatment. This approach leads to long-term survival in 64% of patients, and has been shown in

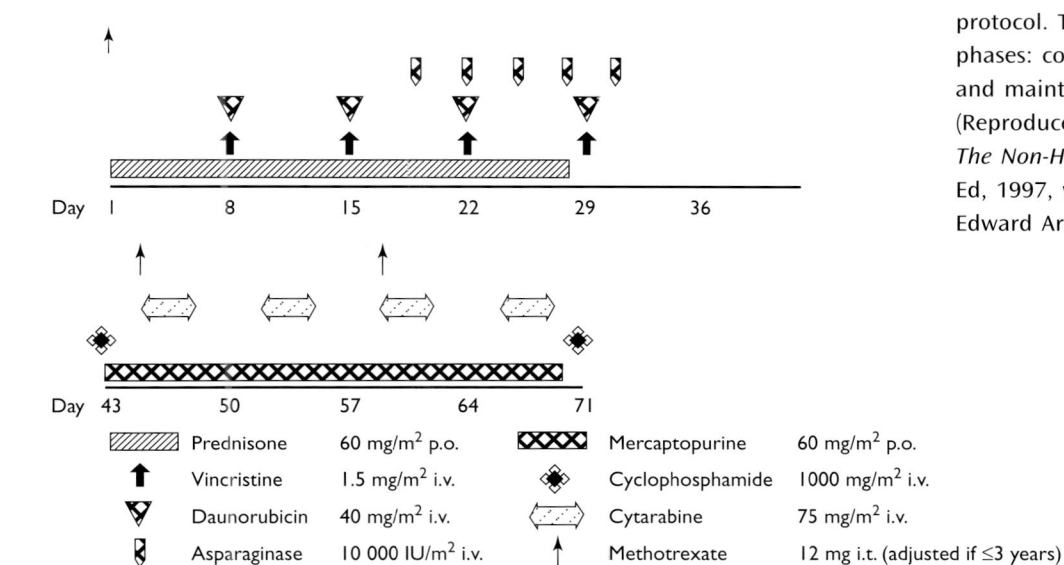

INDUCTION PROTOCOL, I

Figure 11.2
Treatment schema for the BFM 86 protocol. Treatment is given in four phases: consolidation, reinduction and maintenance (not shown). (Reproduced from Magrath IT (ed) *The Non-Hodgkin's Lymphomas*, 2nd Ed, 1997, with permission from Edward Arnold.)

Symbol	Drug	Dose
▨	Prednisone	60 mg/m² p.o.
↑	Vincristine	1.5 mg/m² i.v.
▽	Daunorubicin	40 mg/m² i.v.
▯	Asparaginase	10 000 IU/m² i.v.
⋈	Mercaptopurine	60 mg/m² p.o.
◆	Cyclophosphamide	1000 mg/m² i.v.
⇔	Cytarabine	75 mg/m² i.v.
↑	Methotrexate	12 mg i.t. (adjusted if ≤3 years)

CONSOLIDATION PROTOCOL, M

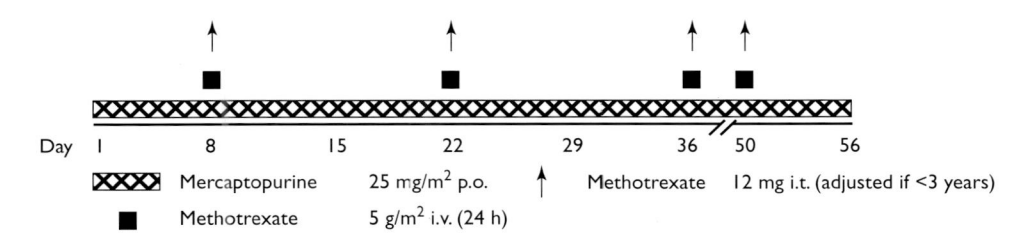

Symbol	Drug	Dose
⋈	Mercaptopurine	25 mg/m² p.o.
■	Methotrexate	5 g/m² i.v. (24 h)
↑	Methotrexate	12 mg i.t. (adjusted if <3 years)

REINDUCTION PROTOCOL, II

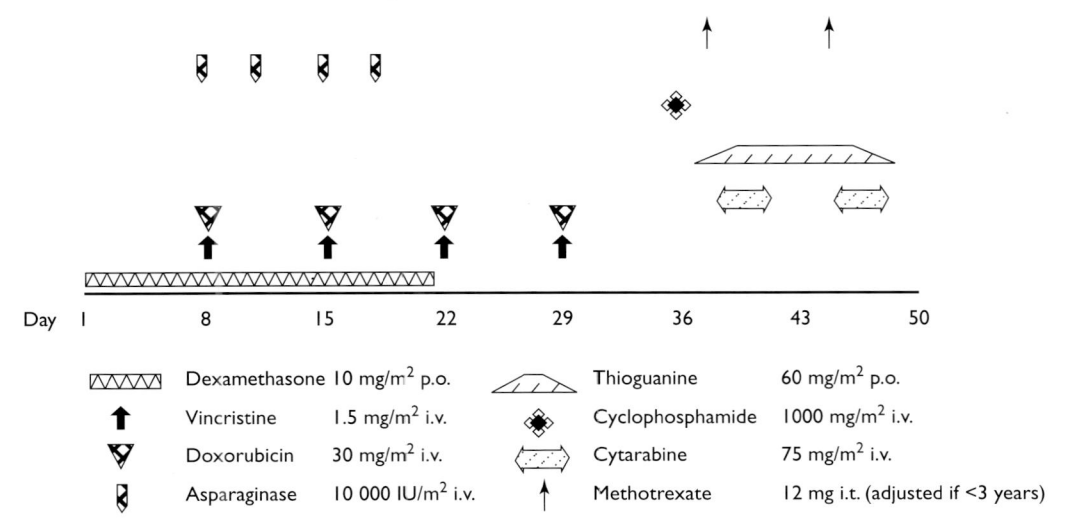

Symbol	Drug	Dose
▨	Dexamethasone	10 mg/m² p.o.
↑	Vincristine	1.5 mg/m² i.v.
▽	Doxorubicin	30 mg/m² i.v.
▯	Asparaginase	10 000 IU/m² i.v.
◿	Thioguanine	60 mg/m² p.o.
◆	Cyclophosphamide	1000 mg/m² i.v.
⇔	Cytarabine	75 mg/m² i.v.
↑	Methotrexate	12 mg i.t. (adjusted if <3 years)

randomized studies to be superior to the use of lymphoma regimens. Cooperative groups based in France (French Society of Pediatric Oncology, SFOP) and Germany (Berlin–Frankfurt–Münster, BFM) have improved on these results. In the LMT 81 protocol, the SFOP added 10 courses of high-dose methotrexate to LSA_2-L_2 and obtained event-free survival of 79% for stage III patients and 72% for stage IV patients. BFM 86 (Figure 11.2) includes an induction phase, a consolidation phase, a second induction phase and maintenance therapy, with a total length of treatment of two years. The seven-year event-free survival for all stages of disease was 82% in 73 treated patients. Outcome of treatment is not improved by using radiation therapy to treat the mediastinum.

Results obtained in adult populations tend to be somewhat inferior to those seen in pediatric populations. Part of the difference is the intensity of the treatment, but the existence of biologic differences between lymphoblastic lymphoma in children and adults cannot be excluded. Aggressive multiagent chemotherapy appears to be capable of achieving complete remission in about 85% of patients. When patients who achieve complete remission receive high-dose therapy and autologous hematopoietic stem cells, six-year actuarial survival is 63% according to the European Group for Bone Marrow Transplantation study. Other series also report long-term survival in about 65% of patients. Patients who remain in remission for more than three years are unlikely to relapse. Relapsed patients can be cured with salvage therapy that includes high-dose therapy and autologous or allogeneic stem cells in about one-third of cases.

Bibliography

Baer R, TAL1, TAL2, and LYL1: A family of basic helix–loop–helix proteins implicated in T cell acute leukemia. *Semin Cancer Biol* 1993; **4:** 341–7.

Bernasconi C, Brusamolino E, Lazzarino M et al, Lymphoblastic lymphoma in adult patients: clinicopathologic features and response to intensive multiagent chemotherapy analogous to that used in acute lymphoblastic leukemia. *Ann Oncol* 1990; **1:** 141–6.

Bouabdalla R, Xerri L, Bardou VJ et al, Role of induction chemotherapy and bone marrow transplantation in adult lymphoblastic lymphoma: a report on 62 patients from a single center. *Ann Oncol* 1998; **9:** 619–25.

Cayuela JM, Hebert J, Sigaux F, Homozygous MTS1 ($p16^{INK4a}$) deletion in primary tumor cells of 163 leukemia patients. *Blood* 1995; **85:** 854–61.

Link MP, Donaldson SS, Berard CW et al, Results of treatment of childhood localized non-Hodgkin's lymphoma with combination chemotherapy with or without radiotherapy. *N Engl J Med* 1990; **322:** 1169–74.

Milpied N, Ifrah N, Kuentz M et al, Bone marrow transplantation for adult poor prognosis lymphoblastic lymphoma in first complete remission. *Br J Haematol* 1989; **73:** 82–87.

Morel P, Lepage E, Brice P et al, Prognosis and treatment of lymphoblastic lymphoma in adults. A report on 80 patients. *J Clin Oncol* 1992; **10:** 1078–85.

Patte C, Kalifa C, Flamant F et al, Results of the LMT81 protocol, a modified LSA2-L2 protocol with high-dose methotrexate, on 84 children with non-B-cell (lymphoblastic) lymphoma. *Med Pediatr Oncol* 1992; **20:** 105–13.

Reiter A, Schrappe M, Parwaresch R et al, Non-Hodgkin's lymphomas of childhood and adolescence: results of a treatment stratified for biologic subtypes and stage – a report of the Berlin–Frankfurt–Münster group. *J Clin Oncol* 1995; **13:** 359–72.

Sweetenham JW, Liberti G, Pearce R et al, High-dose therapy and autologous bone marrow transplantation for adult patients with lymphoblastic lymphoma: results of the European Group for Bone Marrow Transplantation. *J Clin Oncol* 1994; **12:** 1358–65.

Tubergen DG, Krailo MD, Meadows AT et al, Comparison of treatment regimens for pediatric lymphoblastic non-Hodgkin's lymphoma: A Children's Cancer Group Study. *J Clin Oncol* 1995; **13:** 1368–76.

Verdonck LF, Dekker AW, deGast GC et al, Autologous bone marrow transplantation for adult poor-risk lymphoblastic lymphoma in first remission. *J Clin Oncol* 1992; **10:** 644–6.

T-cell lymphoblastic leukemia/lymphoma

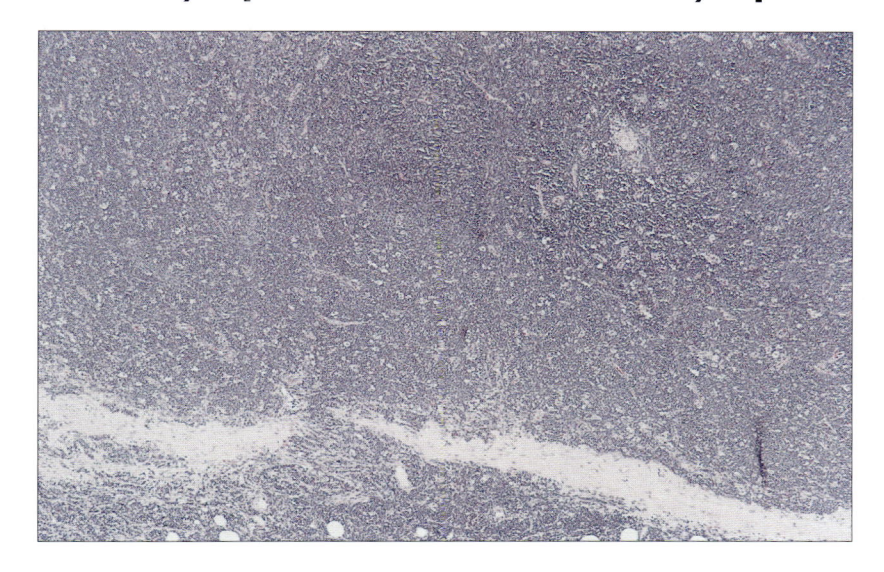

Figure 11.3

T-cell lymphoblastic leukemia/lymphoma – Lymph node:

(a) There is a diffuse cellular infiltrate that replaces the lymph node and extends into perinodal tissue. (H&E stain)

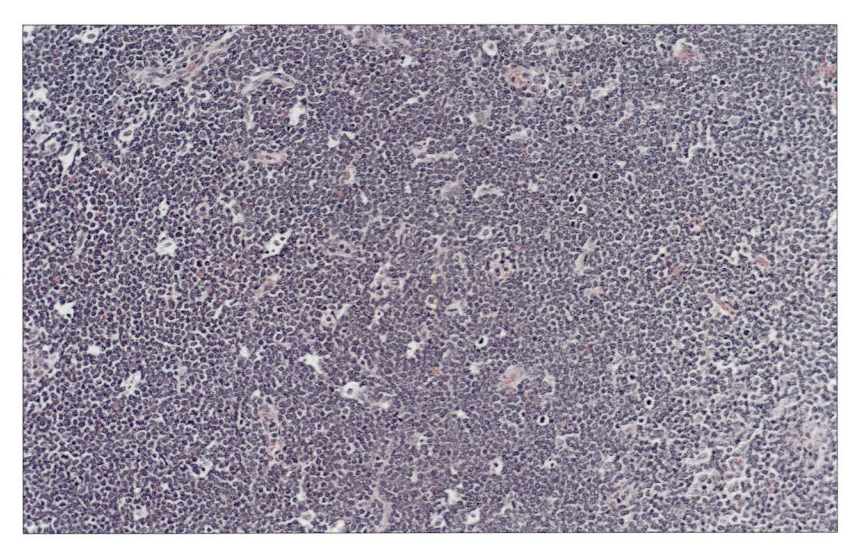

(b) In areas, a 'starry sky' pattern is seen, but it is less striking than that usually seen in Burkitt's lymphoma. (H&E stain)

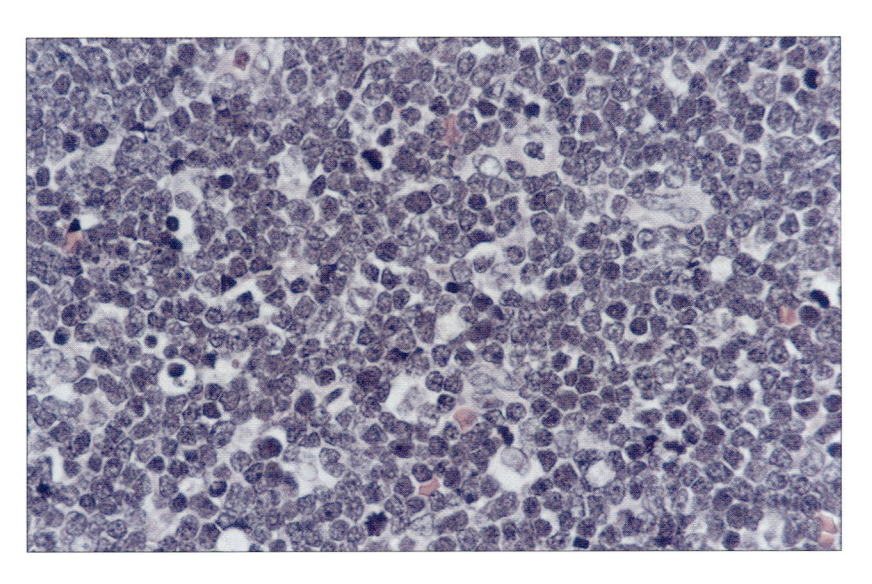

(c) Neoplastic cells are slightly larger than small lymphocytes; they have finely dispersed chromatin and scant cytoplasm. (H&E stain)

Contd

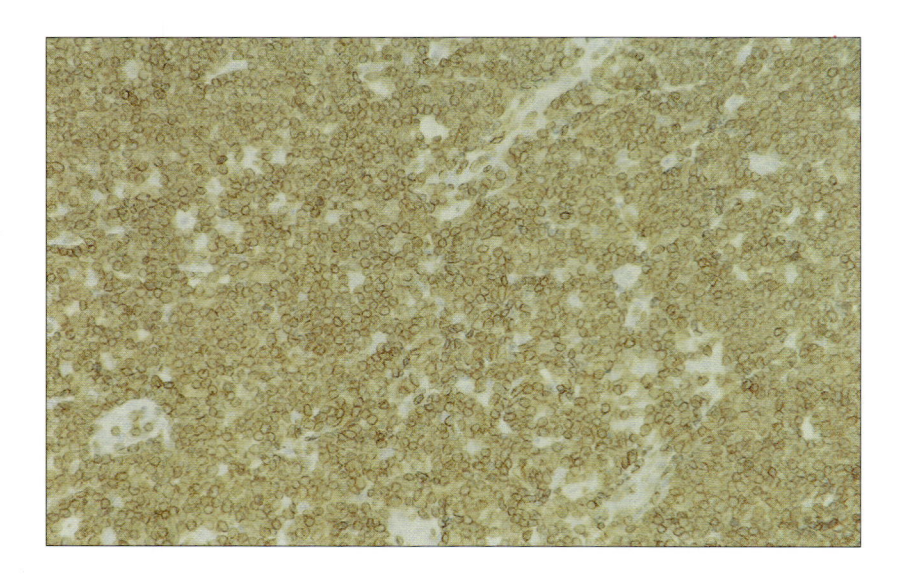

Figure 11.3 *continued*

Neoplastic cells express the T-cell marker CD3 (**d**). Only a few scattered B cells (L26+) (**e**) are present. Many cells show nuclear staining for TdT (**f**). These results confirm the diagnosis of T-cell lymphoblastic lymphoma. (Immunoperoxidase technique on paraffin sections)

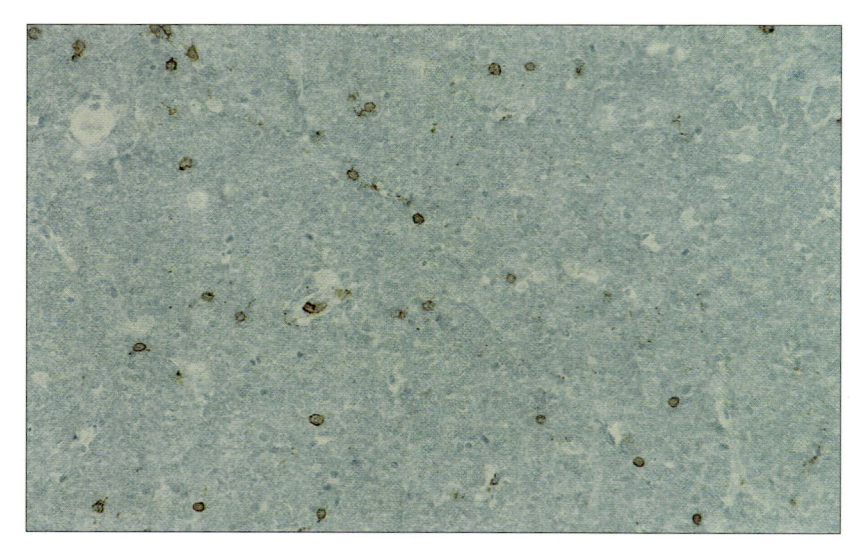

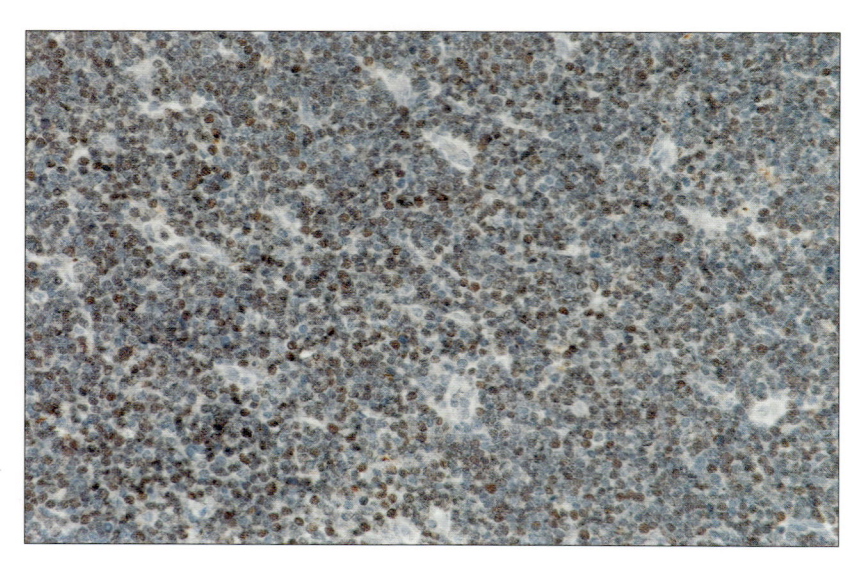

(d)

(e)

(f)

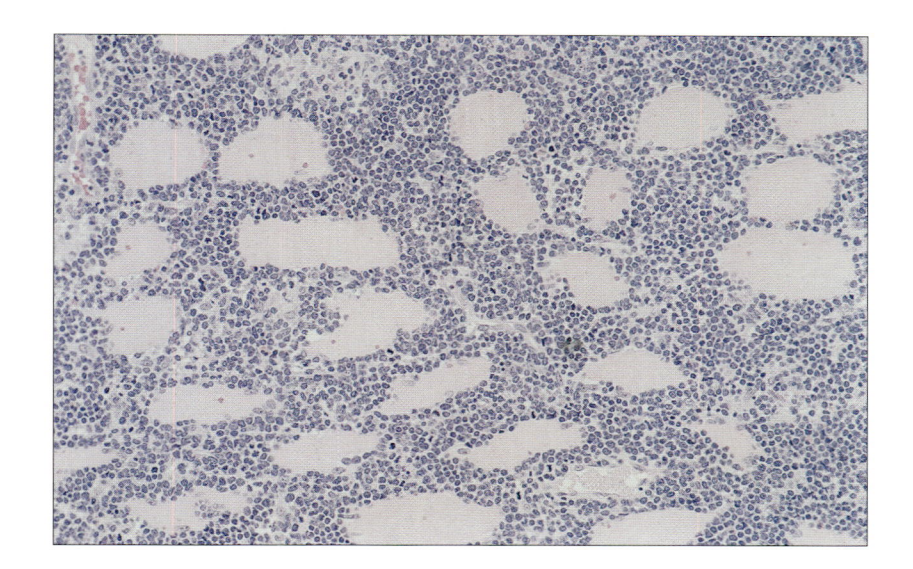

Figure 11.4

T-cell lymphoblastic leukemia/lymphoma – Soft tissue:

(a) In this case, lymphoma infiltrates skeletal muscle. (H&E stain)

(b) The neoplastic cells are small to intermediate in size and have irregular nuclei with finely dispersed chromatin. Mitotic figures are frequent. (H&E stain)

B-cell lymphoblastic leukemia/lymphoma

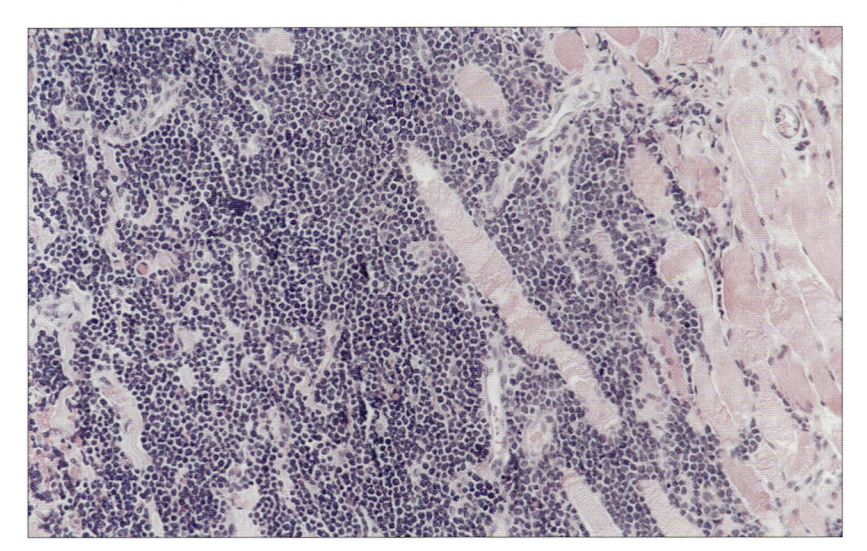

Figure 11.5

B-cell lymphoblastic leukemia/lymphoma:

(a) Lymphoid cells diffusely infiltrate soft tissue. (H&E stain)

(b) Higher power shows a monomorphous population of intermediate-sized cells with finely dispersed chromatin, inconspicuous nucleoli, scant cytoplasm and a high mitotic rate. (H&E stain)

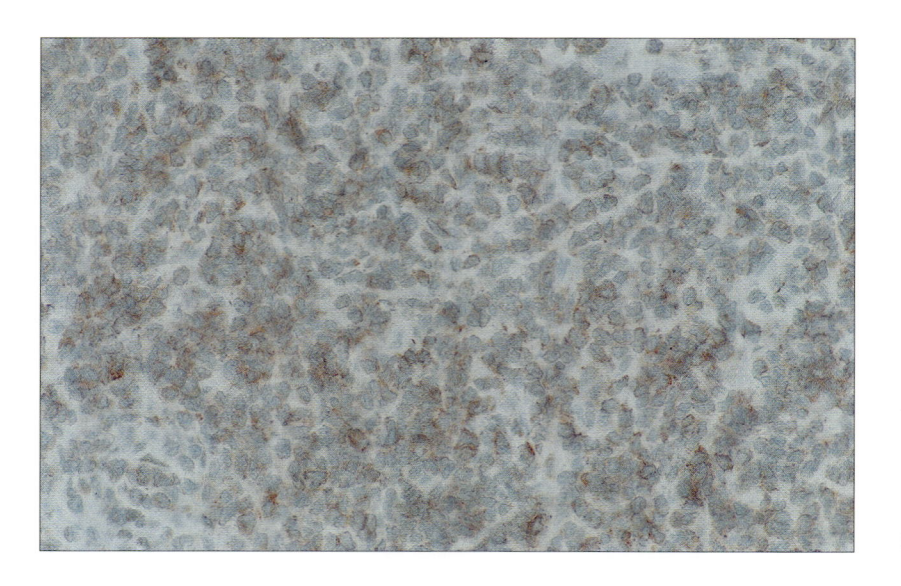

Neoplastic cells express the B-cell antigen CD79a (c), but lack CD20 (d), which is usually absent on precursor B cells. (Immunoperoxidase technique on paraffin sections)

(c)

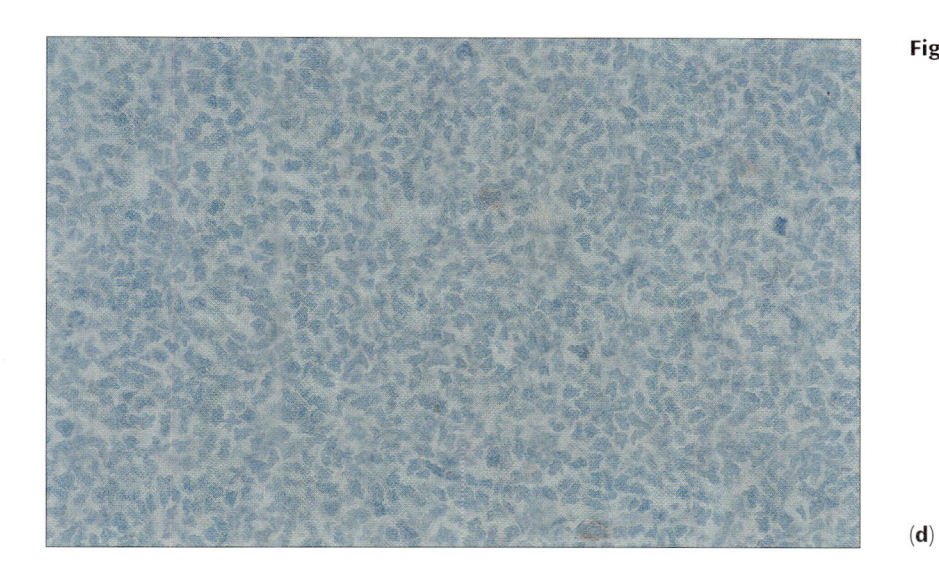

Figure 11.5 *continued*

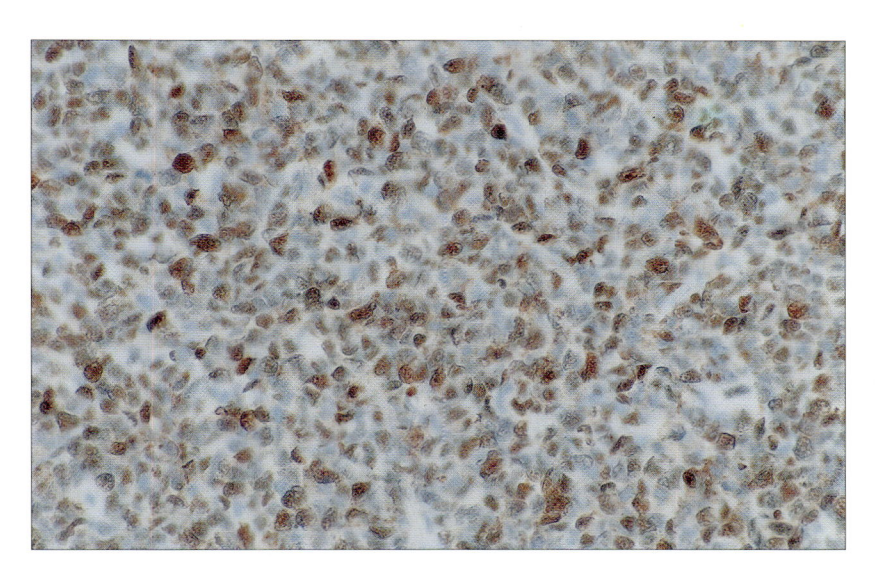

(d)

(e) Neoplastic cells also express TdT. (Immunoperoxidase technique on paraffin sections)

12 Lymphoplasmacytic lymphoma

Definition and classification

Lymphoplasmacytic lymphoma is an unusual type of non-Hodgkin's lymphoma. In the Working Formulation, patients with this disorder were usually classified as having small lymphocytic lymphoma. In the Kiel classification, patients with lymphoplasmacytic lymphoma were often diagnosed as having immunocytomas. Patients with lymphoplasmacytic lymphoma often have the clinical syndrome of Waldenström's macroglobulinemia. When a patient has been diagnosed as having Waldenström's macroglobinemia and a lymph node biopsy is performed, it would be anticipated that this would be the histologic finding.

Lymphoplasmacytic lymphoma could not be diagnosed accurately in the International Non-Hodgkin's Lymphoma Classification Study. The expert pathologists participating in this study were only able to diagnose this lymphoma accurately 50–60% of the time. This suggests that more precise definitions are needed – or that this subgroup of lymphomas represent a mixture of more than one disorder.

Frequency

Lymphoplasmacytic lymphoma occurs infrequently. It represents approximately 1% of non-Hodgkin's lymphomas. There appears to be little geographic variation in the frequency of this lymphoma.

Pathology

Histology (Table 12.1)

Lymphoplasmacytic lymphoma presents a diffuse growth pattern. Cytology includes a mixture of small lymphocytes, plasmacytoid lymphocytes and plasma cells. The latter often contain Dutcher bodies. There is often an interfollicular growth pattern and sparing of the lymph node sinuses. These patients will often have a monoclonal IgM protein and bone marrow infiltration typical of the clinical syndrome of Waldenström's macroglobulinemia.

Table 12.1
Histologic features of lymphoplasmacytic lymphoma

- Diffuse growth pattern
- Admixed small lymphocytes, plasmacytoid lymphocytes and plasma cells (with or without Dutcher bodies)
- Often interfollicular growth pattern with sparing of sinuses
- This is the histologic finding in most cases of Waldenström's macroglobulinemia

Table 12.2 Immunophenotype and genetics of lymphoplasmacytic lymphoma	
Characteristic	Result
Immunophenotype	CD20⁺, cytoplasmic Ig⁺, CD3⁻, CD10⁻, CD5⁻, CD23⁻
Cytogenetics	t(9;14)(p13;q32)
Oncogenes	Not known

Immunophenotype (Table 12.2)

The tumor cells in lymphoplasmacytic lymphoma are malignant B cells. They express the CD20 antigen and are positive for cytoplasmic immunoglobulin. They are CD3⁻, CD10⁻, CD5⁻ and CD23⁻. The negative staining for CD5 helps distinguish this tumor from small lymphocytic lymphoma and mantle-cell lymphoma.

Genetics (Table 12.2)

No consistent cytogenetic abnormality is seen with lymphoplasmacytic lymphoma. Perhaps the most frequently reported cytogenetic abnormality is the t(9;14)(p11;q32). There is no known oncogene that is consistently expressed in lymphoplasmacytic lymphoma.

Clinical characteristics (Table 12.3)

Lymphoplasmacytic lymphoma occurs predominantly in older individuals, and is seen more frequently in males. In the International Lymphoma Classification Study, the median age was 63 years, and 53% of the patients were male. Most patients diagnosed with lymphoplasmacytic lymphoma will have bone marrow involvement and will be stage IV on that basis. In the International Lymphoma Classification Study, 73% of the patients were stage IV and only 20% of the patients were stage I or II. Extranodal involvement is seen in most patients, with the bone marrow being by far the most frequent site.

Table 12.3 Clinical characteristics of lymphoplasmacytic lymphoma	
Characteristic	Result
Median age	63 years
Percent male	53%
Stage I	7%
Stage IE	0%
Stage II	0%
Stage IIE	13%
Stage III	7%
Stage IV	73%
B symptoms	13%
Elevated LDH	15%
Karnofsky ≤ 70%	27%
Tumor mass ≥ 10 cm	25%
Any extranodal site	100%
Bone marrow positive	73%
GI tract involved	7%
IPI score 0/1	16%
2/3	69%
4/5	15%

Systemic symptoms are not typical of lymphoplasmacytic lymphoma, except for those that might be related to an excessive amount of circulating IgM monoclonal protein. Fevers, sweats and weight loss were seen in only 13% of the patients in the International Lymphoma Classification Study and elevated lactate dehydrogenase (LDH) was found in only 15% of patients. Seventy-three per cent of patients were fully active, and large tumor masses were unusual. The gastrointestinal tract was rarely involved.

Most patients with lymphoplasmacytic lymphoma in the International Lymphoma Classification Study had two or three adverse risk factors in the International Prognostic Index. Only 15% of the patients had four or five adverse risk factors.

Treatment and outcome

The prognoses for survival for patients with lymphoplasmacytic lymphoma according to the International Lymphoma Classification Study are

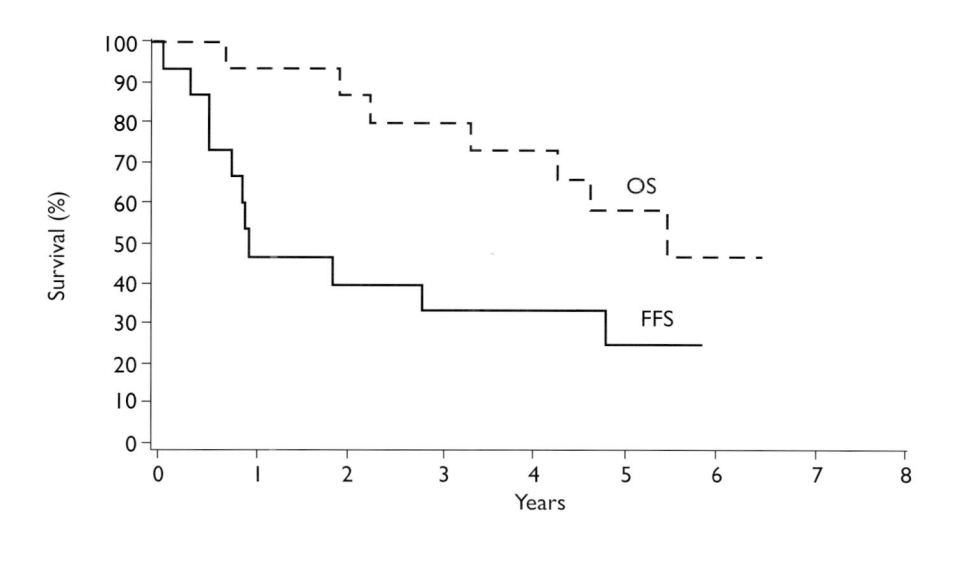

Figure 12.1
Overall survival (OS) and failure-free survival (FFS) of patients with lymphoplasmacytic lymphoma.

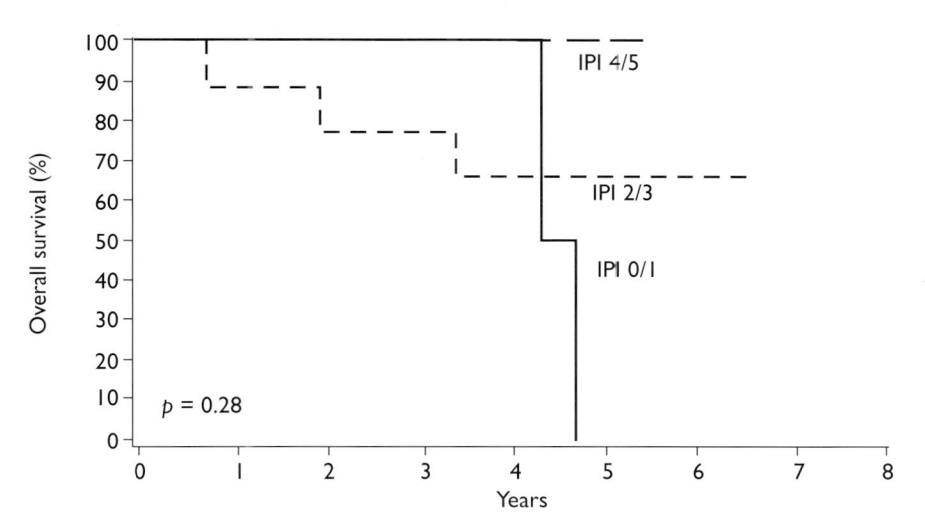

Figure 12.2
Overall survival according to International Prognostic Index (IPI) for patients with lymphoplasmacytic lymphoma.

shown in Figures 12.1 and 12.2. There is no standard therapy for the management of patients with lymphoplasmacytic lymphoma. In the past, chlorambucil was the most common therapy, and is still widely used, with a high response rate. However, this treatment does not produce long-term disease-free survival. It is not clear whether combination chemotherapy improves treatment outcome.

In recent years, purine analogues such as fludarabine and 2-chlorodeoxyadenosine (cladribine) have been shown to have a high level of activity in patients with Waldenström's macroglobulinemia. These agents should be considered in the treatment of patients with lymphoplasmacytic lymphoma, and may become the standard therapy.

It must be remembered that patients who have the syndrome of Waldenström's macroglobulinemia might have other symptoms predominantly related to an excessive amount of circulating IgM monoclonal protein. In these patients, plasmapheresis to reduce the level of IgM in the plasma might be an important and even life-saving treatment. In patients with symptomatic elevation of the level of IgM monoclonal protein, plasmapheresis should be combined with an effective chemotherapeutic agent.

Bibliography

Case DC, Errin TJ, Boyd MA et al, Waldenström's macroglobulinemia: long term results with the M2-protocol. *Cancer Invest* 1991; **9:** 1–7.

Dimopoulos MA, Kantarjian H, Weber D et al, Primary treatment of Waldenström's macroglobulinemia with 2-chlorodeoxyadenosine. *J Clin Oncol* 1994; **12:** 2694–8.

Harris NL, Jaffe ES, Stein H et al, A revised European–American classification of lymphoid neoplasms: a proposal from the International Lymphoma Study Group. *Blood* 1994; **84**: 1361–92.

International Non-Hodgkin's Lymphoma Prognostic Factors Project, A predictive model for aggressive non-Hodgkin's lymphoma. *N Engl J Med* 1993; **329:** 987–94.

Kantarjian HM, Alexanian R, Koller CA et al, Fludarabine therapy in macroglobulinemic lymphoma. *Blood* 1990; **75:** 1928–31.

Leblond V, Ben-Othman T, Deconinck E et al, Activity of fludarabine in previously treated Waldenström's macroglobulinemia: a report of 71 cases. *J Clin Oncol* 1998; **16:** 2060–4.

Lister TA, Cullen MH, Beard ME et al, Comparison of combined and single agent chemotherapy in non-Hodgkin's lymphoma of favourable histological type. *Br Med J* 1978; **i:** 533–7.

Non-Hodgkin's Lymphoma Classification Project, A clinical evaluation of the International Lymphoma Study Group classification of non-Hodgkin's lymphoma. *Blood* 1997; **89:** 3909–18.

Rohatiner AZS, Foran J, Coiffier B et al, Fludarabine in newly diagnosed diffuse low grade non-Hodgkin's lymphoma. *Proc Am Soc Clin Oncol* 1996; **15:** 419.

Waldenström J, Incipient myelomatosis or essential hyperglobulinaemia with fibrinogenopaenia – a new syndrome? *Acta Med Scand* 1944; **117:** 216–22.

Lymphoplasmacytic lymphoma

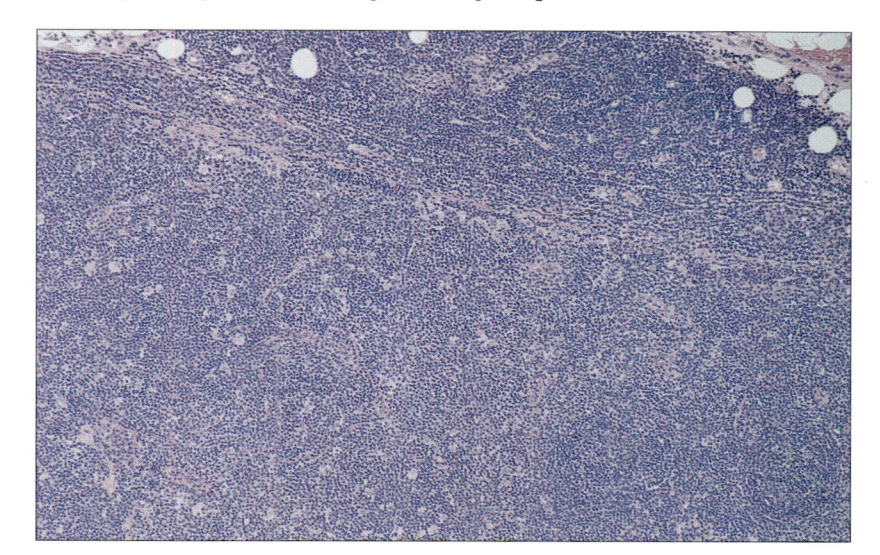

Figure 12.3

Lymphoplasmacytic lymphoma:

(a) Low-power examination shows obliteration of the nodal architecture by a diffuse cellular infiltrate. (H&E stain)

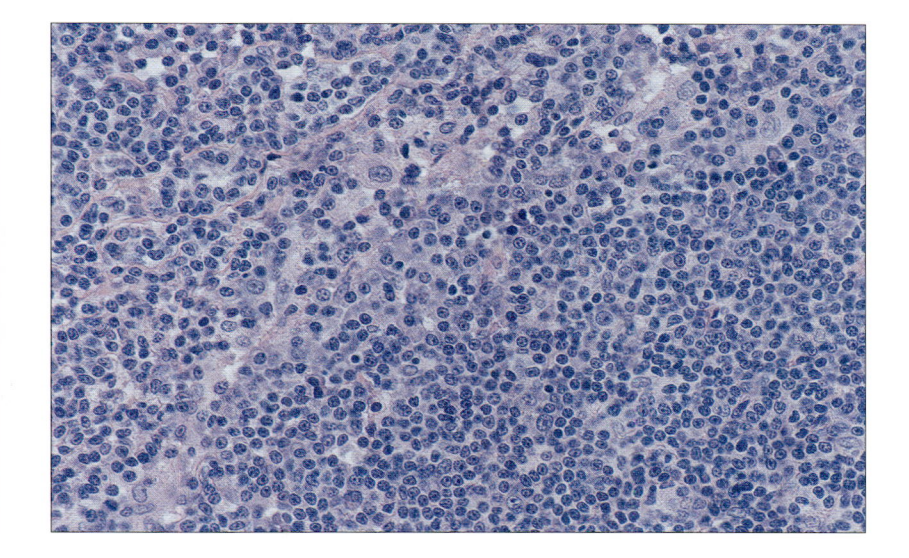

(b) Most cells present are small lymphoid cells. (H&E stain)

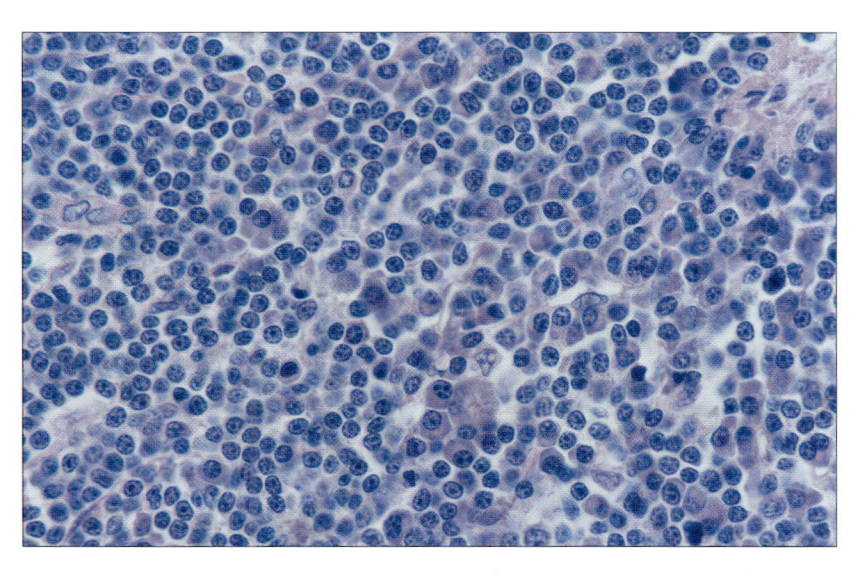

(c) High-power examination shows that, in addition to small lymphocytes, there are aggregates of mature plasma cells. (H&E stain)

Contd

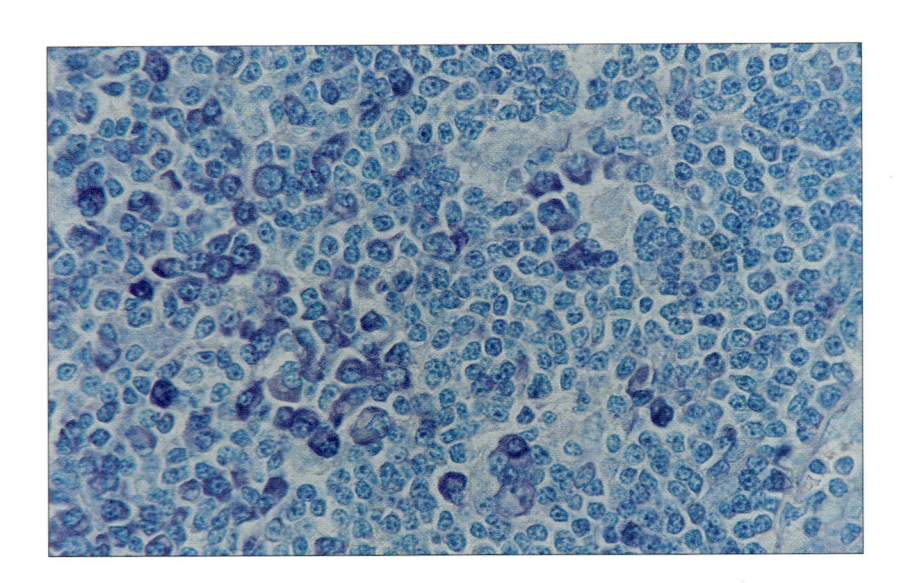

Figure 12.3 *continued*

(d) With a Giemsa stain, the cytoplasm of the plasma cells is deep blue.

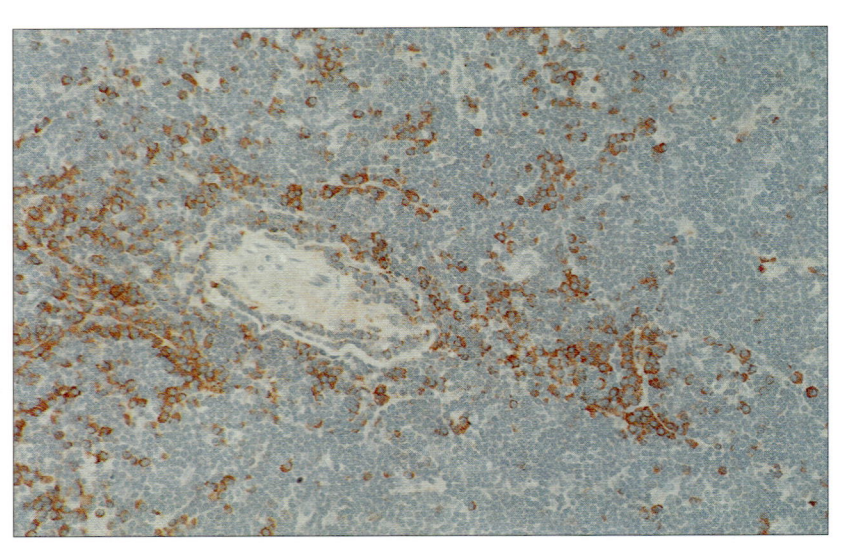

Many plasma cells express cytoplasmic κ light chain (e), but only rare plasma cells are λ⁺ (f). (Immunoperoxidase technique on paraffin sections)

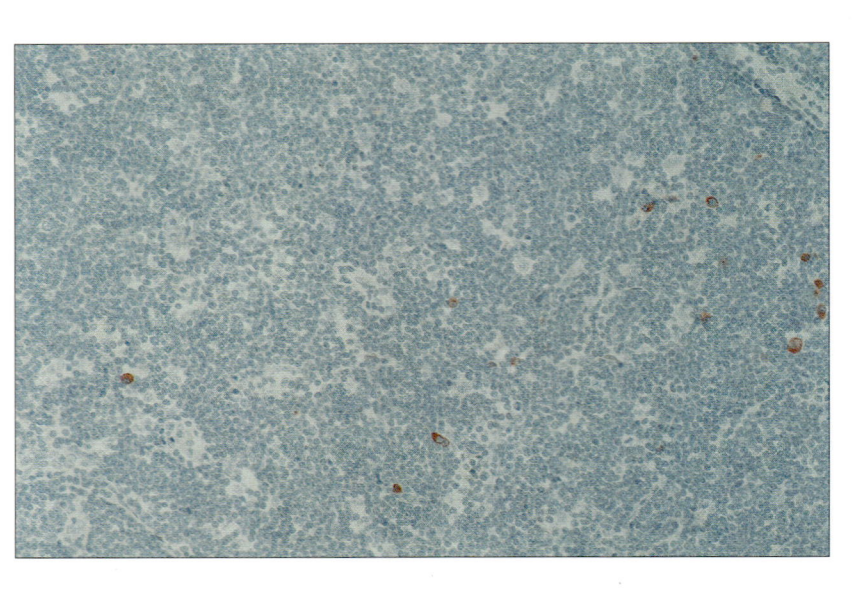

(e)

(f)

13 Nodal and splenic marginal-zone B-cell lymphomas

Nodal marginal-zone B-cell lymphoma

Definition and classification

The terminology 'marginal-zone B-cell lymphoma' (MZBCL) has been proposed in the REAL classification to encompass a group of lymphomas that, despite their different clinical manifestations, appear to have a common origin from the marginal-zone B-cell compartment outside the follicular mantle zone. In addition to low-grade MALT lymphomas (extranodal marginal-zone

Table 13.1
Typical features of monocytoid lymphoma

Histologic features
- Monocytoid B-cells with abundant cytoplasm, reniform or oval nuclei
- Distinctive sinusoidal pattern of spread, with characteristic confluent sinuses filled with monocytoid cells showing secondary follicle invasion

Immunophenotype
- CD19+, CD20+, CD22+, CD11c+
- CD5−, CD10−, CD23−, CD25−
- BCL2 protein overexpression

Genetic characteristics
- Trisomy 3, trisomy 18
- Chromosome 1 structural rearrangements
- BCL1, BCL2, BCL3, BCL6 and c-MYC usually not rearranged

Table 13.2
Typical features of splenic marginal-zone lymphoma

Histologic features
- Nodular lymphoid infiltrate of the splenic white pulp centered on pre-existing follicles; red pulp infiltration is present as well
- Central population of small lymphocytes and peripheral population of medium-sized lymphocytes with slightly irregular nuclei and a moderate amount of pale cytoplasm
- Variable number of interspersed blasts
- Sometimes circulating neoplastic cells with short polar villi

Immunophenotype
- Monotypic surface immunoglobulins (IgM and IgD)
- CD19+, CD20+, CD79a+
- CD5−, CD10−

Genetic characteristics
- Chromosome 1, 3, 7 and 8 abnormalities
- Only a few cases with trisomy 3

B-cell lymphoma of MALT type, described in Chapter 7), this group includes two additional entities: monocytoid B-cell lymphoma (Table 13.1) and splenic marginal-zone lymphoma with or without villous lymphocytes (Table 13.2). These entities have a virtually identical phenotype and have been reported to share some common cytogenetic and molecular features. The principal difference lies in the site of origin; however, whether or not they represent a unique disease entity is still controversial.

The presence of nodal marginal-zone lymphomas with monocytoid B cells was already recognised in the Kiel classification (monocytoid B-cell lymphoma) and the Lukes and Collins classification (parafollicular B-cell lymphoma), but the entity was not included in the Working Formulation, where it may have been placed in any of the subtypes from A to F.

Frequency

Whilst extranodal marginal-zone lymphoma of MALT (mucosa-associated lymphoid tissue) is relatively common (7.6%), its nodal and splenic putative counterparts appear to be quite rare. In a recent evaluation of the clinical significance of the REAL classification in a survey of more than 1400 non-Hodgkin's lymphomas from nine institutions in the USA, Canada, Europe, South Africa and Hong Kong, nodal marginal zone B-cell lymphomas comprised 1.8% and splenic marginal-zone lymphomas 0.8% of all lymphoma cases.

Pathology

Histology

In contrast with mucosa-based extranodal MALT lymphoma, monocytoid B-cell lymphoma is typically lymph-node-based. The tumor cells are usually small- to medium-sized lymphocytes with oval or reniform nuclei, abundant pale cytoplasm and well-defined cell borders, resembling monocytes. There is a distinctive sinusoidal pattern of spread, with characteristic confluent sinuses filled with monocytoid cells showing secondary follicle invasion.

Monocytoid B-cell lymphoma is often seen in association with dissemination of extranodal MALT lymphoma to lymph nodes or spleen; in these cases, the recognition of a primary extranodal disease can be difficult, since the distant spread of MALTomas may occur many years after initial diagnosis. Moreover, the histologic pattern of lymph node involvement by extranodal MALT lymphoma is often indistinguishable from that of primary nodal (monocytoid) marginal-zone lymphomas. This finding further suggests a possible overlap of these entities.

Immunophenotype

The neoplastic cells show typical positivity for surface (and sometimes cytoplasmic) monotypic immunoglobulins and pan-B antigens (CD19, CD20 and CD22), they usually coexpress the monocytic/histiocytic antigen CD11c, and they lack CD5, CD10 and CD23 expression.

Distinction from non-neoplastic monocytoid reactions is based on the greater degree of polymorphism in the lymphomatous lesions, but a search for monotypic surface immunoglobulins may be necessary in order to distinguish between reactive lymphoid infiltrate (e.g. toxoplasmosis lymphadenitis) and monocytoid-B lymphoma in cases where the morphologic pattern is equivocal. Some confusion in the differential diagnosis can arise with hairy cell leukemia, since morphology and phenotype are similar (pan-B and CD11c coexpression); however, in contrast to hairy cell leukemia, marginal-zone lymphomas are usually $CD25^-$, $PCA-1^-$ and tartrate-resistant acid phosphatase (TRAP)-negative.

A further process morphologically resembling a marginal-zone lymphoma is the monocytoid B-cell differentiation that can be seen in other primary low-grade nodal lymphomas, mainly in follicular lymphomas, where a monocytoid component appears to occupy the marginal zone. However, in this phenomenon, the immunophenotypic and genotypic features of the neoplastic cells are those of follicular lymphomas (i.e. $CD10^+/CD11c^-$).

Genetics

Clonal chromosomal abnormalities can be detected in most cases of MZBCL. Recurrent aberrations include whole or partial trisomy 3, trisomy 18, and structural rearrangements of chromosome 1q21 and 1p34 . The *BCL1*, *BCL2*, *BCL3*, *BCL6* and c-*MYC* oncogenes are usually not rearranged.

Clinical characteristics

The clinical data are sparse and have been largely drawn from pathologic series rather than clinical centers. MZBCL is a disease of older people, with the median age at presentation in the sixth decade, and affects both sexes, with an unusual (albeit slight) female predominance. The most common presenting feature is a localized adenopathy – most often in the neck around the parotid gland. Concurrent extranodal involvement, most often of the salivary gland, is not rare, and many patients have a history of Sjögren's syndrome or other autoimmune diseases, further suggesting a possible overlap with extranodal MALT lymphomas. Bone marrow is involved at presentation in less than half of the cases. Transformation to high-grade lymphoma has been described in some cases.

Treatment and outcome

There is at present no consensus about the best treatment, individual cases being managed differently according to site and stage. Indeed, there are very few studies comparing MZBCL with the other low-grade B-cell lymphomas. The most important study was recently published by the Southwest Oncology Group (SWOG), comparing different low-grade lymphomas presenting with advanced disease (stage III–IV). This study reviewed the pathology and clinical course of 376 patients previously classified within the Working Formulation categories A, B, C, D or E and uniformly treated with the standard combination-chemotherapy CHOP regimen. Twenty-one patients with nodal monocytoid B-cell lymphoma and 19 patients with extranodal MALT lymphoma were identified. Advanced-stage extranodal MALT appeared to carry a worse prognosis than nodal MZBCL (10-year actuarial survivals of 21% versus 53% respectively). All MZBCL patients were given full-dose CHOP, and showed a survival pattern superimposable on that of advanced follicular lymphomas, but how they would behave with other treatment strategies frequently employed in low-grade lymphomas (such as watchful waiting, single alkylating agents, or new purine analogues) is still to be ascertained. Moreover, the previously mentioned international collaborative survey for the validation of the REAL classification, which included patients of any stage treated with heterogeneous modalities, showed five-year survivals of 57% for MZBCL and 74% for MALT lymphomas. This discrepancy with the SWOG study might be at least partially due to the higher incidence of advanced disease in the nodal MZBCL group (82%, versus 44% in the extranodal MALT-type group).

Primary splenic marginal-zone B-cell lymphoma with or without villous lymphocytes

Definition and classification

This is a rare (<1% of all lymphoma cases) and recently described entity that was not recognized in either the Working Formulation or the Kiel classification, and has only been included as a provisional entity in the REAL classification. This lymphoma characteristically involves the spleen, and has been regarded as the splenic counterpart of the MALT lymphomas. However, despite the fact that it apparently shares many morphologic, immunophenotypic and genetic features with both extranodal and nodal MZBCL, this lymphoma also presents several other morphologic and biologic features, suggesting that it may not be a 'true' marginal-zone lymphoma (Table 13.2). The distinctive nature and pathology of this still controversial entity have recently been reviewed and discussed by Isaacson and Piris, who proposed that it be considered as a separate new entity.

Pathology

Histology

This disease is characterized by a nodular lymphoid infiltrate of the splenic white pulp that partly or completely invades the pre-existing follicles. In nearly all cases, red pulp infiltration is also present to a varying degree. The tumor cells are usually represented by a central population of small lymphocytes (resembling the mantle-zone cells) that toward the periphery give way to medium-sized lymphocytes with slightly irregular nuclei and a moderate amount of pale cytoplasm, resembling splenic marginal-zone lymphocytes. A variable number of interspersed blasts is usually present in the peripheral zone, and plasma cell differentiation can sometimes be seen. The white blood cell count can be increased, and the circulating cells may have short polar villi on the surface – hence the name of the disease.

Immunophenotype

The white pulp nodules are centered on a $CD21^+$ meshwork of follicular dendritic cells. The neoplastic cells show typical positivity for monotypic immunoglobulins (IgM and, in most but not all cases, IgD) and usually coexpress pan-B antigens (CD19, CD20 and CD79a), and lack CD5, CD10 and CD43 expression. $CD3^+$ non-neoplastic T cells can be numerous within the B-cell neoplastic infiltrate of the white pulp. In the cases defined as splenic lymphomas with villous lymphocytes, flow cytometry can show a much more variable phenotype, sometimes with CD5 expression.

Genetics

A small number of cases have been evaluated in a few series, with partially conflicting results. It appears that the detectable clonal chromosomal abnormalities only partially overlap with those described in extranodal (MALT-type) or nodal (monocytoid B-cell) lymphomas. Very complex karyotypes are often present. The more frequent karyotypic abnormalities appear to involve chromosomes 1, 3 (including trisomy 3, but apparently at a much lower frequency than in extranodal MALT lymphomas), 7 (usually 7q deletions) and 8.

Clinical characteristics

The great majority of patients are aged over 50. Enlargement of the spleen is the most common presenting sign, only rarely accompanied by hypersplenism-associated anemia and thrombocytopenia. Diagnosis is often made at splenectomy performed to establish the cause of unexplained splenomegaly. A modest elevation of absolute blood lymphocyte count is common, and often a neoplastic circulating population of villous lymphocytes can be detected. There may be a paraprotein. Bone marrow is frequently involved at diagnosis – also in cases presenting without peripheral blood involvement. Peripheral lymphadenopathy is uncommon.

Treatment and outcome

Splenic marginal-zone lymphoma appears to have an indolent course, with a reported median survival of approximately 80% at five years. Since the disease is rare and has been described only relatively recently, there are very few data on the results of treatment. Splenectomy seems the therapy of choice – even for cases with blood and bone marrow involvement. Problems associated with bone marrow infiltration may become important after splenectomy, and some patients have been given a single alkylating agent with or without prednisone, as for chronic lymphocytic leukemia. The response to chemotherapy, however, is often poor. Transformation to high-grade lymphoma may occur in a few patients.

Bibliography

Cogliatti SB, Lennert K, Hansmann M et al, Monocytoid B-cell lymphoma: clinical and prognostic features of 21 patients. *J Clin Pathol* 1990; **43**: 619–25.

Dierlamm J, Pittaluga S, Wlodarska I et al, Marginal zone B-cell lymphomas of different sites share similar cytogenetic and morphologic features. *Blood* 1996; **87**: 299–307.

Fisher RI, Dahlberg S, Nathwani BN et al, A clinical analysis of two indolent lymphoma entities: mantle cell lymphoma and marginal zone lymphoma (including the mucosa-associated lymphoid tissue lymphoma and monocytoid B-cell subcategories). A Southwest Oncology Group study. *Blood* 1995; **85**: 1075–82.

Harris NL, Jaffe ES, Stein H et al, A revised European–American classification of lymphoid neoplasms: a proposal from the International Lymphoma Study Group. *Blood* 1994; **84**: 1361–92.

Isaacson PG, Matutes E, Burke M, Catovsky D, The histopathology of splenic marginal zone lymphoma with villous lymphocytes. *Blood* 1994; **84**: 3828–34.

Isaacson PG, Piris MA, Splenic marginal zone lymphoma. *Adv Anatom Pathol* 1997; **4**: 191–201.

Matutes E, Morilla R, Owusu-Ankomah K et al, The immunophenotype of splenic B-cell lymphoma with villous lymphocytes and its relevance to the differential diagnosis with other B-cell disorders. *Blood* 1994; **83**: 1558–62.

Melo JV, Hegde U, Parreira A et al, Splenic B-cell lymphoma with circulating villous lymphocytes: differential diagnosis of B-cell leukemias with large spleen. *J Clin Pathol* 1987; **40**: 642–51.

Mulligan SP, Matutes E, Dearden C, Catovsky D, Splenic lymphoma with villous lymphocytes: natural history and response to therapy in 50 cases. *Br J Haematol* 1991; **78**: 206–9.

Nathwani BN, Mohrmann RL, Brynes RK et al, Monocytoid B-cell lymphoma: an assessment of diagnostic criteria and a perspective on histogenesis. *Hum Pathol* 1992; **23**: 1061–71.

Ngan BY, Warnke R, Wilson M et al, Monocytoid B-cell lymphoma: a study of 36 cases. *Hum Pathol* 1991; **22**: 409–21.

Nizze H, Cogliatti SB, Von Schilling C et al, Monocytoid B-cell lymphoma: morphological variants and relationships to low-grade B-cell lymphoma of the mucosa-associated lymphoid tissue. *Histopathology* 1991; **18**: 403–14.

Non-Hodgkin's Lymphoma Classification Project, A clinical evaluation of the International Lymphoma Study Group classification of non-Hodgkin's lymphoma. *Blood* 1997; **89**: 3909–18.

Ortiz-Hildago C, Wright DH, The morphological spectrum of monocytoid B-cell lymphoma and its relationships to low-grade B-cell lymphomas of mucosa-associated lymphoid tissue. *Histopathology* 1992; **21**: 555–61.

Royer B, Cazals-Hatem D, Sibilia J et al, Lymphomas in patients with Sjögren's syndrome are marginal zone B-cell neoplasms, arise in diverse extranodal and nodal sites, and are not associated with viruses. *Blood* 1997; **90**: 766–75.

Schmid C, Kirkham N, Diss T, Isaacson PG, Splenic marginal zone cell lymphoma. *Am J Surg Pathol* 1992; **16**: 455–66.

Sheibani K, Burke JS, Swartz WG et al, Monocytoid B-cell lymphoma: clinicopathologic study of 21 cases of a unique type of low-grade lymphoma. *Cancer* 1988; **62**: 1531–8.

Shin SS, Sheibani K, Fishleder A et al, Monocytoid B-cell lymphoma in patients with Sjögren's syndrome: a clinicopathologic study of 13 patients. *Hum Pathol* 1991: **22**: 422–30.

Solé F, Woessner S, Florensa L et al, Frequent involvement of chromosomes 1, 3, 7, and 8 in splenic marginal zone lymphoma. *Br J Haematol* 1997; **98**: 446–9.

Zucca E, Roggero E, Pileri S, B-cell lymphoma of MALT type: a review with special emphasis on diagnostic and management problems of low-grade gastric tumours. *Br J Haematol* 1998; **100**: 3–14.

Nodal marginal-zone B-cell lymphoma

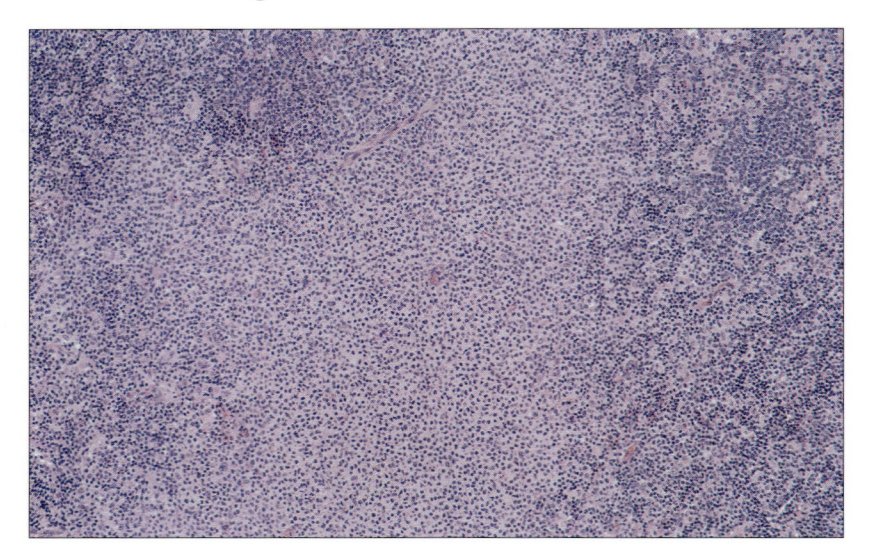

Figure 13.1

Nodal marginal-zone B-cell lymphoma:

(a) Perigastric lymph node in a patient with gastric marginal-zone B-cell lymphoma. Low power shows large zones of the node occupied by monocytoid B cells. (H&E stain)

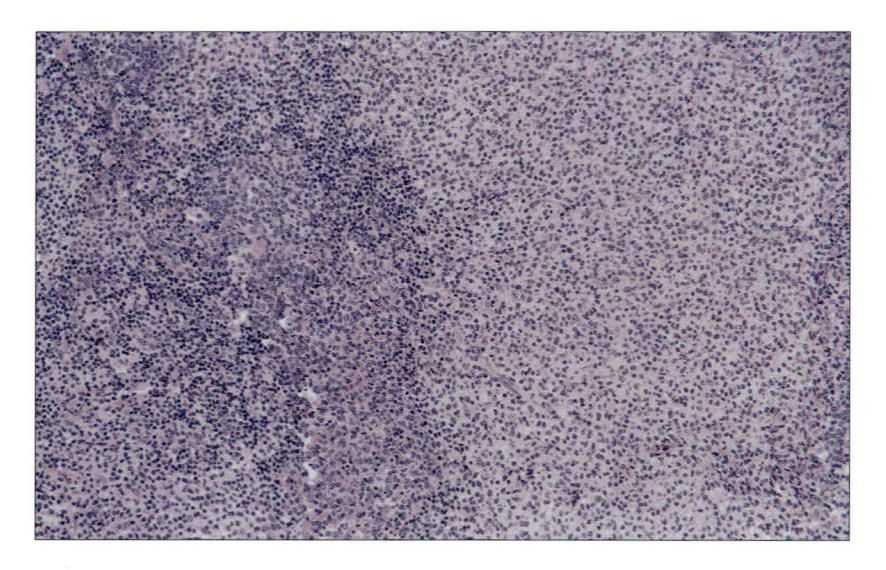

(b) Monocytoid B cells adjacent to a residual reactive follicle. (H&E stain)

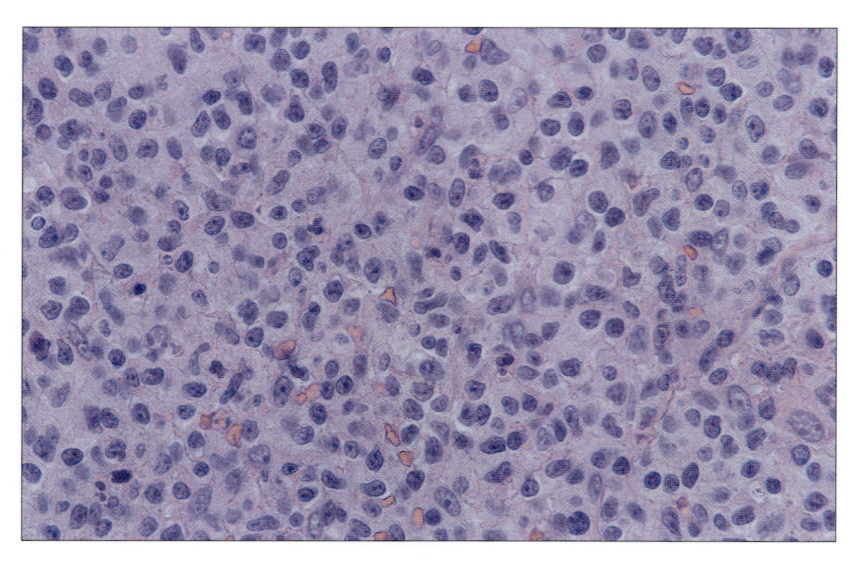

(c) Higher power shows monocytoid B cells with oval to bean-shaped or irregular nuclei and abundant pale cytoplasm; a few admixed neutrophils are present. (H&E stain)

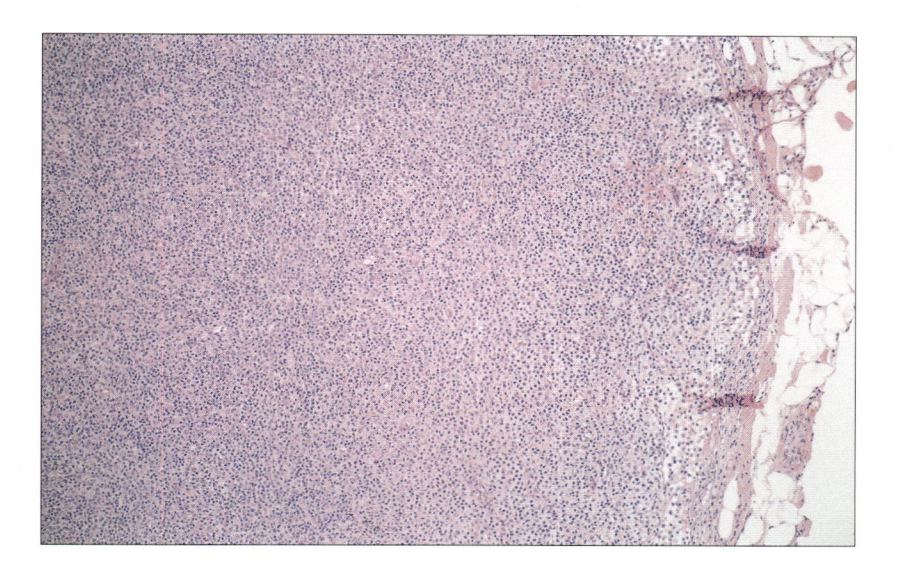

Figure 13.2

Nodal marginal-zone B-cell lymphoma:

(a) Low power shows sheets of pale cells obliterating the normal nodal architecture. (H&E stain)

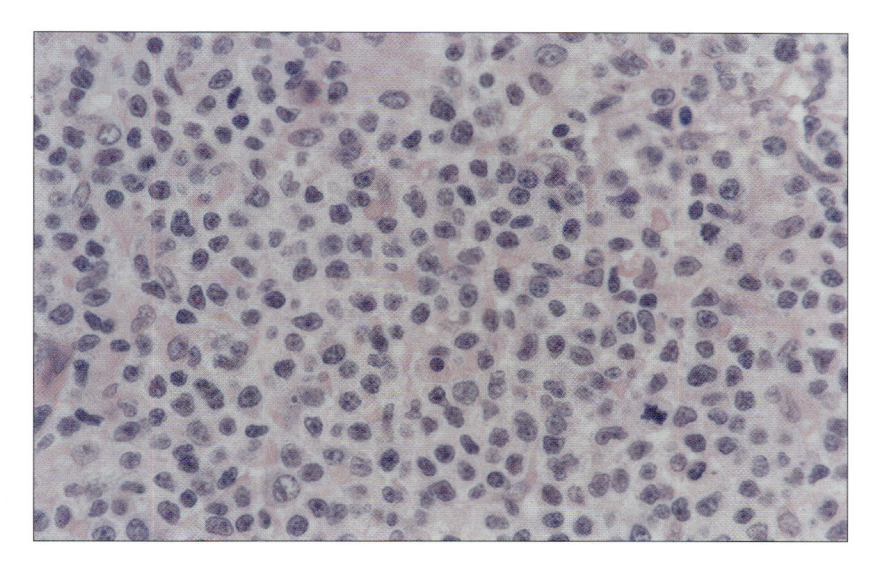

(b) Higher power shows monocytoid B cells with slightly irregular nuclei and abundant pale cytoplasm. Occasional mitotic figures are seen. (H&E stain)

Splenic marginal-zone B-cell lymphoma

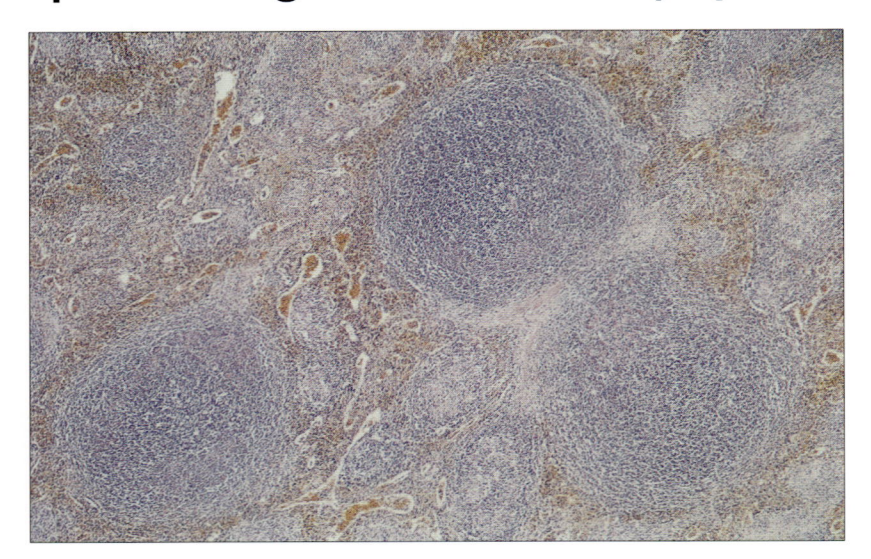

Figure 13.3

Splenic marginal-zone B-cell lymphoma – Spleen:

Lymphoma predominantly involves the white pulp, in the form of large nodules of small lymphoid cells; cells at the periphery of the nodules are slightly paler, because they have more cytoplasm. (H&E stain)

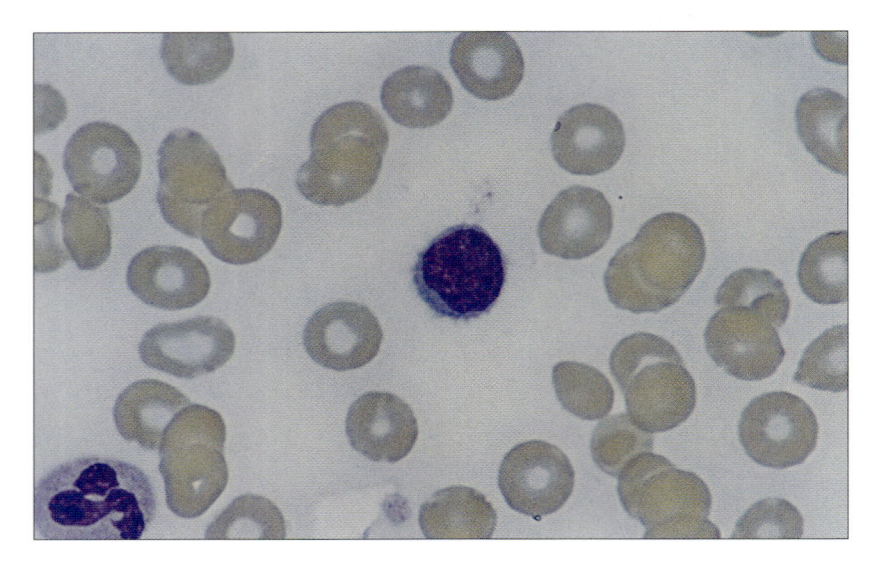

Figure 13.4

Splenic marginal-zone B-cell lymphoma – Peripheral blood:

A villous lymphocyte, a small lymphoid cell with delicate cytoplasmic processes around part of the circumference of the cell, is shown. (Wright stain)

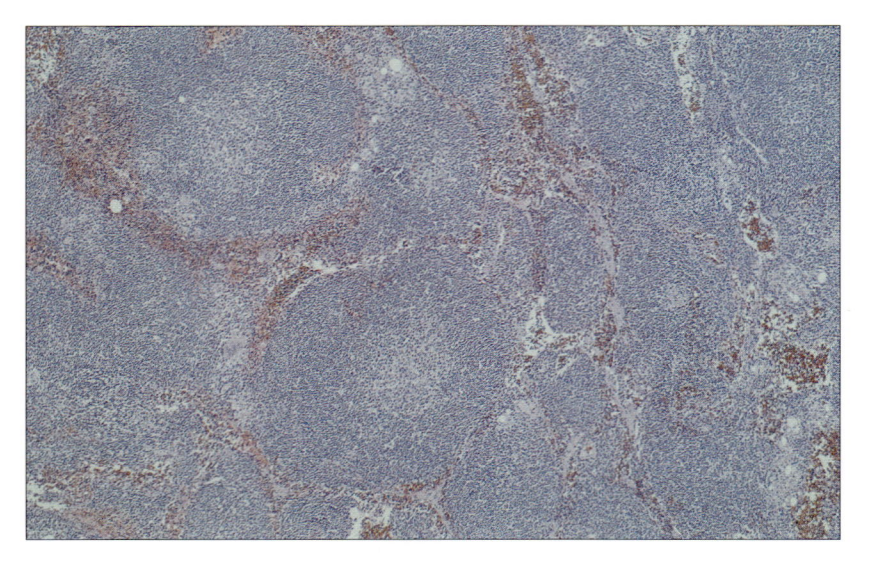

Figure 13.5

Splenic marginal-zone B-cell lymphoma – Periportal lymph node:

(a) Lymphoma partially involves the node in the form of massively expanded marginal zones surrounding reactive follicular centers. (H&E stain)

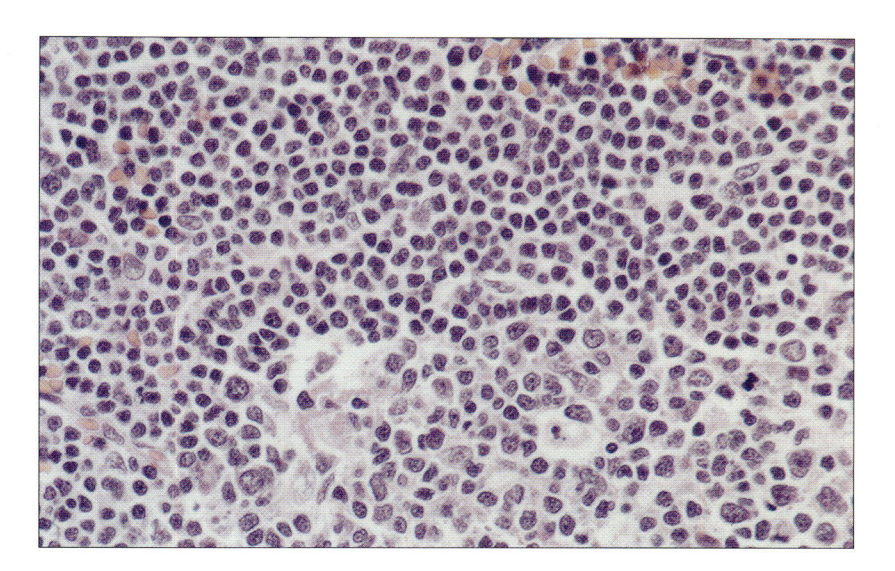

Figure 13.5 *continued*

(b) Higher power shows that the cells in the marginal zone are bland cells that are smaller and more uniform than cells in the adjacent reactive follicular center. (H&E stain)

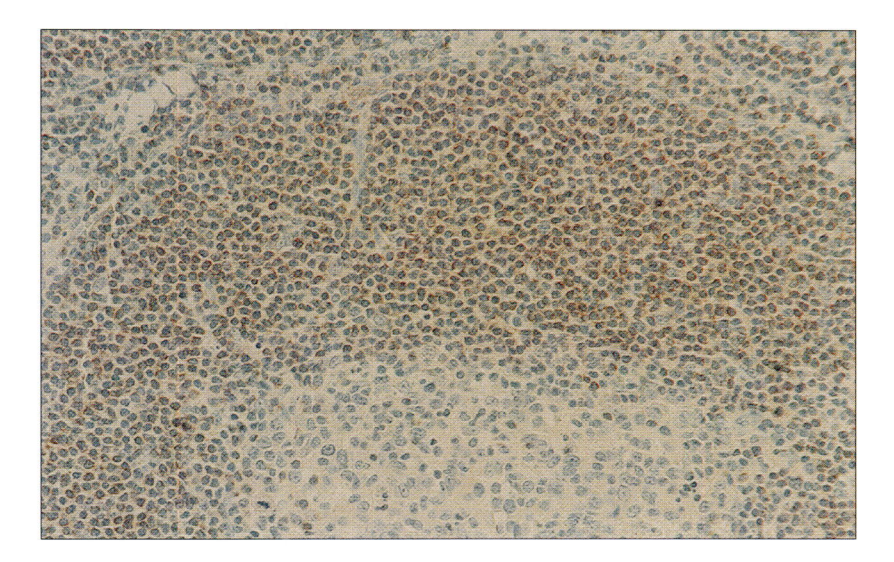

(c) The neoplastic marginal-zone cells are BCL2 protein-positive, in contrast to the BCL2-negative follicular center B cells. (Immunoperoxidase technique on paraffin sections)

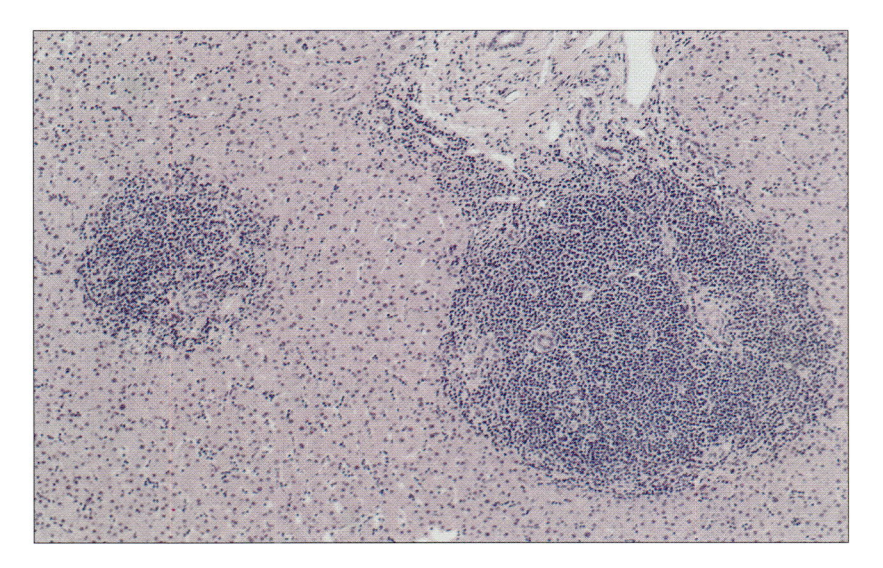

Figure 13.6

Splenic marginal-zone B-cell lymphoma – Liver:

Lymphoma involves the liver in the form of prominent periportal aggregates. (H&E stain)

14 Lymphomas involving extranodal sites

Definition and frequency

At least one-quarter of non-Hodgkin's lymphomas arise from tissue other than lymph nodes, and even from sites that normally contain no lymphoid tissue. These forms are referred to as 'primary extranodal lymphomas'. Since these tumors (which are numerous when considered together) are widely distributed throughout the body, it is difficult to find adequate series for any given site. Moreover, many historical series were published before the recognition of mucosa-associated lymphoid tissue (MALT) as the origin of many extranodal lymphomas, and, in general, the classification of primary extranodal lymphomas was similar to that of nodal lymphomas, without taking account of the fact that their origin could be different. Hence the literature lacks uniformity in histopathologic classification. The first attempt to eliminate this problem was made only very recently with the proposal of the REAL classification.

The definition of primary extranodal lymphoma, particularly in the presence of both nodal and extranodal disease, remains a controversial issue. Operationally, lymphomas can be considered as extranodal when, after routine staging procedures, there is either no or only 'minor' nodal involvement along with a clinically 'dominant' extranodal component, to which primary treatment must often be directed.

There are great differences in the incidence of extranodal lymphomas among countries: USA 24%, Canada 27%, Israel 36%, Lebanon 44%, Denmark 37%, Holland 41%, Italy 48% and Hong Kong 29%. Little is known about the actual incidence in developing countries, which, however, seem to have a high incidence of extranodal forms.

It has recently been demonstrated that non-Hodgkin's lymphomas on the whole are showing a rapid increase in incidence, and during the past 20 years extranodal disease has increased more rapidly than nodal disease. The greatest proportional increases have been observed for lymphomas of the central nervous system (CNS), followed by lymphomas of the gastrointestinal tract and the skin. In addition to the AIDS epidemic, other predisposing factors, such as other viral infections, immunosuppressive treatments and environmental factors (including pesticides and solvents), might explain the increased incidence of extranodal lymphomas.

Clinical characteristics and outcome

Extranodal lymphomas can arise in almost every organ. Gastrointestinal localizations represent the most common form of extranodal lymphoma. Other frequent and clinically important sites include the CNS and the skin.

Signs and symptoms at presentation depend largely on the localization: generally, patients with extranodal lymphomas tend less often to present B symptoms than do patients suffering from lymphomas arising in the nodal regions.

Table 14.1 Localized extranodal lymphoma: survival data from Princess Margaret Hospital, Toronto, 1967–88[a]	
Extranodal site	Five-year survival
Skin	92%
Gastrointestinal	77%
Soft tissue	77%
Orbit	76%
Gastrointestinal	76%
Gynaecological	75%
Waldeyer's	72%
Breast	63%
Genitourinary[b]	52%
Bone	47%
Lung	44%
Brain	24%

[a]Reproduced, with permission, from Cavalli F, Extranodal lymphomas. In: *The Non-Hodgkin's Lymphomas*, 2nd edn (Magrath IT, ed). Arnold: London, 1997: 1007–27.
[b]Includes testes

Survival rates vary among all of the specific sites of primary extranodal lymphomas (Table 14.1). This is partially because of differences in natural history, but is mainly due to differences in management strategy, which are related to organ-specific problems.

Testicular and thyroid lymphomas are more often seen in elderly patients, while the significantly higher incidence of hepatic and intestinal lymphomas is related to lower age. Salivary gland and thyroid lymphomas are significantly more common in females, while intestinal and pulmonary lymphomas are more often found in males. Non-Hodgkin's lymphomas of the stomach, salivary glands and thyroid are more frequently localized, whereas extranodal lymphomas of the lungs, liver, bones and testes are often widespread. With respect to histologic classification, aggressive subtypes (usually diffuse large B-cell lymphomas) are predominant in non-Hodgkin's lymphomas of the CNS, testes, bone, liver and to some extent the stomach. Certain extranodal sites have characteristic patterns of either B-cell disease (such as gastric marginal-zone lymphoma, MALT type) or T-cell disease (for example, cutaneous lymphoma clearly comprises a wide range of lymphomas of T-cell origin, even though a subset of B-cell cutaneous lymphomas does exist).

In this chapter, we shall briefly discuss only the general problems posed by the most common or clinically relevant sites, i.e. gastrointestinal, cutaneous and CNS lymphomas, with special attention to those extranodal clinicopathologic entities that are not described elsewhere in this book.

Primary gastrointestinal lymphomas

Epidemiology and incidence

The gastrointestinal tract is the most frequently involved extranodal localization in non-Hodgkin's lymphoma. In the hospital- and population-based series published thus far, gastrointestinal lymphoma accounts for 4–20% (average 12–13%) of all non-Hodgkin's lymphomas and 30–40% of all extranodal cases. In the Western world, the most common locations are the stomach (approximately 50–60%) and the small intestine (approximately 30%).

Infection by *Helicobacter pylori* has been cited as an environmental factor of possible etiologic relevance in those cases of gastric non-Hodgkin's lymphoma deriving from the MALT. Less epidemiologic information is available on intestinal localizations. Patients with celiac disease have a 200-fold increased risk of developing the so-called 'enteropathy-associated T-cell lymphoma' (EATCL), and some authors even favor the hypothesis that adult-onset celic disease is itself a form of low-grade lymphoma.

Diagnosis, classification and staging

Gastrointestinal lymphomas comprise a number of distinct clinico-pathologic entities (Table 14.2), which have been variously defined according to

Table 14.2
Histologic classification of gastrointestinal lymphomas[a]

B-cell
- Mucosa-associated lymphoid tissue (MALT)-type (extranodal marginal-zone lymphoma):
  Low-grade
  High-grade, with or without a low-grade component
- Immunoproliferative small intestinal disease (IPSID):
  Low-grade
  High-grade, with or without a low-grade component
- Lymphomatous polyposis (mantle-cell lymphoma)
- Burkitt's and Burkitt-like
- Other types of low- or high-grade lymphoma corresponding to lymph node equivalents

T-cell
- Enteropathy-associated T-cell lymphoma (EATCL)
- Other types not associated with enteropathy

[a]Modified, with permission, from Rohatiner et al, *Ann Oncol* 1994; **5**: 397.

Table 14.3
Modified Blackledge staging system for gastrointestinal lymphomas[a]

Stage I	Tumor confined to gastrointestinal tract without serosal penetration: • Single primary site • Multiple, non-contiguous lesions

Stage II	Tumor extending into abdomen from primary site:
	• Nodal involvement
	    II$_1$ Local (gastric/mesenteric)
	    II$_2$ Distant (paraaortic/paracaval)

Stage II$_E$	Penetration of serosa to involve adjacent 'structures': enumerate actual site of involvement, e.g. stage II$_E$ (pancreas), stage II$_E$ (large intestine), stage II$_E$ (post-abdominal wall) Perforation/peritonitis
Stage IV	Disseminated extranodal involvement or a gastrointestinal-tract lesion with supradiaphragmatic nodal involvement

[a]Modified, with permission, from Rohatiner et al, *Ann Oncol* 1994; **5**: 397.

the different histologic classifications in use for nodal lymphomas.

The applicability of the Ann Arbor staging system to gastrointestinal lymphoma has often been questioned, and several alternative staging systems have been proposed. A revised version of the Blackledge staging system has been recently recommended for general use (Table 14.3).

Clinical characteristics, treatment and outcome

Presenting symptoms are generally due to the local lesion (pain, obstruction, hemorrhage). Compared with nodal lymphomas, fewer patients with gastric lymphoma present with bone marrow involvement or elevated lactate dehydrogenase (LDH) levels. Fever and night sweats are uncommon. Weight loss, however, is common, although this is more often a consequence of the localization of the primary lymphoma than a constitutional symptom of the disease.

The optimal method of treatment of gastrointestinal lymphomas is still a controversial issue, and depends on the histologic type and stage of the disease. Here we shall briefly discuss the problems posed by the gastrointestinal lymphomas with aggressive histology; the therapy of MALT lymphomas is discussed in Chapter 7. Advanced gastrointestinal lymphomas appear to behave in the same manner as other advanced lymphomas, with comparable histology and prognostic factors. Therefore combination chemotherapy is the treatment of choice for patients with locally advanced or disseminated aggressive lymphomas. In a prospective study from the French GELA group, including more than 700 patients with aggressive lymphomas treated with intensive chemotherapy, no difference in therapy outcome was observed between patients with an advanced aggressive nodal lymphoma and the subset of patients (approximately 15%) in which the lymphoma was deemed to have arisen in the gastrointestinal tract. The effectiveness of combination chemotherapy in advanced cases of gastrointestinal lymphomas has led to a reconsideration of the role of primary surgery in less advanced cases. The possible advantage of debulking as well as the reduced risk of bleeding and perforation were reasons for advocating surgery as a primary treatment. However, the presence of a bulky mass is sometimes itself an obstacle to surgical intervention, and surgery does not necessarily prevent bleeding or perforation. Moreover, postsurgical complications can delay subsequent chemotherapy or radiotherapy, and can also adversely affect the performance status.

New approaches have therefore been advocated. It has been suggested by the results of some recent gastric lymphoma series that chemotherapy, sometimes combined with radiotherapy, can be curative and that gastrectomy is redundant. For primary intestinal lymphoma, however, there are as yet no studies clearly demonstrating that surgery is unnecessary, and combined-modality treatment is widely considered the procedure of choice.

Immunoproliferative small intestinal disease (IPSID, α-heavy-chain disease)

This condition may be considered as a variant of low-grade MALT lymphoma that is characterized by a diffuse lymphoplasmacytic/plasmacytic infiltrate in the upper small intestine.

The distinguishing feature of IPSID is the synthesis by the plasma cells of α heavy chain with no light chain. This aberrant α heavy chain is secreted and is detectable in the serum, urine, saliva and duodenal fluid in approximately two-thirds of cases; in the remaining cases, the protein is produced but not secreted. Most of the cases have been described in the Middle East, especially in the Mediterranean area, where the disease is endemic.

The natural course of IPSID is usually prolonged, often over many years, and includes a potentially reversible early phase, with the disease usually confined to the abdomen. If untreated, it degenerates, with high-grade transformation, into large-cell lymphoma.

In the early phases, durable remissions can be obtained with sustained antibiotic treatment. However, there is no clear evidence that antibiotics alone are of benefit in the advanced lymphomatous phases, where more recent data suggest that anthracycline-containing regimens may offer the best chance of cure.

Enteropathy-associated T-cell lymphoma (EATCL)

This condition usually develops following a long-standing history of celiac disease and/or dermatitis herpetiformis. It occurs most often in the sixth or seventh decades, but there have been sporadic reports of cases in young adults. The disease is more common in Europe, and relatively rare in North America. Abdominal pain and/or exacerbation of enteropathy-associated symptoms (malabsorption, loss of responsiveness to a gluten-restricted diet) are the most common presentation features. Approximately 25% of cases present with an intestinal perforation. EATCL has been included in the peripheral T-cell lymphoma group of the REAL classification; it usually has high-grade pleomorphic histologic features and its clinical course is often very unfavorable. A variety of combination chemotherapy regimens have been proposed, but responses to the therapy are in general unsatisfactory. Death usually results from multifocal intestinal perforations due to relapsing/refractory ulcerating lymphoma.

Multiple lymphomatous polyposis

This is a peculiar type of lymphoma that presents with multiple lymphomatous polyps of the gastrointestinal tract. In most cases, it represents the intestinal form of mantle-cell lymphoma – only in rare instances does multiple polyposis appear as a clinical syndrome produced by different histologic subtypes other than mantle-cell. Like its nodal counterpart, the disease is often widespread at the time of diagnosis, with frequent bone marrow and spleen involvement and general adenopathy. The prognosis is usually quite poor.

Primary cutaneous lymphomas

Primary cutaneous lymphomas can be defined as the presence of cutaneous localizations alone, with no nodal or systemic disease. Their incidence is estimated at 0.5–1/100 000 per year, and they represent a very numerous group of extranodal lymphomas, accounting for approximately 10% of cases. Moreover, the skin is a relatively common site of dissemination of many nodal non-Hodgkin's lymphomas, especially those of T-cell phenotype. However, the clinical behavior of primary cutaneous lymphomas is usually different from that of primary nodal lymphomas of similar histology, involving the skin secondarily.

It is difficult to properly define the primary cutaneous lymphoma on morphologic grounds alone: several types of primary lymphoma of the skin classified as high grade according to the Kiel classification or the Working Formulation very often show an indolent clinical behavior. Therefore only a combination of histologic, immunologic and clinical data can adequately define the primary cutaneous lymphoma entities. On this basis, a new classification scheme has recently been proposed by the EORTC Cutaneous Lymphoma Study Group (Table 14.4).

Lymphomas of the skin are more often of T-cell type, with mycosis fungoides and Sézary syndrome comprising around 65% of the cases.

Mycosis fungoides is characterized by epidermotropic band-like infiltrates of small- to medium-sized and occasionally large T lymphocytes with cerebriform nuclei involving the papillary dermis. A variable amount of admixed inflammatory cells are usually present. The tumor cells are $CD3^+$, $CD4^-$, $CD45RO^+$, $CD30^-$ and $CD8^-$. The clinical course is indolent, with slow progression over years from patches to more infiltrate plaques. The five-year survival is approximately 90%. Nearly all deaths are due to causes other than mycosis fungoides. In a proportion of patients, lymph nodes and internal organs may be involved in the later stages of disease. Local therapy (e.g. PUVA or radiotherapy) is preferred, as long as the disease remains confined to the skin. Combination chemotherapy can be used in cases with nodal or visceral involvement or widespread disease refractory to skin-targeted treatments.

Sézary syndrome has been considered to be a leukemic variant of mycosis fungoides, and is defined by the triad of erythroderma, generalized lymphadenopathy and the presence of neoplastic T cells (Sézary cells) in skin, lymph nodes and peripheral blood. Histologic and immunohistochemical features are similar to those seen in mycosis fungoides. Chemotherapy and extracorporeal photophoresis have been reported to be effective. However, the disease is aggressive, with a median survival of about three years.

The other types of primary cutaneous T-cell lymphomas (CTCL) are less frequent, and may be further characterized according to the specific expression of cell surface antigens such as CD30. They differ from mycosis fungoides in that the epidermotropism is usually absent (i.e. the neoplastic T cells usually infiltrate the dermis and subcutaneous tissue, but not the epidermis).

The classification of primary cutaneous B-cell lymphomas is particularly controversial. The subtypes 'follicle-center lymphoma of the head and trunk' and 'immunocytoma' of the EORTC classification comprise over 90% of primary cutaneous B-cell lymphomas. This group includes a large percentage of diffuse large cell lymphomas, which, in the scalp and trunk, despite their cytologically and histologically aggressive features, spread only very rarely beyond the skin and have a clinically indolent course. The clinical course of primary cutaneous large B-cell lymphoma of the leg is more aggressive. Moreover, cutaneous follicular lymphoma appears to be distinctly different from the nodal counterpart, both immunophenotypically and genotypically, lacking the chromosomal translocation t(14;18) and the expression of the common leukocyte antigen (CD10). Extranodal marginal-zone lymphomas (MALT type) of the skin have been described. According to some authors – whose view, however, has not been completely accepted – cutaneous immunocytoma should also be interpreted as a low-grade B-cell lymphoma of

Table 14.4
EORTC proposal for a classification of primary cutaneous lymphomas, with relative frequency, survival and equivalents in the Kiel and REAL classifications[a]

EORTC classification	Relative frequency (%)[b]	5-year survival (%)[b]	Equivalent entities Kiel classification	REAL classification
T-cell lymphomas				
Indolent entities				
• Mycosis fungoides (MF)	44	87	Small cell, cerebriform	Mycosis fungoides
• Specific variants of MF:				
MF-associated follicular mucinosis	4	70	Not listed	Not listed
Pagetoid reticulosis	<1	100	Not listed	Not listed
• CTCL, large cell CD30$^+$:	9	90		
Anaplastic			Large T-cell anaplastic (Ki-1$^+$)	Anaplastic large cell
Immunoblastic			T-immunoblastic	PTCL, unspecified
Pleomorphic			Pleomorphic, medium-sized/large T-cell	PTCL, unspecified
• Lymphomatoid papulosis	11	100	Not listed	Not listed
Aggressive entities				
• Sézary syndrome	2	11	Small cell, cerebriform	Sézary syndrome
• CTCL, large cell CD30$^-$:				
Immunoblastic			T-immunoblastic	
Pleomorphic large cell			Pleomorphic, medium-sized/large T-cell	
Provisional entities				
• Granulomatous slack skin	<1	—	Not listed	Not listed
• CTCL, pleomorphic small/medium-sized	3	62	Pleomorphic, small T-cell	PTCL, unspecified
• Subcutaneous panniculitis-like T-cell lymphoma	<1	—	Not listed	Subcutaneous panniculitic T-cell
B-cell lymphomas				
Indolent entities				
• Follicle-center cell lymphoma	13	97	Centroblastic–centrocytic Centroblastic	Follicular center Diffuse large B-cell
• Immunocytoma (marginal-zone B-cell lymphoma)	2	100	Immunocytoma	Extranodal marginal-zone (MALT type)
Entities with intermediate clinical behavior				
• Large B-cell lymphoma of the leg	3	58	Centroblastic B-immunoblastic	Diffuse large B-cell
Provisional entities				
• Intravascular large B-cell lymphoma	<1	50	Not specifically listed[c]	Not specifically listed[c]
• Plasmacytoma	<1	100	Plasmacytoma	Plasmacytoma

CTCL, cutaneous T-cell lymphoma; PTCL, peripheral T-cell lymphoma.
[a]Modified, with permission, from Willemze R, Kerl H, Sterry W et al, EORTC classification for primary cutaneous lymphomas: a proposal from the Cutaneous Lymphoma Study Group of the European Organization for Research and Treatment of Cancer. *Blood* 1997; **90**: 354–71.
[b]The frequency and survival data refer to a large series of 626 patients with primary cutaneous lymphomas registered at the Dutch Cutaneous Lymphoma Working Group between 1986 and 1994.
[c]The rare entity called 'angio-endotheliotropic (intravascular) lymphoma' or 'angiotropic lymphoma', formerly designated as 'malignant angioendotheliomatosis', can usually be classified as a B-immunoblastic lymphoma according to the Kiel classification, and therefore may be considered as a diffuse large B-cell lymphoma within the REAL classification.

MALT type. Since skin-associated lymphoid tissue (SALT) is usually devoid of B cells, in analogy to the MALT concept in the stomach, an acquired SALT could represent the background for the development of the lymphoma.

Furthermore, the historical association of cutaneous B-cell lymphoma with acrodermatitis chronica atrophicans suggests that *Borrelia burgdorferi* might play a role similar to that played by *H. pylori* in the stomach. Interestingly, anecdotal regressions of cases of cutaneous low-grade B-cell lymphoma lesions have recently been reported following antibiotic therapy with anti-*B. burgdorferi* or intralesional interferon-α injection, but the validity of this new approach has still to be confirmed.

Localized cutaneous B-cell lymphomas can be successfully treated with radiation therapy alone, with chemotherapy being reserved for patients with multiple cutaneous or subcutaneous localizations or with diffuse large cell lymphoma of the legs.

Subcutaneous panniculitic T-cell lymphoma

This subtype appears sufficiently distinct from other peripheral T-cell lymphomas, and has been included as a provisional entity in the REAL classification and in the EORTC classification of cutaneous lymphomas. It is characterized by the presence of subcutaneous nodules of variable size, mainly involving the legs. The lesions can be composed of small, medium-sized or large pleomorphic T cells, or an admixture of different cell types. Admixed non-neoplastic macrophages are usually present. Tumor cell necrosis, karyorrhexis and erythrophagocytosis are additional common features. Patients usually present with systemic symptoms such as fever and fatigue. Dissemination to lymph nodes and other organs is uncommon. However, the hemophagocytic syndrome with pancytopenia and hepatosplenomegaly is a frequent complication that often precipitates a rapidly unfavorable clinical course. The prognosis is generally poor, despite aggressive chemotherapy.

Primary central nervous system lymphoma

In its biology, clinical features and response to treatment, primary central nervous system lymphoma (PCNSL) is a disease distinct from other extranodal lymphomas. PCNSL can be defined as lymphoma arising in and confined to the cranial–spinal axis (brain, eye, leptomeninges and spinal cord). Formerly a rare tumor, PCNSL has shown increased incidence both in immunocompromised (congenital, acquired or iatrogenic) high-risk groups and in the general population. The clinical and radiological characteristics of the disease in immunocompetent patients are very different from those observed in AIDS-associated patients, in whom PCNSL often presents with an encephalophatic picture. PCNSL accounts for 1–2% of malignant brain tumors and 2–4% of all extranodal lymphomas. Secondary involvement of the CNS occurs in 5–30% of systemic non-Hodgkin's lymphoma.

Primary lymphoma of the brain

The initial symptomatology encompasses signs of increased intracranial pressure, cranial nerve palsies, neurologic deficits and, fairly often, a significant impairment of mental function.

PCNSL is usually disseminated within the nervous system at diagnosis: in approximately 40–50% of immunocompetent and in nearly 100% of AIDS patients. About 40% of patients have a demonstrable involvement of the spinal fluid and 20% have involvement of the eyes. In addition to the usual procedures, staging requires contrast-enhanced computerized tomography scan and magnetic resonance imaging (MRI) with gadolinium of the brain and orbits, before steroids are started, because of the rapid radiographic disappearance of tumor following the administration of steroids ('ghost tumor') – a peculiar feature of PCNSL, not shared by any other intracranial malignant tumor. Most typically, PCNSL appears as a mass in the supratentorial white matter. An ophthalmologic evaluation with split-lamp examination should also be performed. Histologic confirmation is essential, by stereotactic biopsy, lumbar puncture demonstrating a frank positive cytology, or vitreous biopsy. Histologically, the vast majority of lymphomas are of diffuse large B-cell type, but small non-cleaved cell (Burkitt's) histology is not uncommon in immunocompromised patients.

A surgical procedure more extensive than stereotactic biopsy is rarely indicated. Aggressive surgical decompression with partial or gross total removal of the tumor is of no benefit. Historically, whole-brain radiation has been the treatment of choice, but, despite different radiation schedules with good initial responses, over 90% of patients have recurrences in the brain, often in sites remote from the initial ones. Systemic dissemination occurs in only 10% of cases, and many of these have single localizations. The prognosis for unselected patients with immunocompetent PCNSL treated with radical irradiation alone is very poor, the five-year survival rate being 5–10%, with a median survival between 12 and 18 months. Because of the poor results obtained with radiation therapy alone, new approaches have been developed. Several single-institution studies have reported encouraging results with systemic chemotherapy alone or combined with radiotherapy, with five-year projected overall survival of 30–50% and median survival of two to three years. In general, the most recent studies seem to indicate that radiation therapy alone is unable to provide significant long-term survival, it may interfere with later chemotherapy, and it may increase the risk of treatment-induced dementia. There is mounting evidence that initial chemotherapy should be the treatment of choice, with irradiation being reserved for resistant or relapsing disease.

Primary ocular lymphoma

It should be noted that primary orbital and ocular adnexa lymphomas represent a different entity, most often of extranodal marginal-zone histotype, and must not be confused with lymphoma of the eye. Primary ocular lymphoma (i.e. restricted to the globe, usually the vitreous, retina and chorioid) is exceedingly rare. Ocular involvement is often bilateral, and more than half of the patients will later develop brain lesions. Radiotherapy to both eyes has been the standard treatment, and, as in other PCNSL, combination with systemic chemotherapy is being investigated.

Primary leptomeningeal lymphoma

In rare instances, PCNSL presents as a localized leptomeningeal disease in the absence of parenchymal brain involvement. Diagnosis is commonly obtained by positive cerebrospinal fluid (CSF) cytology or on meningeal biopsy. The therapeutic approach is similar to that for primary brain lymphomas. Prognosis is usually poor.

Primary extradural lymphoma

Primary extradural lymphoma represents approximately 1% of all localized non-Hodgkin's lymphomas, most often presenting with spinal-cord compression at the thoracic level. The diagnosis is generally obtained at the time of decompressive surgery, with diffuse large cell lymphoma being the most common histology. Its inclusion as a PCSNL is controversial. CNS relapses seem to be uncommon, and the good results obtained with radiotherapy and systemic chemotherapy seem to indicate that the natural history of primary extradural lymphoma is different from that of PCSNL.

Other particular entities arising at extranodal sites

Many non-Hodgkin's lymphoma entities may specifically arise at extranodal sites. Most of them (e.g. MALT lymphomas and Burkitt's lymphoma) are described in other chapters of this book. A few additional entities will be briefly mentioned here.

Angiocentric nasal/nasal-type T/NK-cell lymphoma (NTNKL)

NTNKL has been referred in the past as 'lethal midline granuloma' and, more recently, as 'angiocentric T/NK-cell nasal lymphoma'. Lymphomas with characteristics similar to those of nasal T/NK-cell lymphoma can be identified at other extranodal sites. This entity is strongly associated with Epstein–Barr virus (EBV) infection, and usually presents with a destructive midline facial tumor. The available literature concerning the treatment of T/NK-cell nasal/nasal type lymphoma is poor, with some groups using localized radiotherapy alone, and others multiagent chemotherapy with or without additional radiation therapy. Prognosis is usually poor once dissemination occurs. Moreover, the hemophagocytic syndrome (hepatosplenomegaly, liver function abnormalities, thrombocytopenia and erythrophagocytosis) is a common clinical complication that adversely affects survival.

Hepatosplenic $\gamma\delta$ lymphoma

This disease affects young patients – commonly with bone marrow involvement and without lymphadenopathy or significant peripheral blood lymphocytosis. The clinical course is usually very aggressive, median survival being less than one year, despite the possibility of initial response to chemotherapy. A subset of non-hepatosplenic $\gamma\delta$ T-cell lymphomas have recently been described that are characterized by an aggressive clinical course with involvement of extranodal (mucosal or cutaneous) sites without peripheral lymphadenopathy or bone marrow localizations.

Primary body-cavity-based lymphomas

Two distinct clinicopathologic entities with particular epidemiologic, molecular and clinical features, showing a particular tropism for body cavities, have recently been described.

Primary effusion lymphoma

This rare entity occurs predominantly in HIV-seropositive patients, and typically presents as lymphomatous effusions (pleural, pericardial or ascitic), usually without a solid tumor mass. The histologic features comprise large or anaplastic B cells. DNA sequences from Kaposi's sarcoma-associated herpesvirus/human herpesvirus 8 (KSHV/HHV-8) and from EBV are detectable in tumor cells in the large majority of cases. Prognosis appears to be dismal and, because of the small numbers of reported cases, no exact treatment rules can be given.

Pyothorax-associated lymphoma

Principally reported in Japan, this rare disease affects elderly patients with a more than 20-year history of pyothorax, usually related to chronic tuberculosis. Histologically, this extranodal lymphoma is usually of the large B-cell type. EBV genome is found in the lymphoma cells in approximately 85% of cases, but KSHV/HHV-8 DNA is usually absent. The clinical manifestations very often comprise a neoplastic mass associated with the pleural effusion.

Bibliography

Aozasa K, Ohsawa M, Kanno H, Pyothorax-associated lymphoma: a distinctive type of lymphoma strongly associated with Epstein–Barr virus. *Adv Anat Pathol* 1997; **4:** 58–63.

Arnulf B, Copie-Bergman C, Delfau-Larue MH et al, Nonhepatosplenic gamma/delta T-cell lymphoma: a subset of cytotoxic lymphomas with mucosal or skin localization. *Blood* 1998; **91:** 1723–31.

Bessel EM, Graus F, Punt JAG et al, Primary non-Hodgkin's lymphoma of the CNS treated with BVAM or CHOD/BVAM chemotherapy before radiotherapy. *J Clin Oncol* 1996; **14:** 945–54.

Blay JY, Bouhour D, Carrie C et al, The C5R protocol: a regimen of high-dose chemotherapy and radiotherapy in primary cerebral non-Hodgkin's lymphoma of patients with no known cause of immunosuppression. *Blood* 1995; **86:** 2922–9.

Cavalli F, Extranodal lymphomas. In: *The Non-Hodgkin's Lymphomas*, 2nd edn (Magrath IT, ed). Arnold: London 1997: 1007–27.

Cheung MM, Chan JK, Lau WH et al, Primary non-Hodgkin's lymphoma of the nose and nasopharynx: clinical features, tumor immunophenotype, and treatment outcome in 113 patients. *J Clin Oncol* 1998; **16:** 70–7.

Coiffier B, Salles G, Does surgery belong to medical history for gastric lymphoma? *Ann Oncol* 1997; **8:** 419–21.

Cooke CB, Krenacs L, Stetler-Stevenson M et al, Hepatosplenic T-cell lymphoma: a distinct clinicopathologic entity of cytotoxic γδ T-cell origin. *Blood* 1996; **88:** 4265–74.

De Angelis LM, Yahalom J, Primary central nervous system lymphoma. In: *Cancer: Principles and Practice of Oncology*, 5th edn (De Vita VT Jr, Hellman S, Rosenberg SA, eds). Lippincott–Raven: Philadelphia, 1997: 2233–42.

Diamandidou E, Cohen PR, Kurzrock R, Mycosis fungoides and Sézary syndrome. *Blood* 1996; **88:** 2385–409.

Fine HA, Loeffler JS, Primary central nervous system lymphoma. In: *The Lymphomas* (Canellos GP, Lister TA, Sklar JL, eds). WB Saunders: Philadelphia, 1998: 481–94.

Harris NL, Jaffe ES, Stein H et al, A revised European–American classification of lymphoid neoplasms: a proposal from the International Lymphoma Study Group. *Blood* 1994; **84:** 1361–92.

Isaacson PG, Norton AJ, Malignant lymphoma of the gastrointestinal tract. In: *Extranodal Lymphomas* (Isaacson PG, Norton AJ, eds). Churchill Livingstone: Edinburgh, 1994: 15–65.

Jaffe ES, Chan JKC, Su IJ et al, Report of the workshop on nasal and related extranodal angiocentric T/natural killer cell lymphomas. Definitions, differential diagnosis, and epidemiology. *Am J Surg Pathol* 1996; **20:** 103–11.

Kim YH, Hoppe RT, Cutaneous T-cell lymphomas. In: *The Non-Hodgkin's lymphomas*, 2nd edn (Magrath IT, ed). Arnold, London: 1997: 907–26.

Kütting B, Bonsmann G, Metze D et al, *Borrelia burgdorferi*-associated primary cutaneous B cell lymphoma: complete clearing of skin lesions after antibiotic pulse therapy or intralesional injection of interferon alfa-2a. *J Am Acad Dermatol* 1997; **36:** 311–14.

Lachance TH, O'Neill BP, MacDonald DR et al, Primary leptomeningeal lymphoma: report of 9 cases, diagnosis with immunocytochemical analysis and review of the literature. *Neurology* 1991; **41:** 95–100.

Nador RG, Cesarman E, Chadburn A et al, Primary effusion lymphoma: a distinct clinicopathologic entity associated with the Kaposi's sarcoma-associated herpes virus. *Blood* 1996; **88:** 645–56.

Rohatiner A, d'Amore F, Coiffier B et al, Report on a workshop convened to discuss the pathological and staging classifications of gastrointestinal tract lymphoma. *Ann Oncol* 1994; **5:** 397–400.

Salles G, Herbrecht R, Tilly H et al, Aggressive primary gastrointestinal lymphomas: review of 91 patients treated with the LNH-83 regimen. A study of the GELA. *Am J Med* 1991; **90:** 77–84.

Shultz C, Scott C, Sherman W et al, Preirradiation chemotherapy with cyclophosphamide, doxorubicin, vincristine, and dexamethasone for primary CNS lymphomas: initial report of Radiation Therapy Oncology Group Protocol 88-06. *J Clin Oncol* 1996; **14:** 556–64.

Slater DN, MALT and SALT: the clue to cutaneous B-cell lymphoproliferative disease. *Br J Dermatol* 1994; **131:** 557–61.

Willemze R, Kerl H, Sterry W et al, EORTC classification for primary cutaneous lymphomas: a proposal from the Cutaneous Lymphoma Study Group of the European Organization for Research and Treatment of Cancer. *Blood* 1997; **90:** 354–71.

Zucca E, Cavalli F, Gut lymphomas. *Baillière's Clin Haematol* 1996; **9:** 727–41.

Zucca E, Roggero E, Bertoni F, Cavalli F, Primary extranodal non-Hodgkin's lymphomas. Part 1: Gastrointestinal, cutaneous and genitourinary lymphomas. *Ann Oncol* 1997; **8:** 727–37.

Intestinal T-cell lymphomas

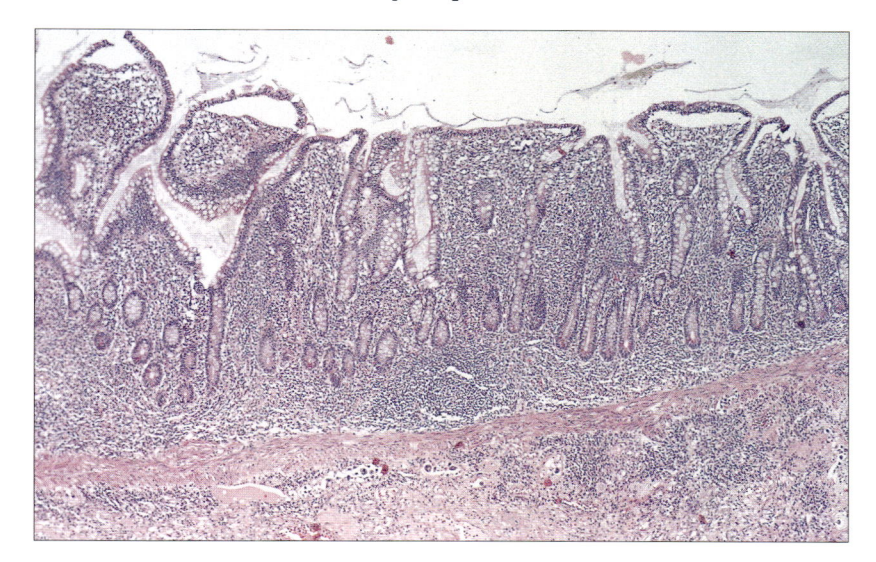

Figure 14.1

Intestinal T-cell lymphoma:

(a) Away from the lymphoma, the small intestine shows areas of villous blunting. (H&E stain)

(b) The villi contain increased numbers of intraepithelial lymphocytes. (H&E stain)

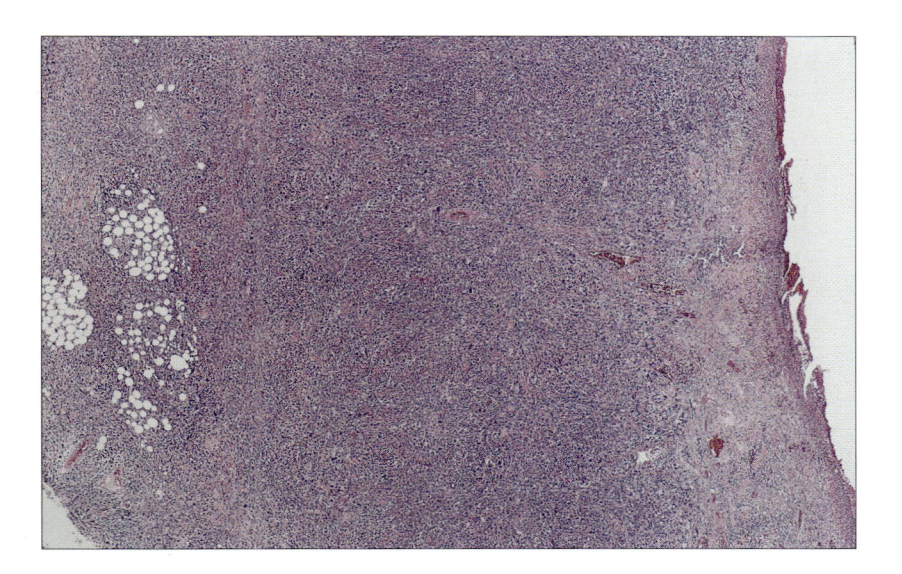

(c) The lymphoma is transmurally invasive into subserosal fat; the mucosa is ulcerated.

Contd

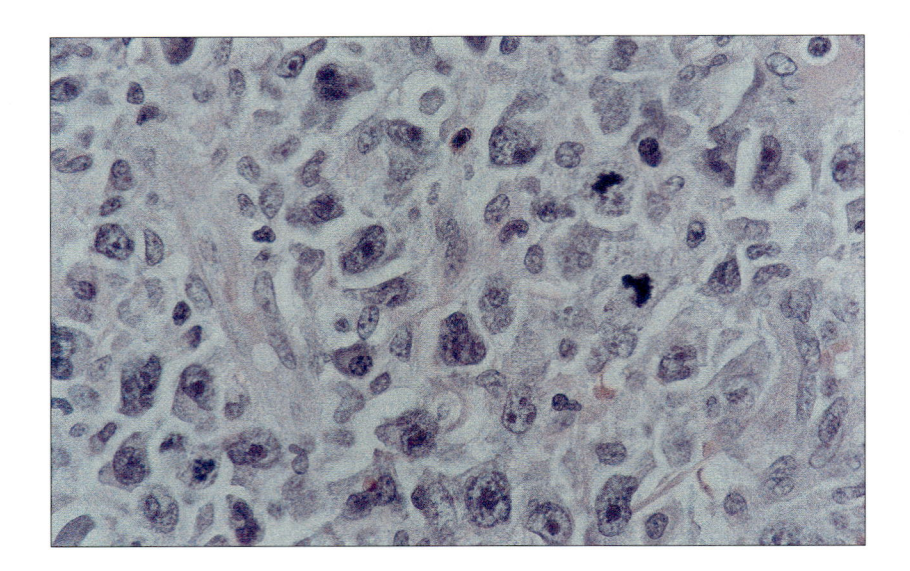

Figure 14.1 *continued*

(d) The lymphoma is composed of large atypical cells with a high mitotic rate. (H&E stain)

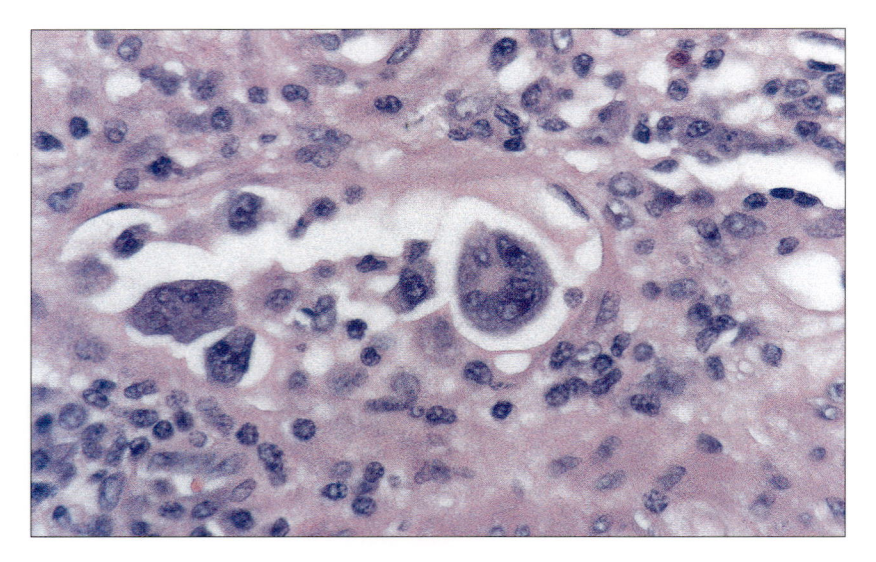

(e) Neoplastic cells in a small vascular space. (H&E stain)

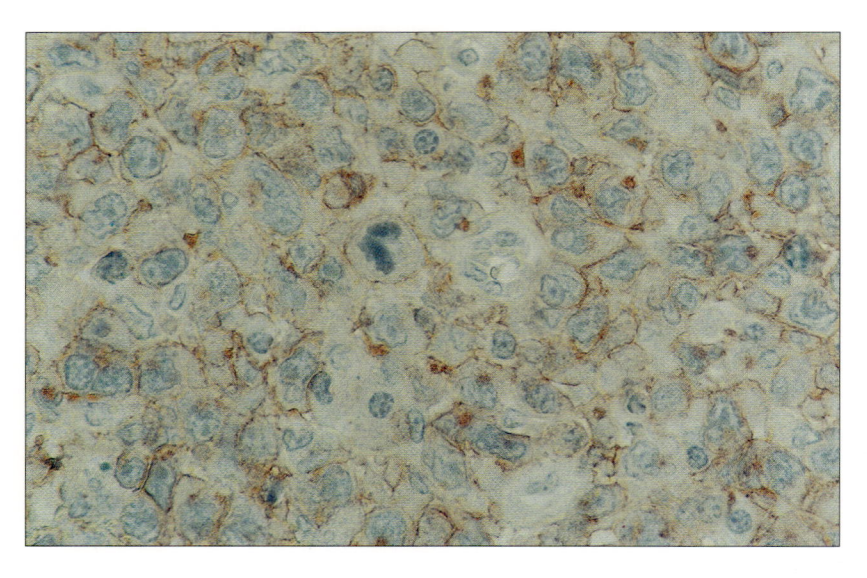

(f) The lymphoma is CD8+ (shown here); the neoplastic cells also express CD3 and CD45RO. (Immunoperoxidase technique on paraffin sections)

Mycosis fungoides/Sézary syndrome

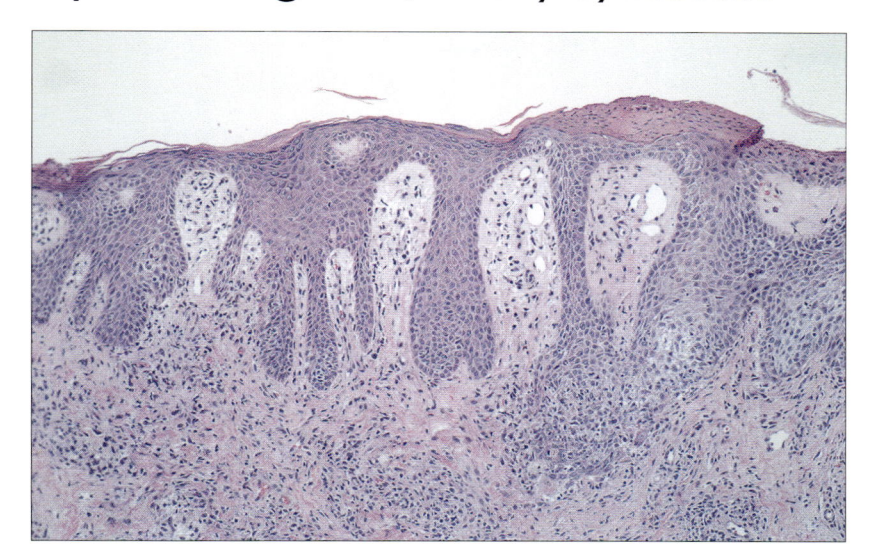

Figure 14.2

Mycosis fungoides/Sézary syndrome:

(a) The epidermis shows parakeratosis and elongate rete pegs. The dermis contains an infiltrate of lymphoid cells that extends to involve the epidermis. (H&E stain)

(b) Lymphoid cells in the epidermis are slightly larger and have more irregular nuclei than normal lymphocytes. They are surrounded by narrow haloes. Focally, clusters of atypical lymphoid cells are found (Pautrier's collections). (H&E stain)

Subcutaneous panniculitis-like T-cell lymphoma

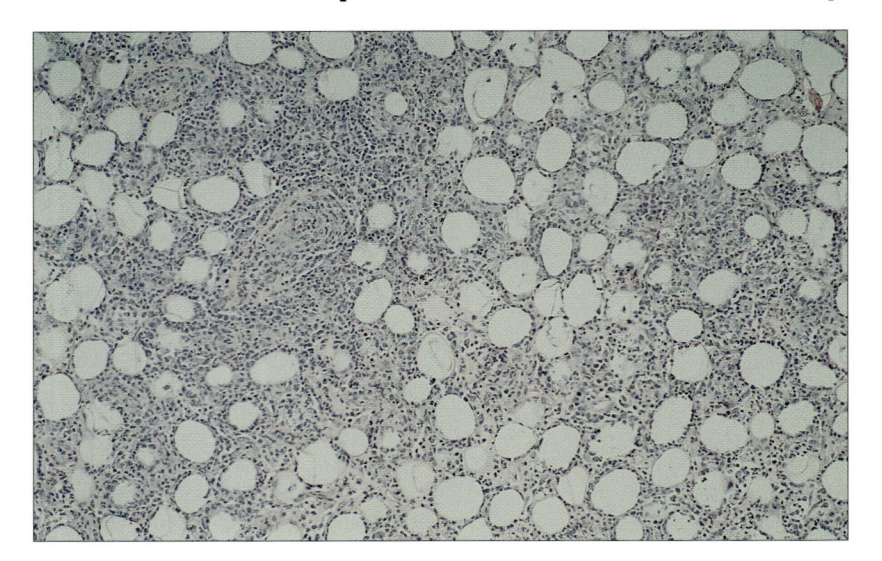

Figure 14.3

Subcutaneous panniculitis-like T-cell lymphoma:

(a) The subcutis contains a dense infiltrate of lymphoid cells. (H&E stain)

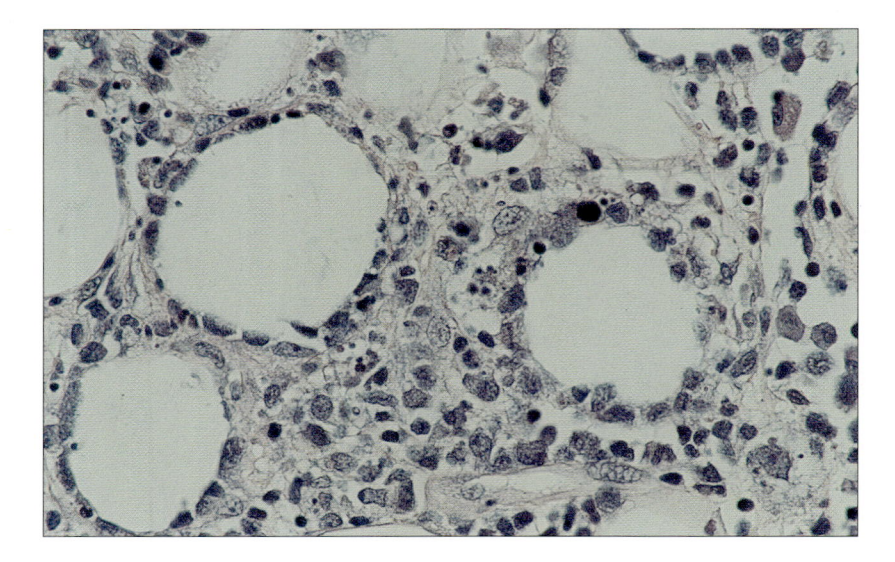

(b) Higher power shows atypical lymphoid cells and abundant cellular debris. The lymphoid cells surround the fat cells; the plasma membrane of many of these fat cells is difficult to recognize. (H&E stain)

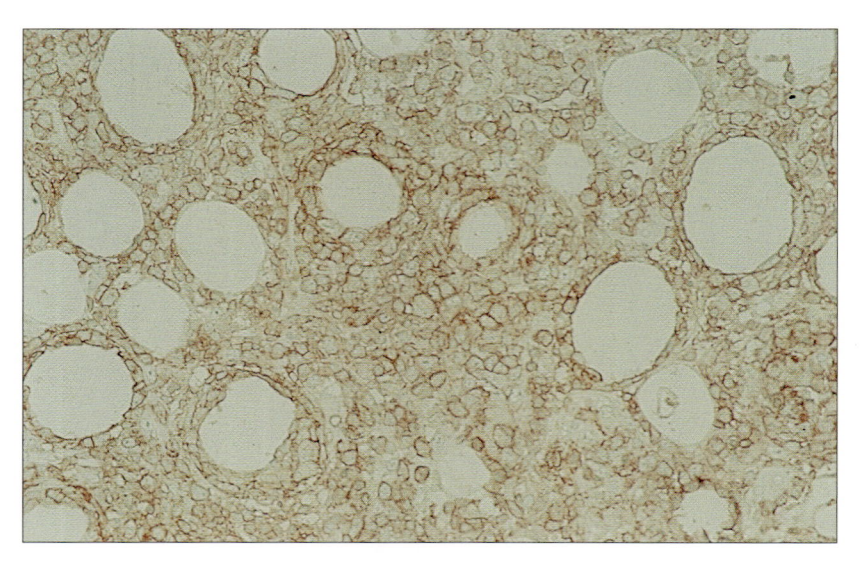

(c) The atypical cells express T-cell-associated antigens: CD43 is shown here. (Immunoperoxidase technique on paraffin sections)

Angiocentric nasal/nasal-type T/NK-cell lymphoma

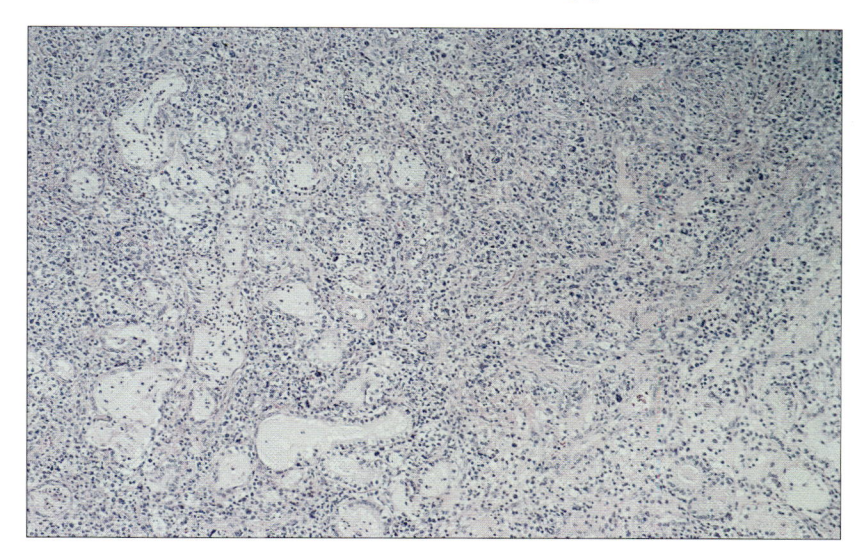

Figure 14.4

Angiocentric nasal/nasal-type T/NK-cell lymphoma:

(a) There is a dense diffuse cellular infiltrate extensively involving nasal tissue. (H&E stain)

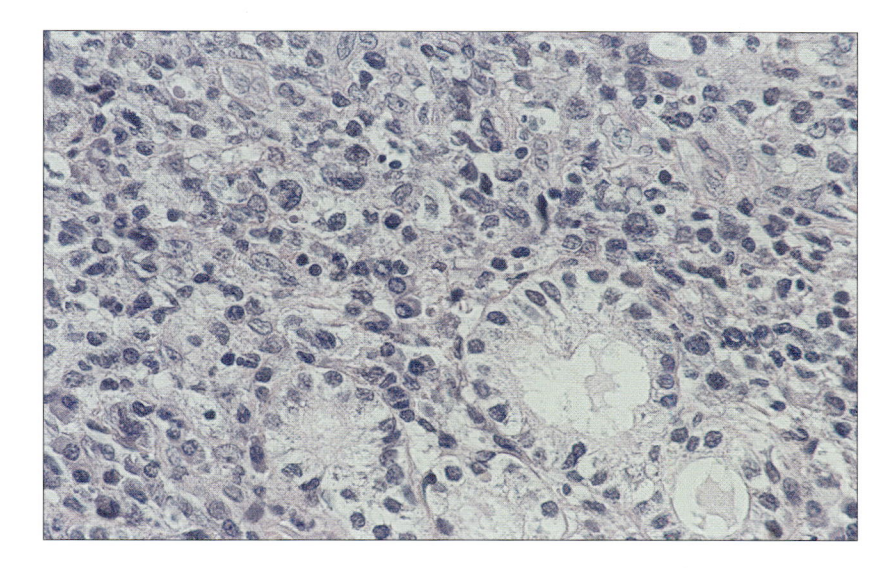

(b) Small, intermediate-sized and large atypical lymphoid cells surround submucosal glands. (H&E stain)

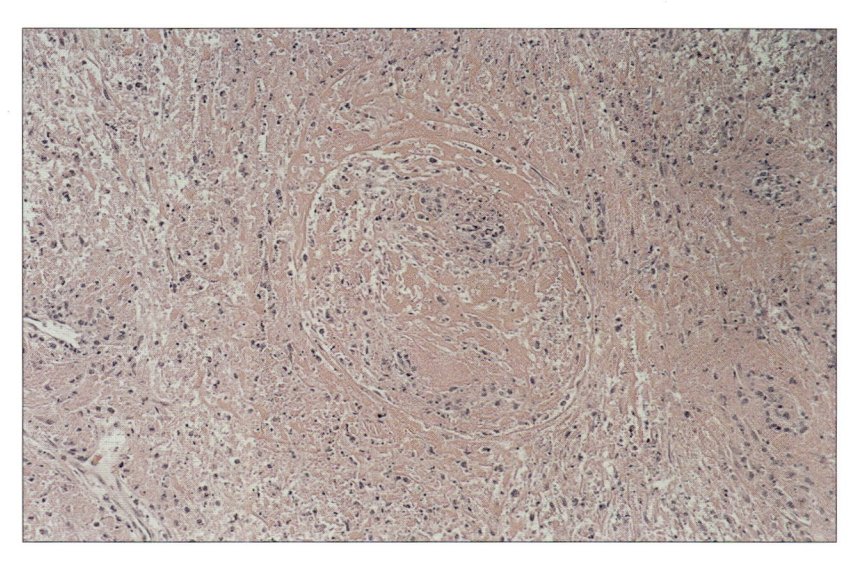

(c) In areas, there is extensive necrosis; centrally the outline of an oval necrotic structure, possibly a large blood vessel, can be seen. (H&E stain)

Contd

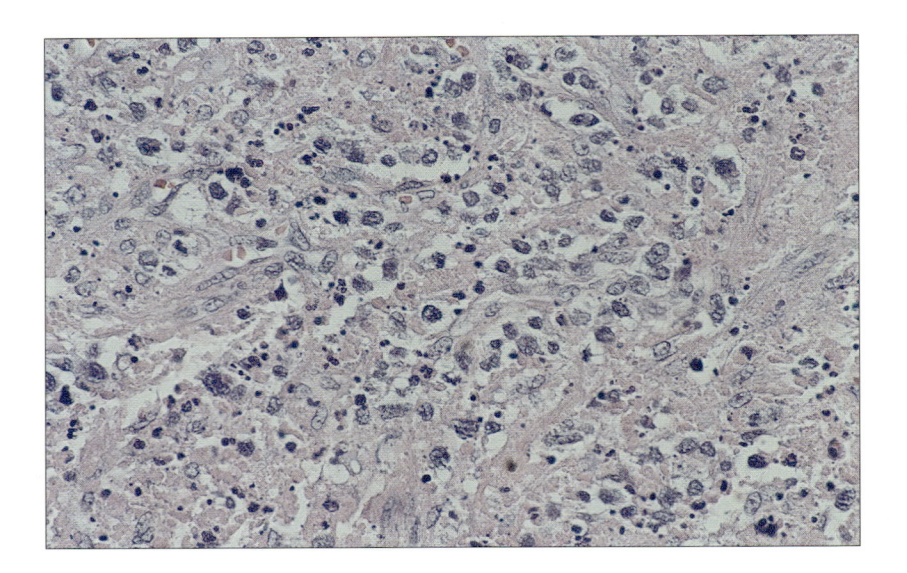

Figure 14.4 *continued*

(d) Atypical lymphoid cells scattered in necrotic tissue. (H&E stain)

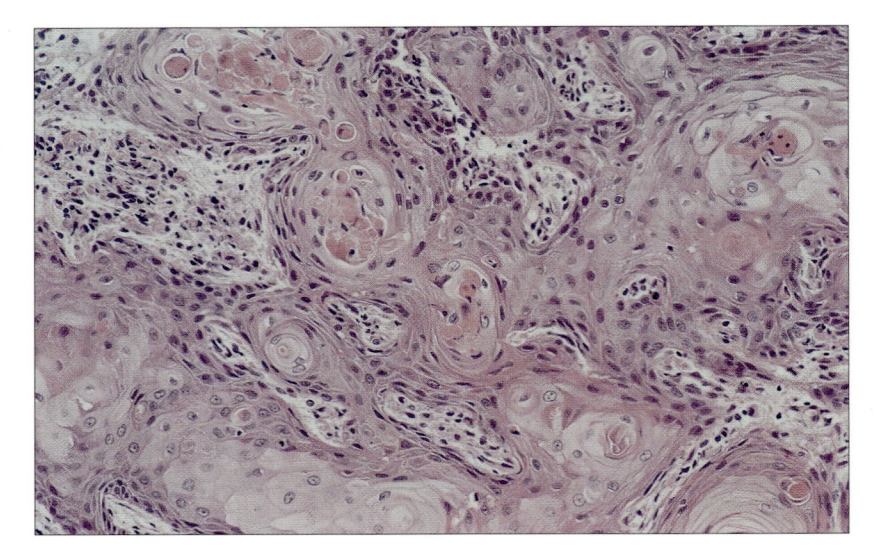

(e) In this case, there is associated striking pseudoepitheliomatous hyperplasia of the overlying squamous epithelium. (H&E stain)

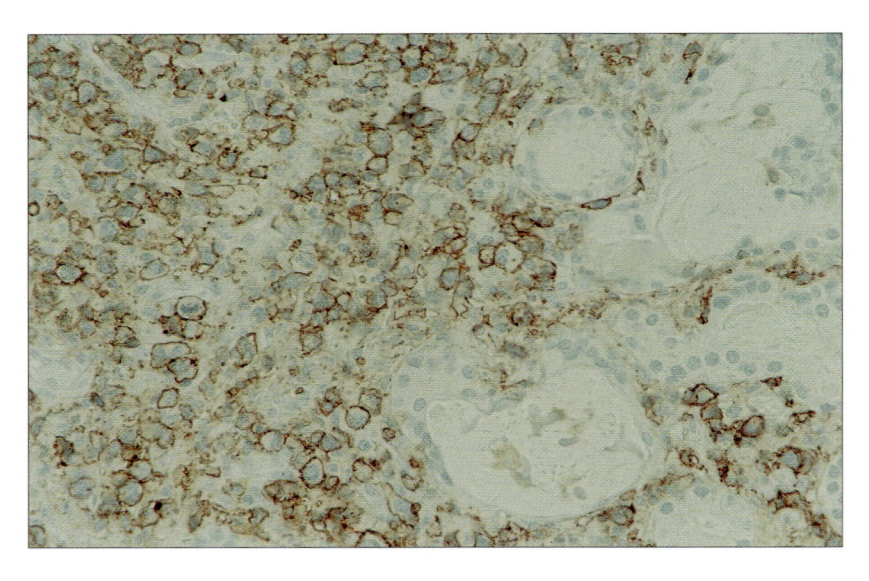

The lymphoma expresses T/NK-cell-associated antigens (CD45RO shown in **f**) as well as CD56 (**g**). (Immunoperoxidase technique on paraffin sections)

(f)

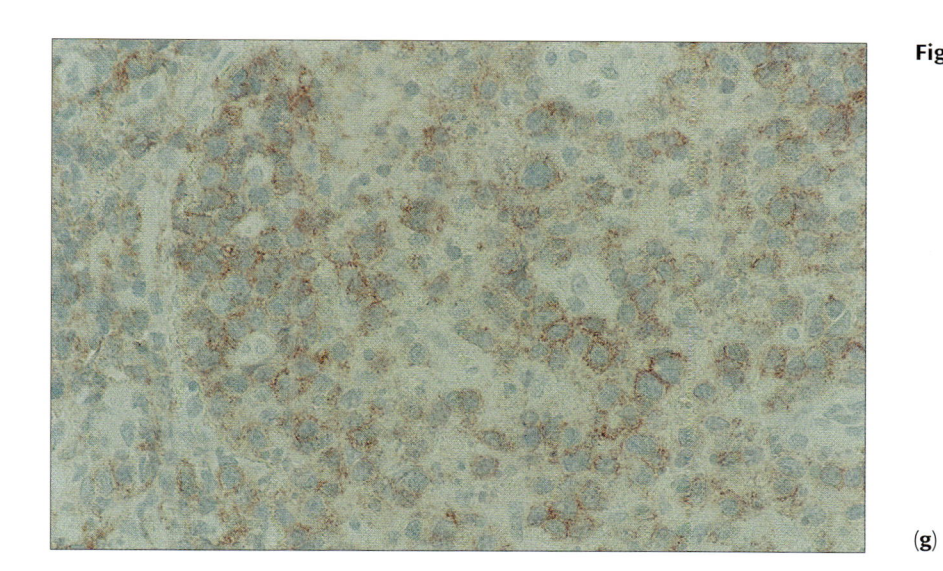

Figure 14.4 *continued*

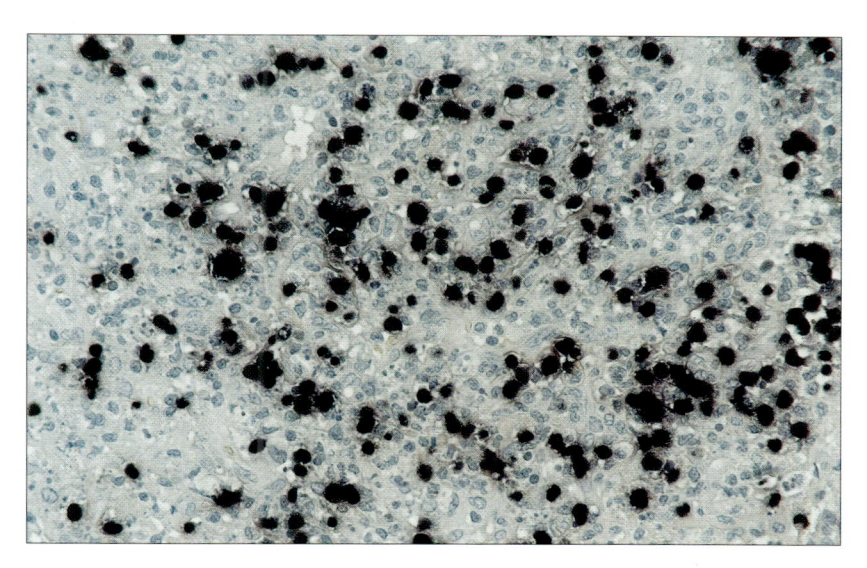

(g)

(h) The neoplastic cells are EBER+. (In situ hybridization on paraffin sections)

Hepatosplenic γδ T-cell lymphoma

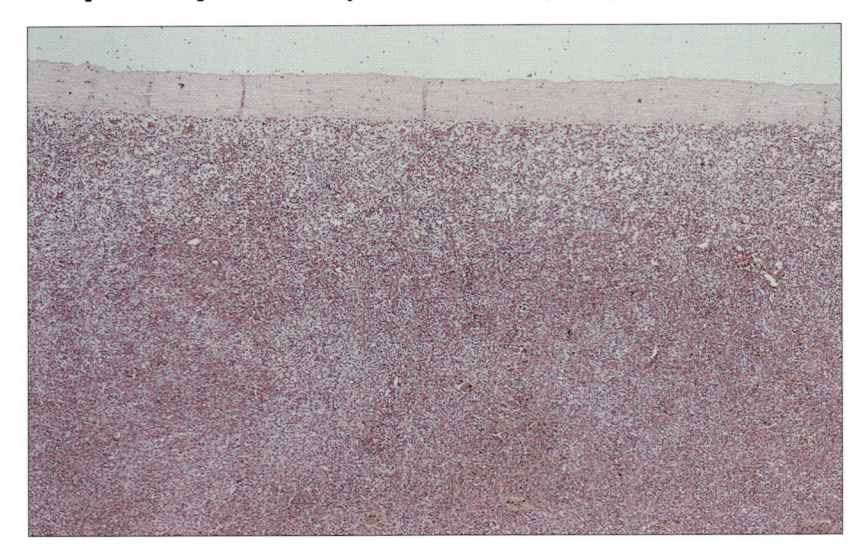

Figure 14.5

Hepatosplenic γδ T-cell lymphoma – Spleen:

(a) The spleen weighed more than 2 kg. Microscopic examination reveals marked red pulp expansion with inconspicuous white pulp. (H&E stain)

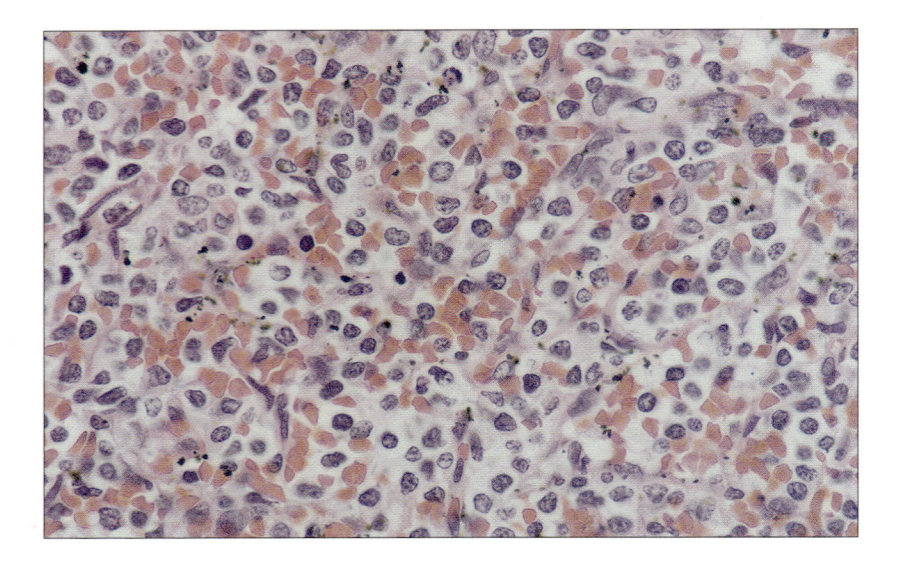

(b) Higher power shows sheets of intermediate-sized lymphoid cells with uniform oval nuclei and abundant pale cytoplasm. (H&E stain)

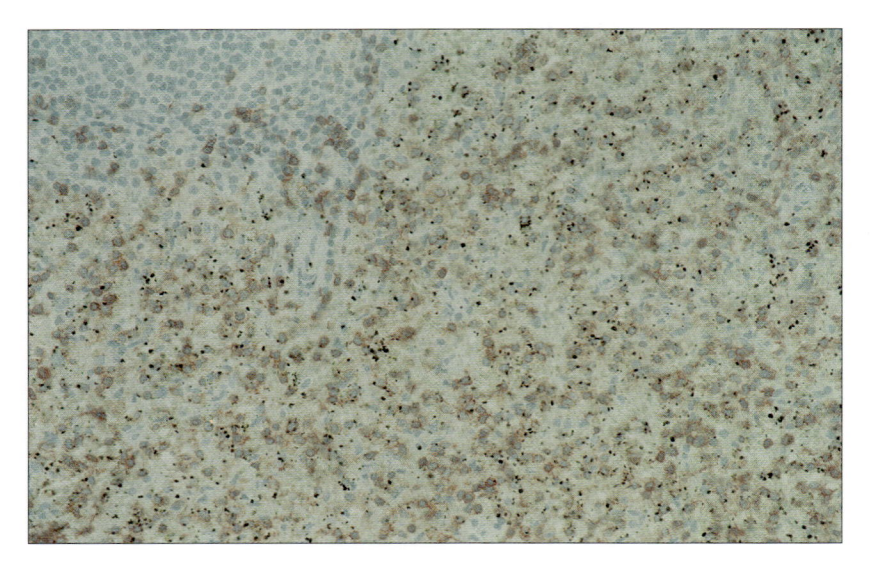

(c) The neoplastic cells are T cells (CD3+). (Immunoperoxidase technique on paraffin sections)

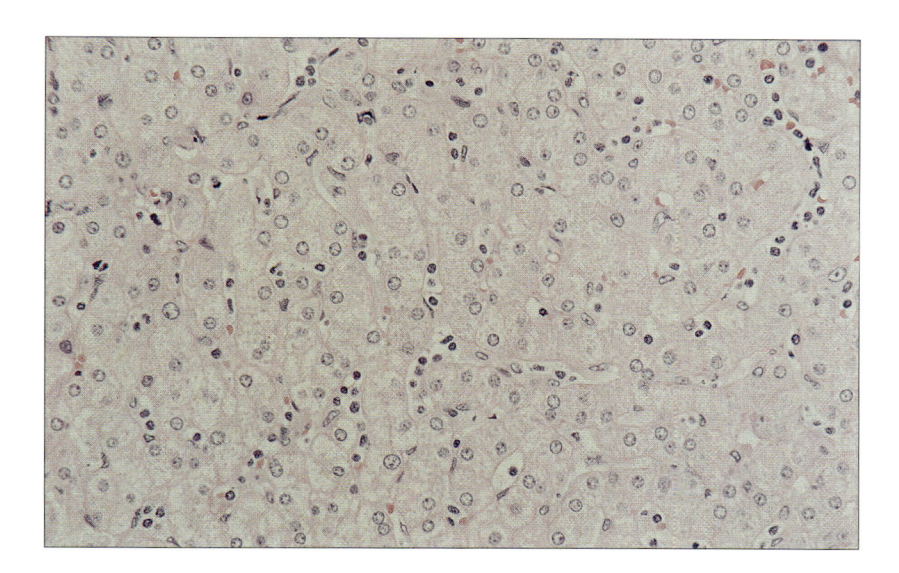

Figure 14.6

Hepatosplenic γδ T-cell lymphoma – Liver:

(a) The hepatic sinuses contain increased numbers of lymphoid cells. (H&E stain)

(b) The lymphoid cells are slightly larger than normal lymphocytes, and also have more cytoplasm. (H&E stain)

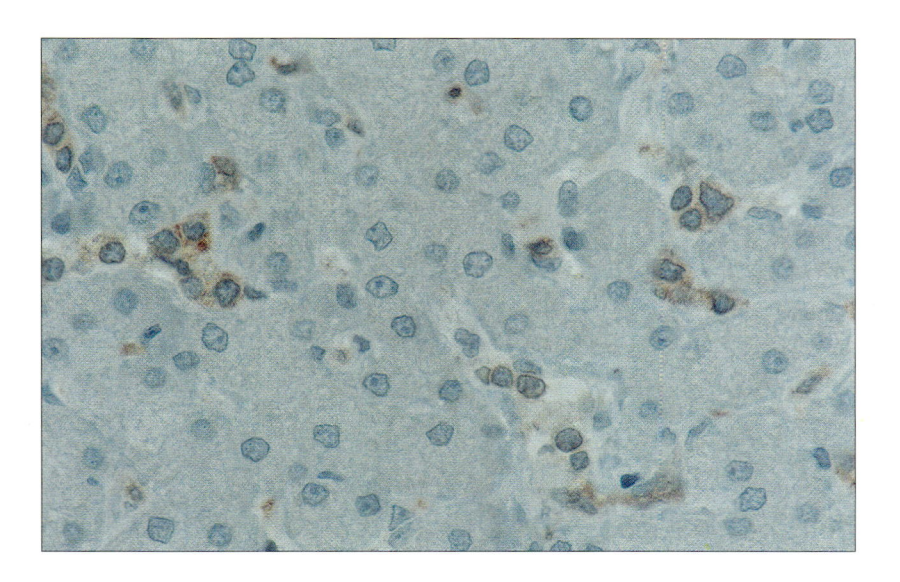

(c) The lymphoid cells express CD3, consistent with T lineage. (Immunoperoxidase technique on paraffin sections)

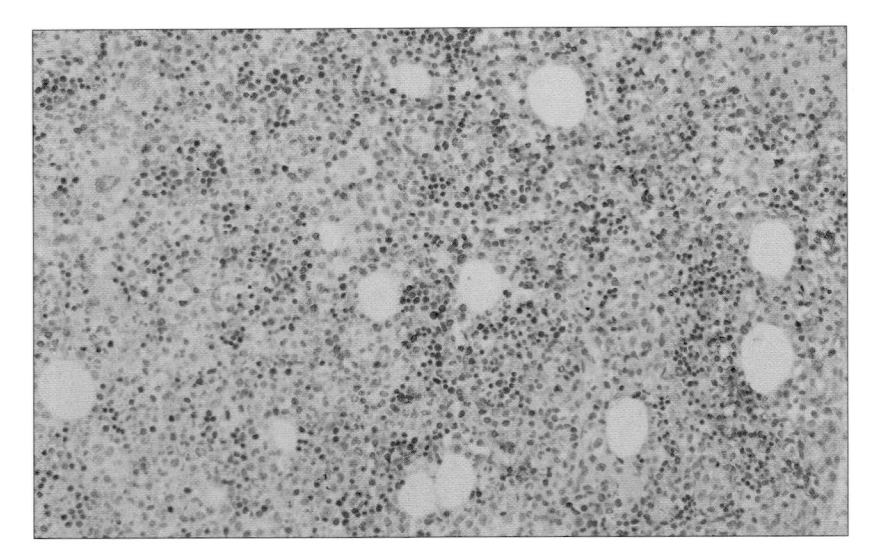

Figure 14.7

Hepatosplenic γδ T-cell lymphoma – Bone marrow:

On routinely stained sections, an atypical lymphoid infiltrate could not be discerned. However, with antibodies to CD3, many small clusters of cells are stained, consistent with subtle marrow involvement by lymphoma (**a**, low power; **b**, higher power). The distribution of these cells suggests that they occupy vascular sinusoids. (Immunoperoxidase technique on paraffin sections)

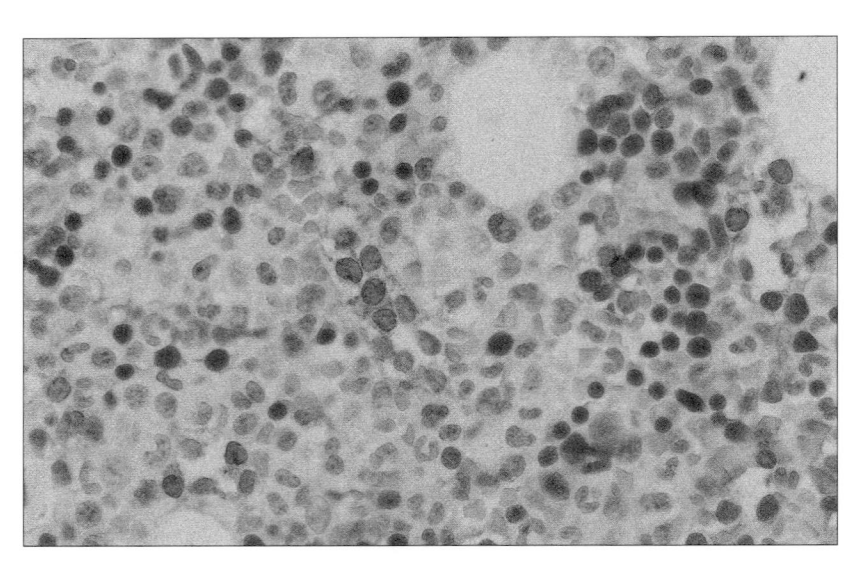

(a)

(b)

15 Hodgkin's disease

Definition and classification

Hodgkin's disease is a malignant lymphoproliferative disorder, but fundamental questions regarding its cell of origin and clonality remain unanswered or answered only with uncertainty. The disease has characteristic clinical and morphologic features. On morphologic grounds, at least five different subtypes have been defined: nodular-sclerosis, mixed-cellularity, lymphocyte-depleted, lymphocyte-predominant and lymphocyte-rich classic Hodgkin's disease. The subtypes are not readily distinguishable on clinical grounds. The interrelationship among these entities is unknown, but they each have distinctive histologic features. In general, the malignant cell (the Reed–Sternberg cell or one of its variants) represents a minor subset of the tumor mass. The malignant cells are scattered throughout the tumor in a sea of normal reactive lymphoid and inflammatory cells, and it is these normal infiltrating cells that constitute the major portion of tumor masses.

Frequency

About 8000 cases are diagnosed in the USA each year. Hodgkin's disease represents about 14% of all lymphoid malignancies. The annual incidence is about 2.9/100 000 population. The incidence of other lymphomas, particularly diffuse lymphomas, is increasing, while that of Hodgkin's disease is stable or slightly declining. Therefore Hodgkin's disease is falling as a fraction of all lymphoid tumors. Hodgkin's disease is rare in the Orient. The distribution of the histologic subtypes varies in different countries. Nodular-sclerosis Hodgkin's disease predominates in the USA, while the mixed-cellularity type is more common in Central and South America.

Pathology

Histology

The histologic classification of Hodgkin's disease that is in general use is a modification of the original scheme of Lukes and Butler (1966). Six entities in the Lukes and Butler classification became four by consensus at the Rye Conference in 1971. The REAL classification and the WHO classification recognize five entities, as noted above. The malignant cell is a Reed–Sternberg cell, whose nature remains a topic of scientific debate. It appears in various forms in distinct Hodgkin's disease subtypes. The malignant cell is associated with a florid inflammatory background of phenotypically normal lymphocytes, eosinophils, neutrophils, macrophages and plasma cells in varying patterns and proportions.

Nodular-sclerosis (NS) Hodgkin's disease. This accounts for about 75% of Hodgkin's disease in the

USA; it is slightly more common in women than in men and it is more common in younger patients. The critical histologic features are a nodular growth pattern, broad bands of fibrosis separating cellular areas, and the presence of a typical Reed–Sternberg cell variant called a lacunar cell. Lacunar cells have abundant clear cytoplasm and a distinct cell membrane. The name derives from a fixation artifact in which the cytoplasm retracts, leaving a clear space surrounding a single or multi-lobated nucleus. The nucleolus is not as prominent as in the Reed–Sternberg cells of mixed-cellularity Hodgkin's disease. Efforts to subdivide NS Hodgkin's disease into cellular and lymphocyte-depleted variants have not been reproducible, nor have they been shown to be of prognostic significance. The lymphocyte-depleted variant is said to have a higher number of malignant cells, often occurring in sheets with fewer inflammatory cells and containing areas of necrosis.

Mixed-cellularity (MC) Hodgkin's disease. This accounts for about 20% of cases in the USA. MC Hodgkin's disease has a diffuse pattern of growth that usually effaces the lymph node architecture but occasionally spares hyperplastic follicles. It has the most cellular inflammatory background. The Reed–Sternberg cells are usually binucleated (but there may be more nuclei or nuclear lobes), with each nucleus containing a single prominent nucleolus, giving the cell the classic 'owl's eyes' appearance. MC Hodgkin's disease is the subtype most often associated with clonal Epstein–Barr virus (EBV) infection.

Lymphocyte-depleted (LD) Hodgkin's disease. This is the least common form of Hodgkin's disease, accounting for 1–2% of cases. It can mimic diffuse large cell lymphoma. LD Hodgkin's disease is associated with classic-looking Reed–Sternberg cells (often in clusters or in sheets), a paucity of inflammatory cells, and a prominent fibroblastic proliferation, often with areas of necrosis.

Lymphocyte-predominant (LP) Hodgkin's disease. This is an unusual form of Hodgkin's disease, accounting for about 3–5% of all cases. LP Hodgkin's disease differs from other forms in its histologic characteristics, the immunophenotype of the malignant cells, and its clinical behavior. Classic Reed–Sternberg cells are usually absent or exceedingly rare in LP Hodgkin's disease. The neoplastic cells are called L&H or 'popcorn' cells; they have a lobulated nuclear contour that looks like popcorn, dispersed chromatin, and vague or inconspicuous nucleoli. The malignant cells may grow in clusters or nodules within a background of lymphocytes and macrophages. Most cases have a nodular growth pattern, but a small number of cases show a diffuse growth pattern. In both forms, the morphology of the cells is similar.

Lymphocyte-rich classic Hodgkin's disease. This rare form of Hodgkin's disease resembles LP Hodgkin's disease, but the malignant cells look like classic Reed–Sternberg cells rather than popcorn cells. The background contains small lymphocytes and scattered eosinophils and plasma cells. Recognition of this form of Hodgkin's disease is felt to be important, because it behaves much more like classic Hodgkin's disease than does LP (see below).

Immunophenotype

In NS, MC and LD Hodgkin's disease, the malignant cell is a Reed–Sternberg cell or a morphologic variant. It usually expresses CD30, CD15 (typically a myeloid cell antigen) and the transferrin receptor. In some cases (about 20%), the cell expresses B-cell markers, and in some cases (about 20%), T-cell markers. Rarely (in about 3% of cases) the cells express both B- and T-cell markers. In most cases (about 57%), the cells express neither B- nor T-cell markers. Immunohistologic analysis is difficult, because the malignant cells are surrounded by normal T and B cells, and the localization of any particular marker can be difficult to ascertain with certainty. Examination of DNA extracted from Hodgkin's disease-involved tissues has occasionally revealed clonal immunoglobulin gene arrangements, clonal T-cell receptor gene (*TCR*) re-arrangements, both, or neither. However, this technique was suboptimal for the analysis of genetic changes in rare cells within a tumor mass. More recent experiments have involved the isolation by micromanipulation of single Reed–Sternberg cells, the isolation of cDNA from single cells, and the analysis of rearrangements in the immunoglobulin genes. These experiments, too, have yielded some conflicting results. However, it appears that Reed–Sternberg cells that express B-cell markers such as CD20 contain clonally rearranged immunoglobulin genes and thus are derived from B cells. Not all cases express B-cell markers, so it is not clear whether Reed–Sternberg cells can only be derived from B cells.

In contrast to the situation with the classic Hodgkin's disease subtypes (NS, MC and LD), the immunophenotype of LP Hodgkin's disease is less ambiguous. LP popcorn cells do not express CD30 and CD15, they do express B-cell markers such as CD20 and CD9a, and in most cases, they contain J chain, a B-cell component. They express epithelial membrane antigen (EMA), which is not expressed on any normal B cells. In addition, the non-neoplastic cells in LP Hodgkin's disease have some interesting features. The T cells that cluster around the neoplastic cells often express CD57, a natural killer (NK)-cell marker. Within the vague nodules of tumor is a meshwork of follicular dendritic cells that express CD21. A summary of immunophenotype data is presented in Table 15.1.

Table 15.1
Immunophenotype in Hodgkin's disease

	Classic (NS, MC, LD) Hodgkin's disease	LP Hodgkin's disease
CD30	+	–
CD15	+	–
EMA	–	+
CD45	–	+
CD20, CD79	+ in 25%	+ in 100%
CD3	+ in 20%	–
J chain	–	+

	Patterns of marker expression	
Percent of cases of classic Hodgkin's disease (NS, MC, LD)	CD20 and CD79a	CD3 and TCRβ
20	+	–
20	–	+
3	+	+
57	–	–

NS, nodular-sclerosis; MC, mixed cellularity; LD, lymphocyte-depleted; LP, lymphocyte-predominant.

Genetics

Unlike many other lymphoid neoplasms, there is no genetic lesion that is characteristic of Hodgkin's disease. The cells are aneuploid, and interphase cytogenetics on numerous single Reed–Sternberg cells from a single mass tends to support the notion that the cells are clonally derived. Although there is controversy about the lineage of NS, MC and LD Hodgkin's disease, many cases express clonally rearranged immunoglobulin genes that contain point mutations suggesting the possibility that they are derived from follicular center B cells that have undergone somatic mutation. Even in those cases where the genes are rearranged, immunoglobulin molecules are generally not detected. Often the messages contain stop codons, deletions or frame shifts introduced by mutations that prevent translation. In some cases the immunoglobulin genes appear to be polyclonally rearranged, while in some cases immunoglobulin genes are not rearranged.

Genetic lesions affecting many chromosomes and regions have been identified in Reed–Sternberg cells. None of the many abnormalities qualify as recurring lesions, and the genes disrupted have not yet been identified to the extent that putative involvement in pathogenesis can be inferred. The aneuploidy results in variable numbers of individual chromosomes being present in the cells. In one study, Reed–Sternberg cells contained between two and eight copies of individual chromosomes.

Mutations in *p53* have been identified in some cases, and, depending upon the technique used to examine the cells, 30–60% of cases contain evidence of EBV infection. When EBV is present, it is usually in the form of a clonal episome. However, few viral antigens are expressed: LMP1 is the only viral gene product that has been consistently found in the cases containing EBV genomes.

Clinical characteristics/natural history

Patients most often present with painless swelling of a lymph node. When only a single site is involved, it is usually the left cervical/supraclavicular region. However, presentation of a nodal mass in the high neck, axilla and inguinal region may also be seen. Hodgkin's disease almost never involves the epitrochlear nodes or Waldeyer's ring. There are two peaks in the age distribution: one at age 27 years and another after age 80 years. Males are affected somewhat more commonly than females (M:F 1.4:1). If the patient does not notice lymph node swelling, it is common for the diagnosis to be pursued because a mediastinal mass was noted on a routine chest radiograph. About two-thirds of patients have a mediastinal mass at presentation, and it may be very large (more than one-third of the greatest chest diameter) in about one-quarter of patients. Large mediastinal masses are most common in NS histology. The development of B symptoms – fever, night sweats and unexplained weight loss of greater than 10% of the body weight over the last six months – can be the initial indication of underlying disease. Even without overt manifestations of B symptoms, patients may feel fatigued and anorexic.

The pattern of the fever has been noted to be intermittent in some patients, not occurring daily but in cycles of more or less continuous fever lasting one or two weeks separated by afebrile periods of similar duration. However, this classic manifestation of Hodgkin's disease, which is called Pel–Ebstein fever, is rare. It is more common for the fever to peak in the evening and break precipitously in the early morning hours, leading to night sweats. The patient is often unaware of the fever until it breaks. Pruritis is common, but is not considered a B symptom. The occurrence of lymph node pain as a consequence of ingesting alcohol occurs rarely, but is highly suggestive of Hodgkin's disease. This is thought to be related to the alcohol-induced degranulation of eosinophils. Usually Hodgkin's disease does not grow rapidly enough to produce painful adenopathy, but the release of eosinophil granule components may produce pain in nodes involved with Hodgkin's disease. Other rare manifestations of Hodgkin's disease include pericardial tamponade from a pericardial effusion, bone pain from bony involvement, superior vena caval obstruction, or flank or back pain from retroperitoneal adenopathy. Paraneoplastic syndromes may also be seen, including hypercalcemia, dermatologic lesions (erythema nodosum, dermatomyositis), and neurologic syndromes (Guillain–Barré, inflammatory brachial plexopathy). Laboratory abnormalities may include thrombocytosis, granulocytosis, eosinophilia, elevated erythrocyte sedimentation rate and anemia.

Hodgkin's disease tends to spread from one lymph node group to another in a contiguous fashion. It is unusual for involvement to skip lymph node-bearing sites. Thus certain patterns of disease have been noted. If disease is noted in the neck and groin, it is most likely that abdominal nodes are also involved. The liver is not involved unless the spleen is involved. The lung parenchyma is nearly never involved without involvement of ipsilateral hilar nodes. When only a single site in the abdomen is involved, it is usually the spleen, which is involved in about 30% of patients. Because the spleen lacks lymphatic afferents, this has been used to argue for hematogenous spread of disease in addition to lymphatic spread. If the disease does spread hematogenously then Reed–Sternberg cells must be restricted in the sites where they can grow, because other extranodal sites are rarely involved until very late in the course of disease.

Because of the orderly progression of Hodgkin's disease, the staging classification that emerged to identify patients of distinct risk is an anatomically based system. Originally devised at a conference in Ann Arbor in 1966, the staging classification was revised in 1988 at a meeting in the Cotswolds in the UK (Table 15.2). Once a diagnosis of Hodgkin's disease has been made – usually on the basis of the histology of an excised lymph node – additional testing is required to determine the stage of disease (Table 15.3). With improvements in treatment, stage of disease is mainly useful in determining what treatment to use. Stage has lost its impact on survival, because the outcome from treatment of all stages of disease is now similar; at least 80% of patients below 50 years old can expect to be cured by their initial treatment regardless of stage (see below). LP may be distinct from

Table 15.2
Staging classification for Hodgkin's disease

Stage	Definition
I	Involvement of a single lymph node region or lymphoid structure (e.g. spleen)
II	Involvement of two or more lymph node regions on the same side of the diaphragm
III	Involvement of lymph node regions or lymphoid structures on both sides of the diaphragm:
	III_1 involvement limited to spleen, splenic hilar nodes, celiac nodes or portal nodes
	III_2 involvement includes paraaortic, iliac or mesenteric nodes plus those in III_1
IV	Involvement of extranodal site(s) beyond that designated as 'E', more than one extranodal deposit at any location, any involvement of liver or bone marrow
A	No symptoms
B	Unexplained weight loss of more than 10% of body weight in the last 6 months,
	Unexplained fever >38°C in the previous month
	Recurrent drenching night sweats in the previous month
X	Bulky disease:
	≥10 cm maximum diameter of a nodal mass
	Mediastinal mass greater than one-third the transverse chest diameter at T5–6 level on chest radiograph
E	Localized, solitary involvement of extra lymphatic tissue, except liver and bone marrow:
	If this is the only site of disease, it is stage IE
	By limited direct extension from a known nodal site
	Single discrete site proximal to a regional involved nodal site (IIE)

Table 15.3
Recommended staging evaluation for patients with Hodgkin's disease.

Mandatory procedures
Excisional biopsy of involved lymph node
History with attention to B symptoms
Physical examination, record bidirectional dimensions of any adenopathy, look for splenomegaly, tenderness
Laboratory tests:
 Complete blood count
 Chemistry panel, liver and renal function tests
 Erythrocyte sedimentation rate
Radiographic tests:
 PA and lateral chest radiograph
 Abdominal and pelvic computed tomography
 Bipedal lymphangiogram
Bilateral bone marrow biopsies and aspirates

Procedures useful under certain circumstances
Thoracic computed tomography if chest radiograph is abnormal
Staging laparotomy if there is clinical early-stage disease and radiation therapy is the treatment of choice
Liver biopsy if there is evidence of splenic or hepatic involvement
Bone scan if bone pain is present
Echocardiography if pericardial disease is suspected on chest radiograph or by clinical examination

Procedure especially useful in restaging
Double-dose gallium-67 scan

the other histologic subtypes in this regard. It is difficult to draw firm conclusions because the disease is rare, but LP Hodgkin's disease tends to present in early stage with high neck nodes and responds well to therapy. However, its natural history is marked by patterns of disease recurrence and response to subsequent therapy without achieving prolonged disease-free survival; however, the natural history is indolent and prolonged survival is common.

Treatment

Successful treatment for Hodgkin's disease has been available for the past 30 years. The treatment strategies emerged as a consequence of carefully controlled clinical trials, and were based upon surgical staging and stage-related interventions. With long-term follow-up of patients cured in the 1960s and 1970s, we have learned that the original successful approaches to staging and treatment have produced late sequelae, often life-threatening or fatal, and therefore the original approaches are being reexamined in an effort to maintain high cure rates from primary treatment and reduce late staging- and treatment-related complications. In particular, staging laparotomy and splenectomy lead to increased susceptibility to infection, and splenectomy may increase the risk of some second malignancies. Combination chemotherapy regimens involving alkylating agents and nitrosoureas are associated with infertility and an increased risk of acute leukemia. Regimens containing bleomycin may lead to pulmonary fibrosis, especially if given together with radiation therapy. Radiation therapy is associated with second solid tumors, hypothyroidism, pulmonary fibrosis and premature atherosclerotic coronary artery disease. Secondary aggressive lymphomas also occur in about 4% of patients, but this is not clearly related to the form of treatment, and may be a consequence of the long-lasting immune deficits that persist even after the cure of Hodgkin's disease.

No consensus has emerged about the best way to control late complications. If staging laparotomy is omitted from the workup, most clinicians employ systemic chemotherapy so that sites of disease not looked for are nonetheless treated. Some have advocated using combined-modality therapy in all stages of the disease, with the goal of avoiding late complications by using lower total doses of drugs and radiation therapy. The author's view (DLL) is that combining chemotherapy and radiation therapy leads to synergistic toxicities not seen in patients in whom only one modality is used, and the author is not convinced by any published data that 2400 cGy of radiation therapy is less carcinogenic than 3600–4000 cGy of radiation therapy. For these reasons, the author advocates an approach that employs clinical staging followed by combination chemotherapy for all stages of disease except peripheral IA disease. Radiation therapy is used in addition to chemotherapy in two subsets of patients: those with large mediastinal masses and those who do not achieve a complete response with chemotherapy alone. Only patients with peripheral IA disease receive regional radiation therapy without systemic therapy.

The earliest successes came from using staging laparotomy to define the extent of disease and from employing total lymphoid irradiation in patients with stage I and II disease and combination chemotherapy in stages III and IV disease. Of 100 patients presenting with a diagnosis of Hodgkin's disease, 90 will have clinical early-stage disease after physical examination and chest radiography. Bipedal lymphography results in the detection of paraaortic node involvement in one-third of the remaining early-stage patients (30%), and most of these cases would not be detected by abdominal computed tomography. Of the remaining 60 patients with early-stage disease after lymphography, another one-third (20%) will be found to have intraabdominal disease at laparotomy. When staging laparotomy is omitted, patients run a significant risk of intraabdominal sites of disease remaining undetected. However, a small subset of patients with clinical early-stage disease have a particularly low likelihood of having intraabdominal disease, and in this subset (women with clinical stage IA disease, men with high cervical disease or non-massive mediastinal mass as the only site of involvement, or LP histology), laparotomy may be safely omitted.

Total lymphoid radiation therapy as delivered at Stanford University resulted in long-term control of Hodgkin's disease in about 80% of patients with early-stage Hodgkin's disease. Unfortunately, the same success rate has not been seen universally – often as a consequence of technical failures in radiation planning. In one Patterns of Care Study, a retrospective examination of portal films that document the radiation field found that more than one-third of them failed to encompass the known extent of disease. The relapse rates in these inadequately treated individuals were significantly higher than those in patients whose radiation port adequately incorporated the disease sites. The typical radiation dose was 3600–4000 cGy delivered in 200 cGy fractions. Many efforts have been made to improve the success of radiation therapy in early-stage disease by the addition of combination chemotherapy. However, meta-analysis of these combined-modality studies fails to demonstrate an improvement in overall survival. In general, the control of the Hodgkin's disease is about 10% improved, but deaths from treatment-related complications counterbalanced the small decrease in deaths from Hodgkin's disease.

The death rate of patients who received radiation therapy for their Hodgkin's disease is significantly higher than that of age-matched controls. The deaths are not from uncontrolled Hodgkin's disease. In fact, by 25 years after treatment, deaths from treatment-related problems outnumber deaths from Hodgkin's disease. The causes of death are overwhelmingly related to second solid tumors, premature coronary atherosclerosis (*fatal* myocardial infarction is more than three times more likely in patients who received mediastinal radiation therapy than in age-matched controls), and serious infections (related to disease-related immunosuppression and splenectomy). In view of this excess in deaths related to the standard treatment approach, splenectomy is now used extremely rarely to stage patients, and many groups are attempting to reduce the radiation risk by giving lower total doses of radiation to smaller fields and incorporating chemotherapy. It seems clear that the control of Hodgkin's disease will not be compromised by this approach. However, it remains unclear whether late complications of treatment will be significantly reduced by this approach. An alternative approach to reducing the late complication rate is to use chemotherapy alone in patients with early-stage disease.

Advanced-stage disease is routinely treated with combination chemotherapy. The choice of regimen is somewhat controversial. Most often ABVD (doxorubicin, bleomycin, vinblastine, dacarbazine) is the first choice. However, fatal pulmonary fibrosis from the bleomycin has been noted in as many as 3% of patients. This rate of treatment-related fatality is comparable to the 2.2% risk of acute leukemia from MOPP (nitrogen mustard, vincristine, procarbazine, prednisone) – a complication that has prompted a major decline in the use of alkylating agent-containing regimens. The main clear advantage of ABVD over MOPP is that ABVD does not induce infertility. Alternating (e.g. MOPP alternating with ABVD) or hybrid (e.g. MOPP/ABV) programs are also effective. It is not entirely clear that the seven-drug and eight-drug regimens are more effective than ABVD alone; however, these regimens are very effective, and they result in the delivery of half the total dose of agents given when four-drug regimens are used alone. To the extent that toxicities are dose-related, it is expected that the late toxicities from hybrid or alternating regimens will be lower than from four-drug regimens. In general, either with four-drug or with seven- or eight-drug regimens, complete response rates should be around 90% and about 75–80% of patients are long-term disease-free survivors. Older patients, particularly those over 70 years, appear to have a poorer outcome – for reasons that are not completely defined.

Although retrospective studies have suggested that adding radiation therapy to involved sites of disease after chemotherapy improves disease control in patients with advanced-stage disease, randomized studies have not supported this notion, and a meta-analysis has suggested that advanced-stage patients treated with combined-modality therapy have poorer long-term survival than those treated with chemotherapy alone based upon an increase in late treatment-related deaths.

Efforts to improve the treatment of advanced-stage disease have involved the development of new combination chemotherapy programs. The Stanford V regimen uses a short total course of chemotherapy (12 weeks), with radiation therapy given to previous sites of disease. With short follow-up, this regimen is very effective; however, it remains to be seen whether late effects are reduced. The BEACOPP regimen (bleomycin, etoposide, doxorubicin, cyclophosphamide, vincristine, procarbazine, prednisone) is a dose-intensified treatment program that also shows excellent antitumor efficacy. Follow-up here is also too short to assess late effects. It is not clear whether all patients with advanced disease require a dose-intensive regimen to optimize their chances for disease control. However, these regimens obtain complete responses in more than 90% of patients, and the responses appear durable at early follow-up times.

Patients not cured by their initial treatment have a legitimate opportunity to be cured by salvage therapy. The success of salvage therapy depends on the clinical situation. Patients with early-stage Hodgkin's disease relapsing after treatment with radiation therapy are rescued with combination chemotherapy in about two-thirds of cases. Patients relapsing with B symptoms or extranodal disease are somewhat less likely to be rescued successfully with standard-dose combination chemotherapy. Patients who were not cured by their initial combination-chemotherapy program fall into three groups: primary induction failure, relapse after short initial remission (<12 months), and relapse after long initial remission (>12 months). Patients relapsing after long initial remissions often retain chemotherapy responsiveness, but the duration of second remissions is usually shorter than that of the first. The success of high-dose therapy with autologous stem cell transplantation has led to the recommendation that any patient relapsing from a chemotherapy-induced complete remission should have high-dose therapy as the first choice of salvage therapy. Patients who had long initial remissions have a very high rate of salvage with such an approach (78% in one series). Patients who had short initial remissions have a 40–50% chance of achieving long-term disease-free survival from high-dose salvage therapy. Patients whose disease grows through conventional-dose chemotherapy are unlikely to benefit from high-dose therapy.

Although most patients who do not achieve a complete response to initial chemotherapy have disease that grows through treatment, a fraction of these patients have one or two sites of persistent disease that responded partially to chemotherapy. Such patients may be converted to durable complete responders by the use of radiation therapy to the residual sites of disease. Another group of patients who appear to benefit from the addition of radiation therapy to chemotherapy comprises those presenting with large mediastinal masses. Patients with massive mediastinal disease treated with combined-modality therapy have an 80% chance of long-term disease-free survival.

In summary, patients with clinical early-stage disease should probably not be taken to exploratory laparotomy unless it is intended that radiation therapy alone be a treatment option. Patients with LP histology and peripheral IA disease may be clinically staged (i.e. no laparotomy) and treated with radiation therapy to the involved fields with a high rate of success. Patients with massive mediastinal involvement should probably receive combined-modality therapy, with combination chemotherapy followed by mantle-field radiation therapy. All other patients may be treated using combination chemotherapy alone following clinical staging. The few percent (5% or fewer) of patients who obtain an excellent partial response to chemotherapy may be converted to complete responders with involved-field radiation therapy. Other experts may recommend that these patients receive combined-modality therapy as standard treatment. Patients relapsing after radiation therapy may be rescued with standard-dose combination chemotherapy. Those relapsing after chemotherapy generally receive high-dose therapy with autologous stem cell support. With the use of state-of-the-art therapies available today, long-term survival is possible in 80–90% of patients with Hodgkin's disease.

Bibliography

Armitage JO, Bierman PJ, Vose JM et al, Autologous bone marrow transplantation for patients with relapsed Hodgkin's disease. *Am J Med* 1991; **19:** 605–11.

Bartlett NL, Rosenberg SA, Hoppe RT et al, Brief chemotherapy, Stanford-V, and adjuvant radiotherapy for bulky or advanced-stage Hodgkin's disease. A preliminary report. *J Clin Oncol* 1995; **13:** 1080–8.

Blayney DW, Longo DL, Young RC et al, Decreasing risk of leukemia with prolonged follow-up after chemotherapy and radiotherapy for Hodgkin's disease. *N Engl J Med* 1987; **316:** 710–14.

Bonadonna G, Valagussa P, Santoro A, Alternating non-cross-resistant combination chemotherapy or MOPP in stage IV Hodgkin's disease. A report of 8-year results. *Ann Intern Med* 1986; **104:** 739–46.

Bookman MA, Longo DL, Concomitant illness in patients treated for Hodgkin's disease. *Cancer Treat Rev* 1986; **13:** 77–109.

Canellos GP, Anderson JR, Propert KJ et al, Chemotherapy of advanced Hodgkin's disease with MOPP, ABVD, or MOPP alternating with ABVD. *N Engl J Med* 1992; **327:** 1478–84.

Connors JM, Klimo P, Adams G et al, Treatment of advanced Hodgkin's disease with chemotherapy – comparison of MOPP/ABV hybrid regimen with alternating courses of MOPP and ABVD: a report from the National Cancer Institute of Canada Clinical Trials Group. *J Clin Oncol* 1997; **15:** 1638–45.

DeVita VT Jr, Simon RM, Hubbard SM et al, Curability of advanced Hodgkin's disease with chemotherapy. Long-term follow-up of MOPP-treated patients at the

National Cancer Institute. *Ann Intern Med* 1980; **92:** 587–95.

Diehl V, Sieber M, Ruffer U et al, BEACOPP: an intensified chemotherapy regimen in advanced Hodgkin's disease. The German Hodgkin's Lymphoma Study Group. *Ann Oncol* 1997; **8:** 143–8.

Hancock SL, Tucker MA, Hoppe RT, Breast cancer after treatment of Hodgkin's disease. *J Natl Cancer Inst* 1993; **85:** 25–31.

Hasenclever D, Diehl V, Armitage JO et al, A prognostic score for advanced Hodgkin's disease. *N Engl J Med* 1998; **339:** 1506–14.

Hummel M, Ziemann K, Lammert H et al, Hodgkin's disease with monoclonal and polyclonal populations of Reed–Sternberg cells. *N Engl J Med* 1995; **333:** 901–6.

Kaplan HS, *Hodgkin's Disease*, 2nd edn. Harvard University Press: Cambridge, MA, 1980.

Kuppers R, Rajewsky K, Zhao M et al, Hodgkin's disease: Hodgkin and Reed–Sternberg cells picked from histological sections show clonal immunoglobulin gene rearrangements and appear to be derived from B cells at various stages of development. *Proc Natl Acad Sci USA* 1994; **91:** 10962–6.

Lister TA, Crowther D, Staging for Hodgkin's disease. *Semin Oncol* 1990; **17:** 696–703.

Loeffler M, Brosteanu O, Hasenclever D et al, Meta-analysis of chemotherapy versus combined modality treatment trials in Hodgkin's disease. International Database on Hodgkin's Disease Overview Study Group. *J Clin Oncol* 1998; **16:** 818–29.

Longo DL, Duffey PL, Young RC et al, Conventional-dose salvage combination chemotherapy in patients relapsing with Hodgkin's disease after combination chemotherapy: the low probability for cure. *J Clin Oncol* 1992; **10:** 210–18.

Longo DL, Glatstein E, Duffey PL et al, Radiation therapy versus combination chemotherapy in the treatment of early-stage Hodgkin's disease: seven-year results of a prospective randomized trial. *J Clin Oncol* 1991; **9:** 906–17.

Longo DL, Glatstein E, Duffey PL et al, Alternating MOPP and ABVD chemotherapy plus mantle-field radiation therapy in patients with massive mediastinal Hodgkin's disease. *J Clin Oncol* 1997; **15:** 3338–46.

Lukes RJ, Butler JJ, Therr pathology and nomenclature of Hodgkin's disease. *Cancer Res* 1966; **26:** 1063–81.

Macfarlane GJ, Evstifeeva T, Boyle P, Grufferman S, International patterns in the occurrence of Hodgkin's disease in children and young adult males. *Int J Cancer* 1995; **61:** 165–9.

Mauch PM, Kalish LA, Marcus KC et al, Long-term survival in Hodgkin's disease. *Cancer J Sci Am* 1995; **1:** 33–43.

Rappaport H, Berard CW, Butler JJ et al, Report of the committee on histopathological criterial contributing to staging of Hodgkin's disease. *Cancer Res* 1971; **31:** 1864–5.

Reece DE, Connors JM, Spinelli JJ et al, Intensive therapy with cyclophosphamide, carmustine, etoposide, ± cisplatin and autologous bone marrow transplantation for Hodgkin's disease in first relapse after combination chemotherapy. *Blood* 1994; **83:** 1193–9.

Regula DP, Hoppe RT, Weiss LM, Nodular and diffuse types of lymphocyte predominance Hodgkin's disease. *N Engl J Med* 1988; **318:** 214–9.

Specht L, Gray RG, Clarke MJ, Peto R, Influence of more extensive radiotherapy and adjuvant chemotherapy on long-term outcome of early-stage Hodgkin's disease: a meta-analysis of 23 randomized trials involving 3,888 patients. International Hodgkin's Disease Collaborative Group. *J Clin Oncol* 1998; **16:** 830–43.

Stein H, Hummel M, Marafioti T et al, Molecular biology of Hodgkin's disease. *Cancer Surv* 1997; **30:** 107–23.

Tucker MA, Coleman CM, Cox RS et al, Risk of second cancers after treatment for Hodgkin's disease. *N Engl J Med* 1988; **318:** 76–81.

Weiss LM, Arber DA, Chang KL, Clonality in lymphocyte predominance Hodgkin's disease. *Cancer Surv* 1997; **30:** 125–41.

Weiss LM, Movahed AM, Warnke RA, Sklar J, Detection of Epstein–Barr viral genomes in Reed–Sternberg cells of Hodgkin's disease. *N Engl J Med* 1989; **320:** 502–6.

Nodular-sclerosis Hodgkin's disease

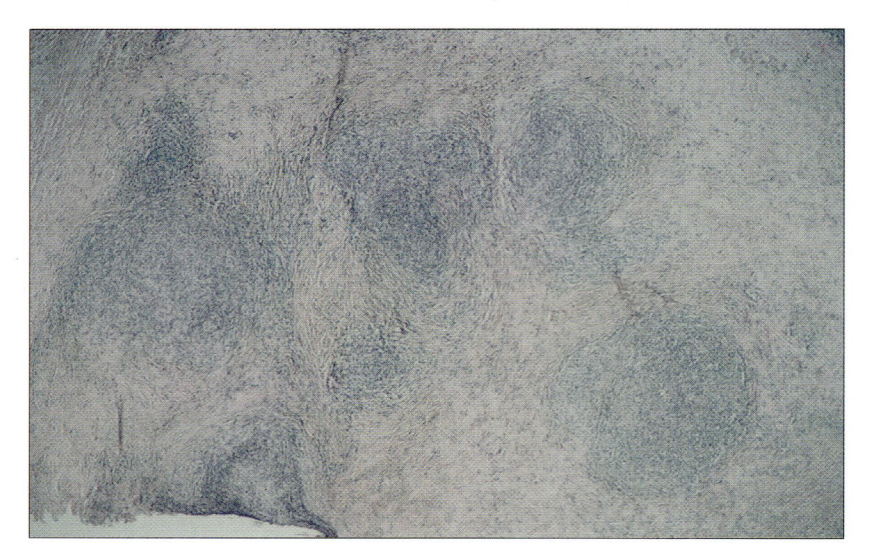

Figure 15.1

Nodular-sclerosis Hodgkin's disease:

(a) Low-power examination shows cellular nodules in a sclerotic background. (H&E stain)

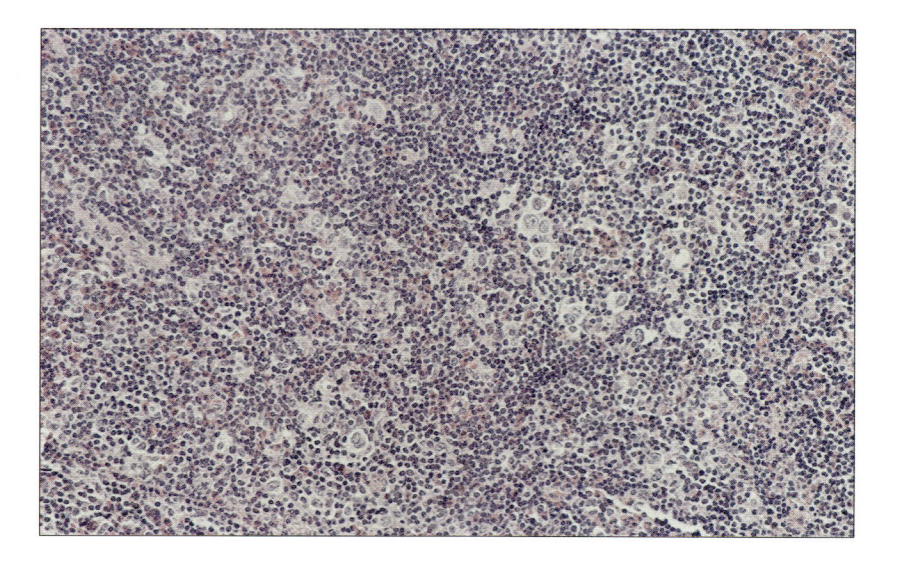

(b) Most cells in the nodules are lymphocytes; also present are scattered pale lacunar cells. (H&E stain)

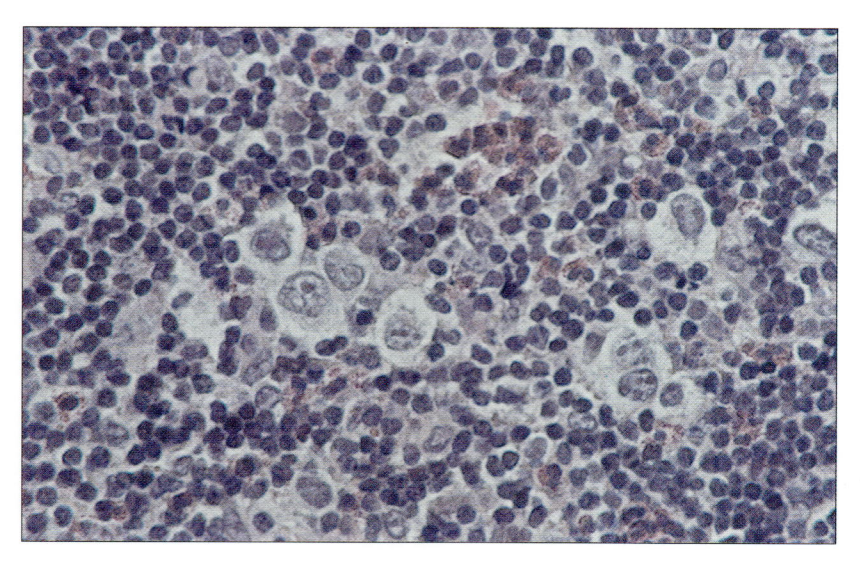

(c) Lacunar cells, with pale, oval to lobated nuclei and abundant cytoplasm that retracts following formalin fixation, are present in a background of lymphocytes and eosinophils. (H&E stain)

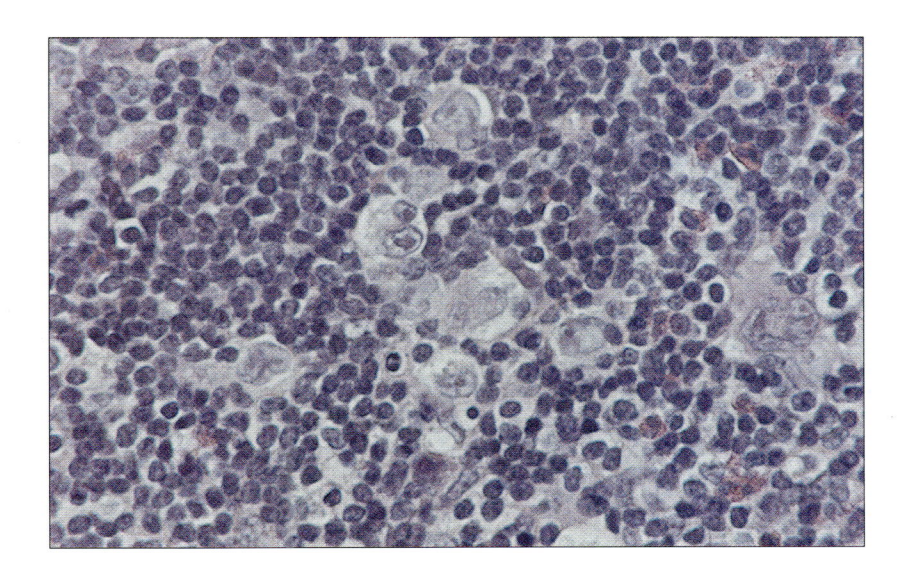

Figure 15.1 *continued*

(d) Occasional diagnostic Reed–Sternberg cells and neoplastic cells with wreath-like nuclei are present. (H&E stain)

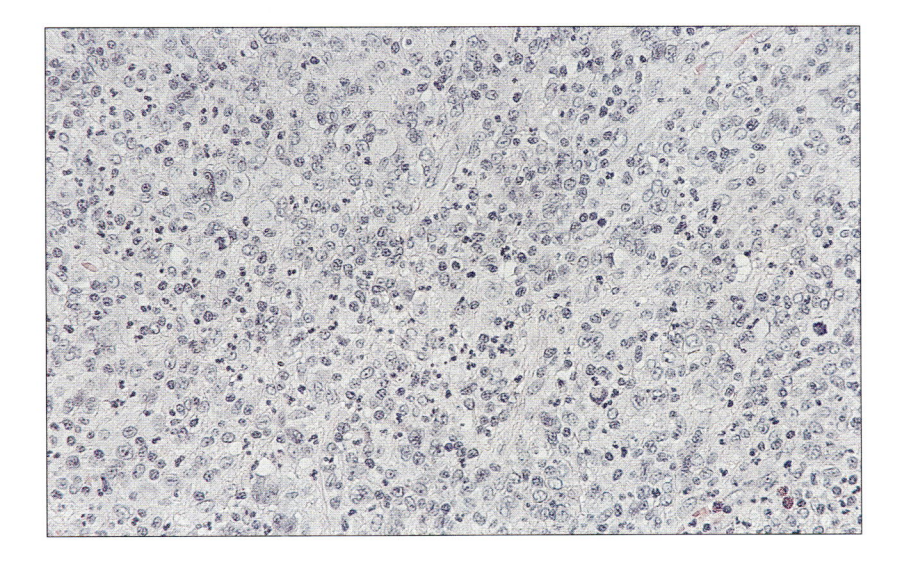

(e) In this case, there are sheets of neoplastic cells, consistent with the syncytial variant. (H&E stain)

Mixed-cellularity Hodgkin's disease

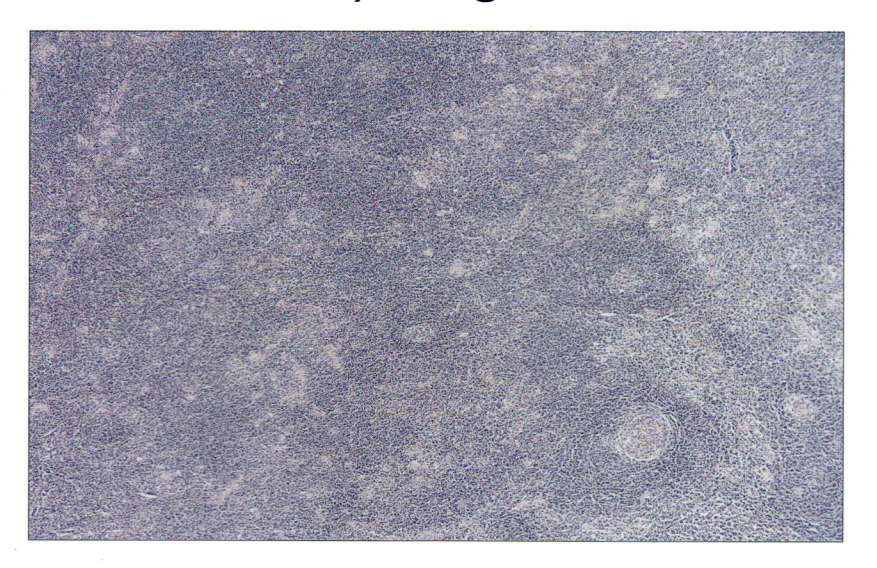

Figure 15.2

Mixed-cellularity Hodgkin's disease:

(a) Much of the lymph node is replaced by Hodgkin's disease, but residual reactive follicles can be found. (H&E stain)

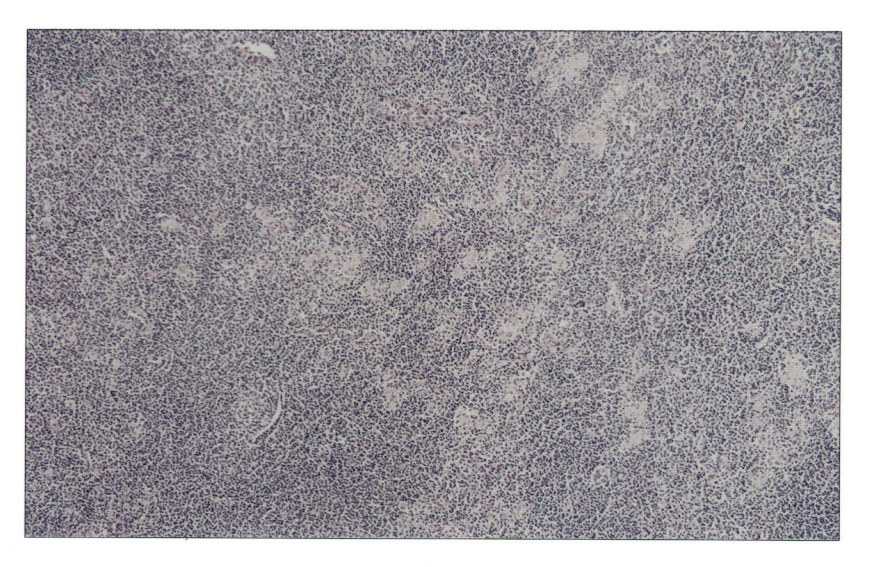

(b) In some areas, small clusters of epithelioid histiocytes with eosinophilic cytoplasm are present. (H&E stain)

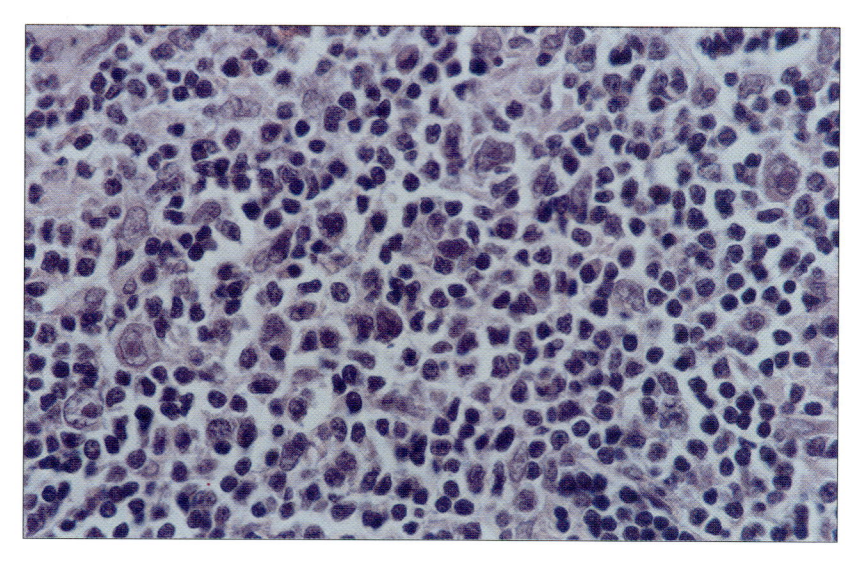

(c) Mononuclear Reed–Sternberg variants are present in a background that is composed predominantly of lymphocytes in this field. (H&E stain)

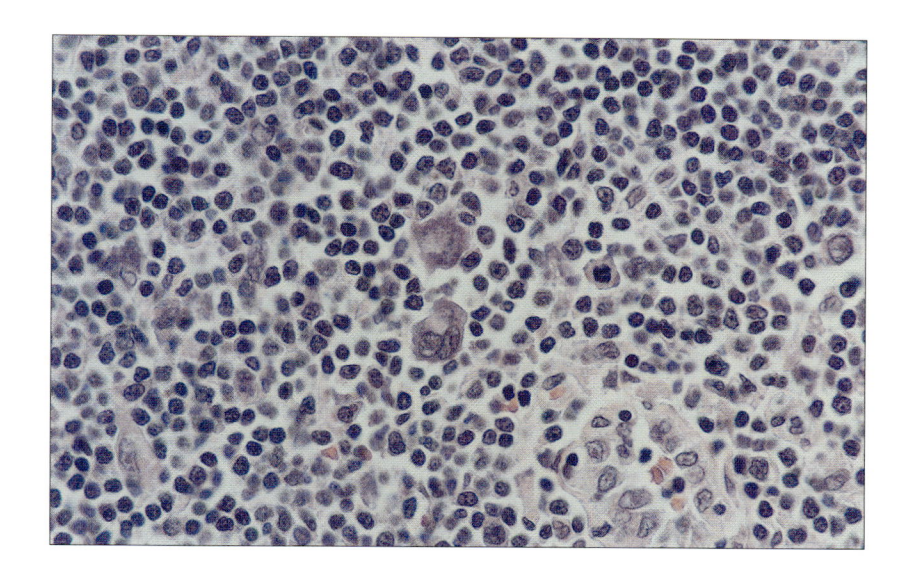

Figure 15.2 *continued*

(d) Occasional diagnostic Reed–Sternberg cells are present. (H&E stain)

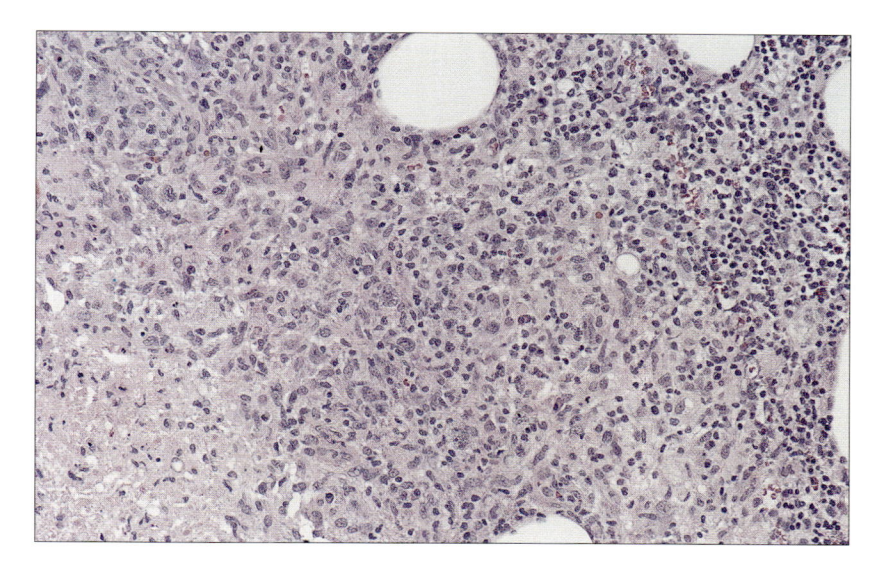

(e) In another case, there is necrosis, and neoplastic cells are more abundant. (H&E stain)

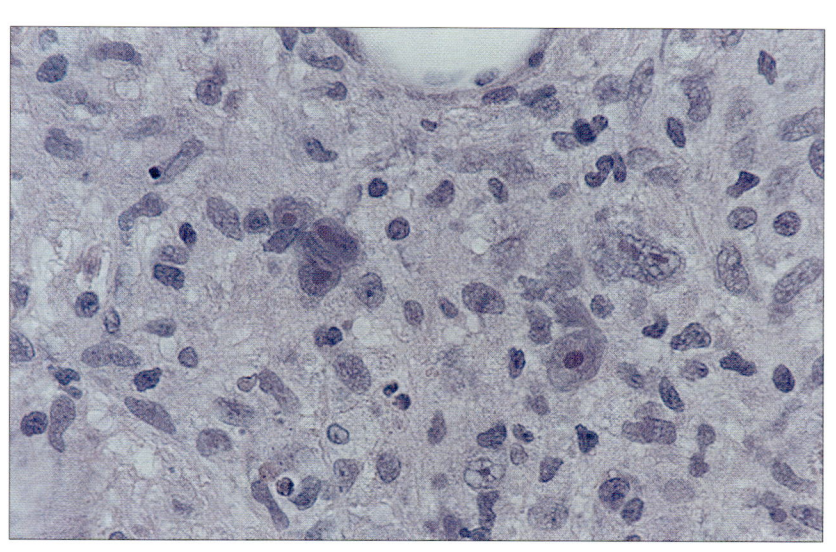

(f) Higher power shows Reed–Sternberg variants admixed with histiocytes and a few lymphocytes. In areas of this case, the proportion of neoplastic cells approached that found in lymphocyte-depleted Hodgkin's disease. (H&E stain)

Contd

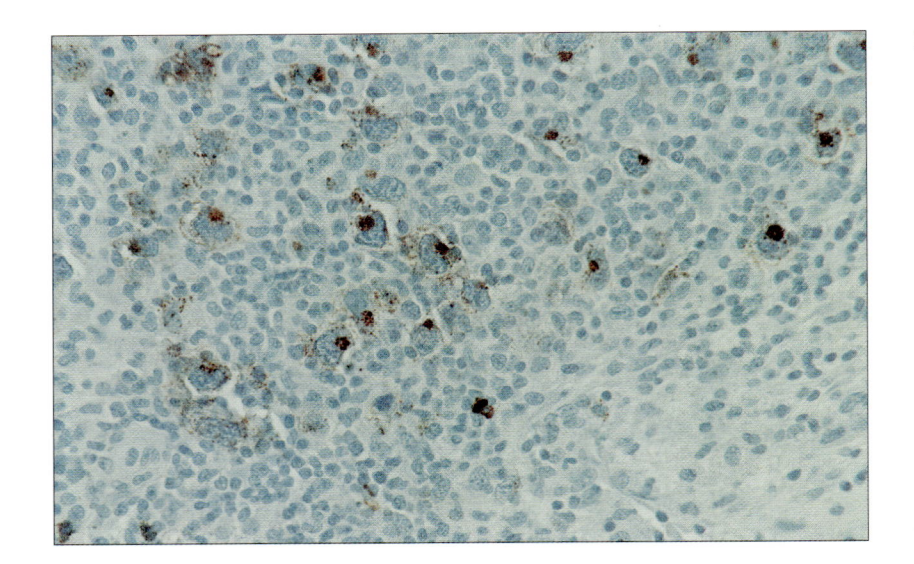

Figure 15.2 *continued*

Reed–Sternberg cells and variants expressing CD15 (**g**) and Epstein–Barr virus latent membrane protein (**h**). (Immunoperoxidase technique on paraffin sections)

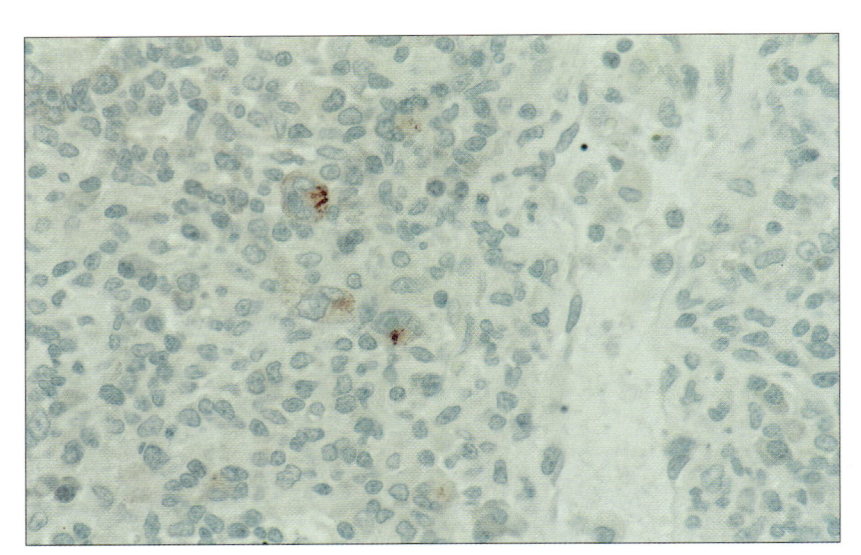

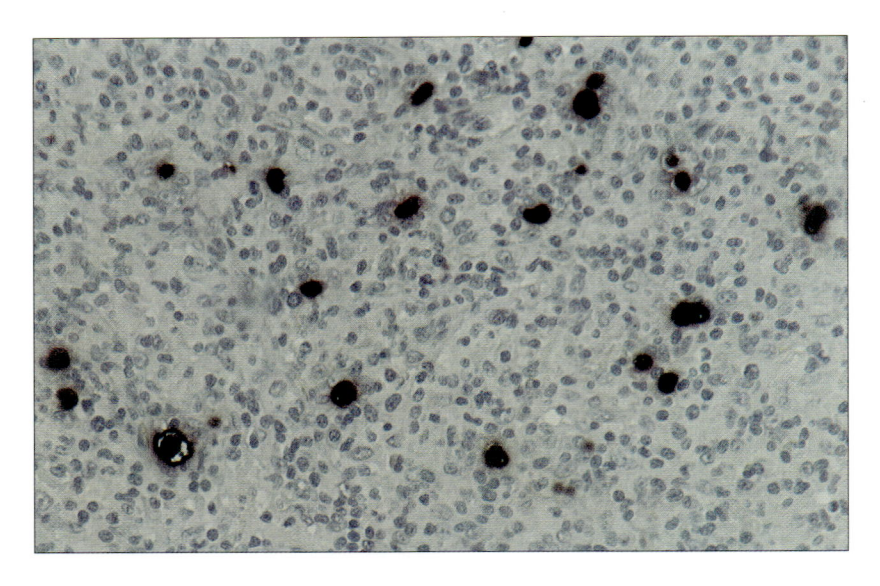

(g)

(h)

(i) Reed–Sternberg cells and variants are EBER+. (In situ hybridization on paraffin sections)

Lymphocyte-depleted Hodgkin's disease, reticular subtype

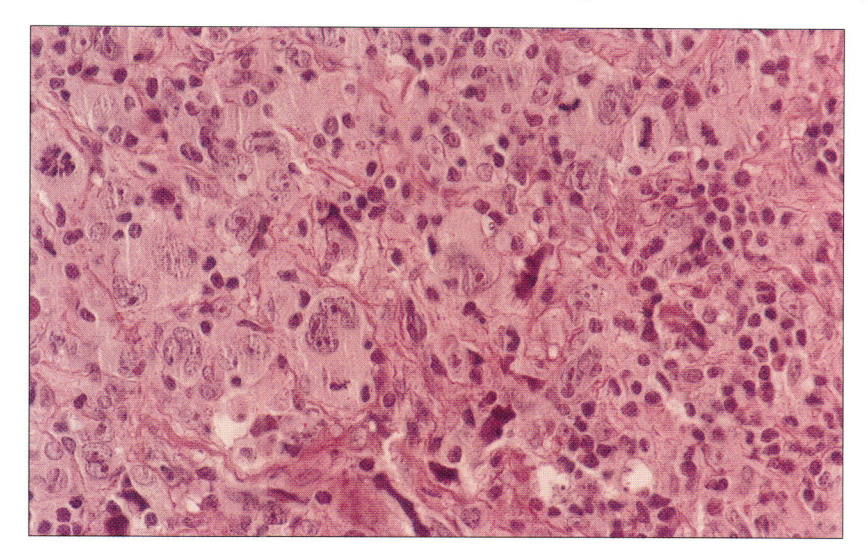

Figure 15.3

Lymphocyte-depleted Hodgkin's disease, reticular subtype – Lymph node:

In a paraaortic lymph node from an elderly patient with B symptoms, there are sheets of large atypical cells with an appearance consistent with Reed–Sternberg cells and variants. (H&E stain)

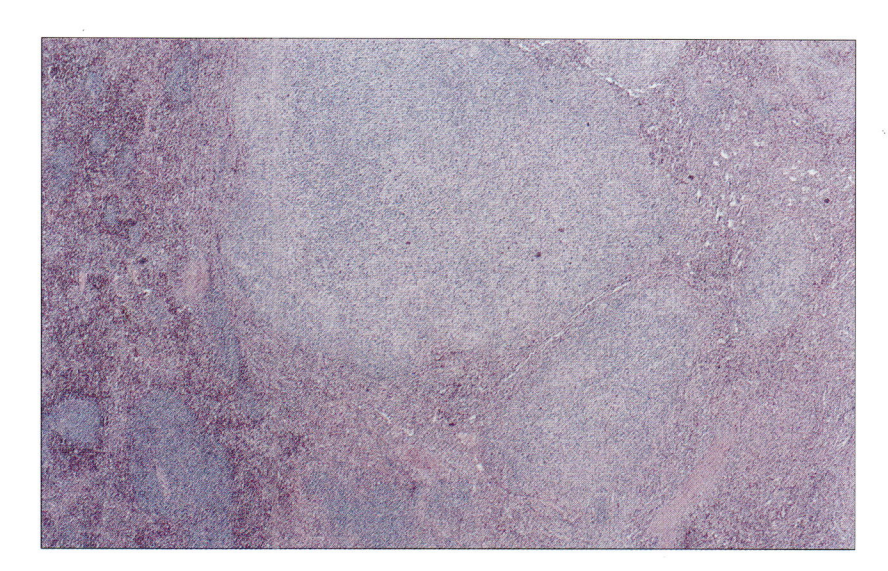

Figure 15.4

Lymphocyte-depleted Hodgkin's disease, reticular subtype – Spleen:

(a) The spleen contains large nodules that were easily identified on gross examination. (H&E stain)

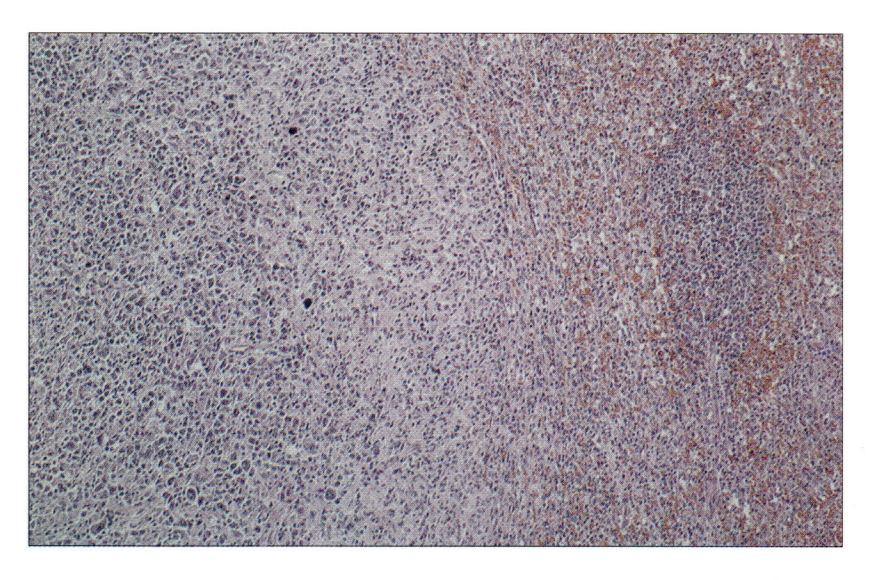

(b) The abnormal nodules are much larger than normal white pulp. (H&E stain)

Contd

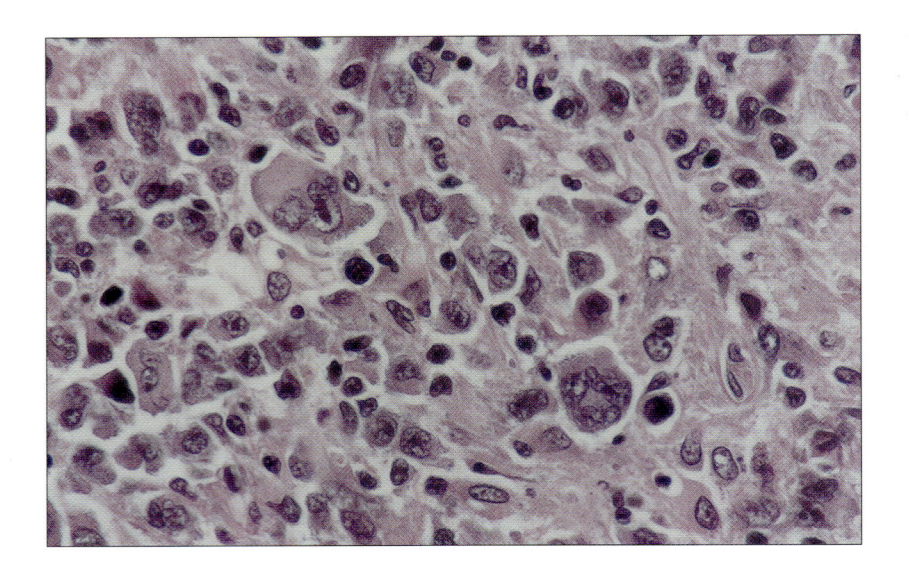

Figure 15.4 *continued*

(c) The nodules contain numerous Reed–Sternberg cells and variants.

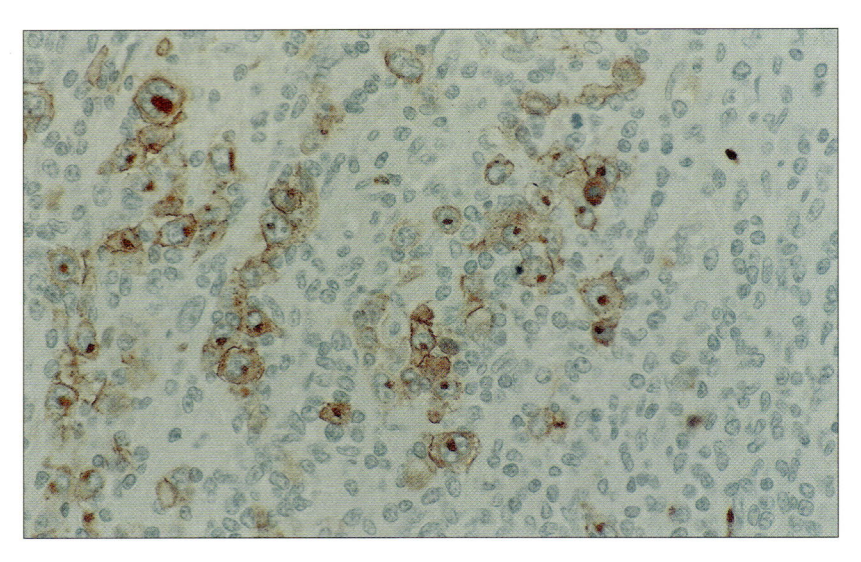

The neoplastic cells are CD15+ (**d**), CD30+ (**e**) and CD45− (**f**). (Immunoperoxidase technique on paraffin sections)

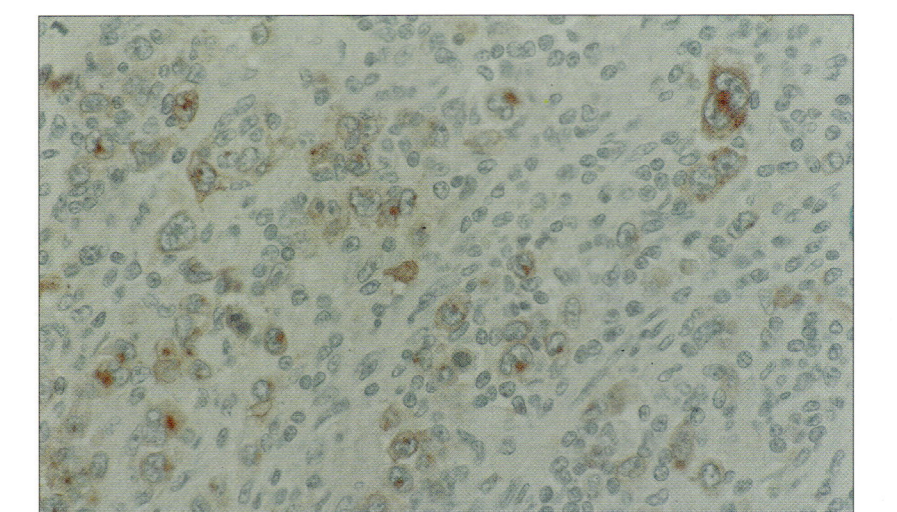

(d)

(e)

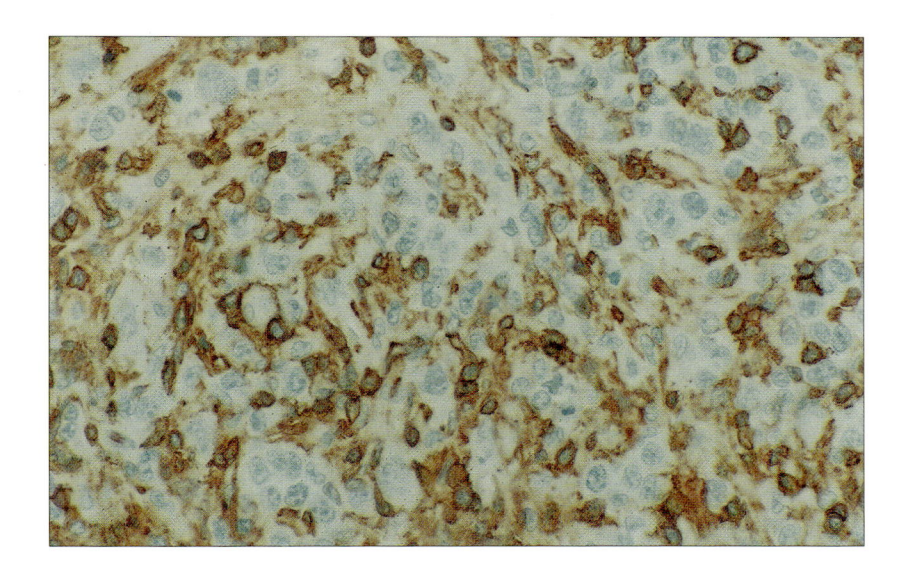

Figure 15.4 *continued*

(f)

Lymphocyte-depleted Hodgkin's disease, diffuse-fibrosis subtype

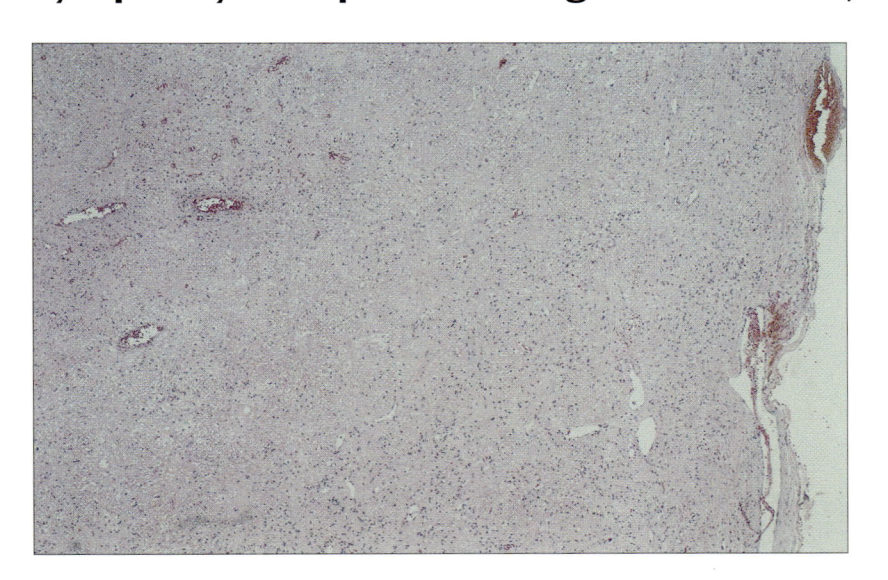

Figure 15.5

Lymphocyte-depleted Hodgkin's disease, diffuse-fibrosis subtype:

(a) The normal lymph node architecture is obliterated. (H&E stain)

Contd

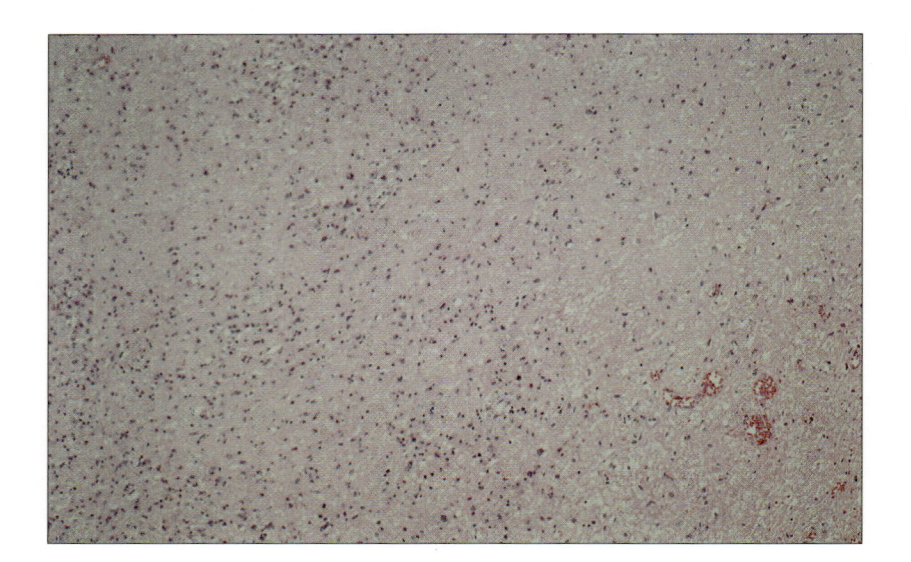

Figure 15.5 *continued*

(b) The proliferation within the node is hypocellular; the abundant eosinophilic material is collagen. (H&E stain)

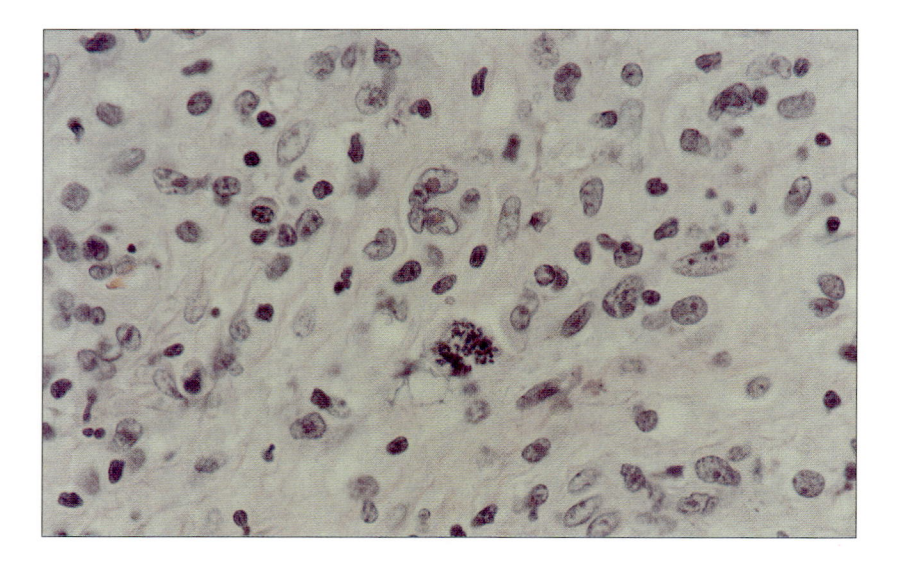

(c) High power shows small lymphocytes, plasma cells, histiocytes and occasional Reed–Sternberg cells and variants in a sclerotic background. (H&E stain)

Lymphocyte-predominant Hodgkin's disease

Figure 15.6

Lymphocyte-predominant Hodgkin's disease:

(a) Microscopic examination shows a lymph node with a nodular proliferation of lymphoid cells and histiocytes. (H&E stain)

(b) Individual nodules are large and poorly circumscribed. (H&E stain)

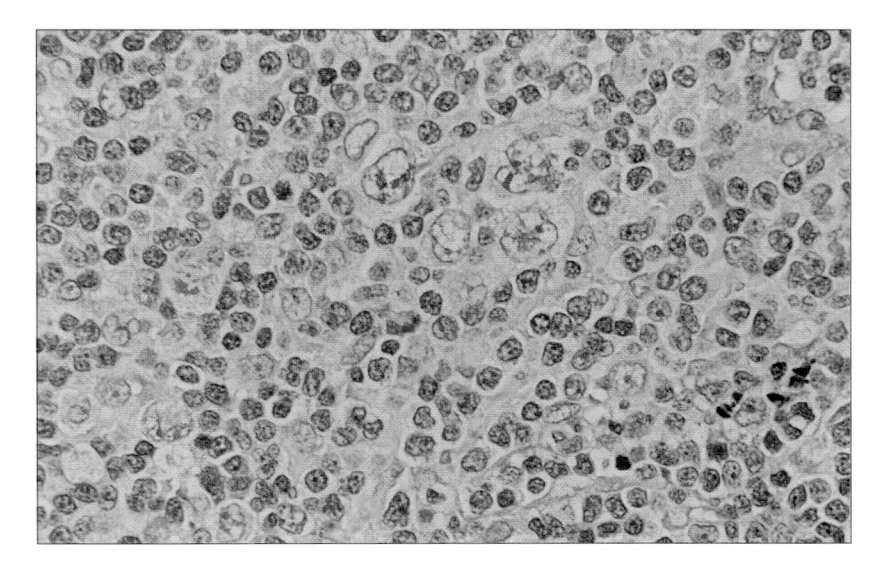

(c) The nodules contain lymphocytes, histiocytes and large atypical cells with pale, lobated nuclei, small nucleoli and relatively scant cytoplasm (L&H cells or 'popcorn' cells). (H&E stain)

Contd

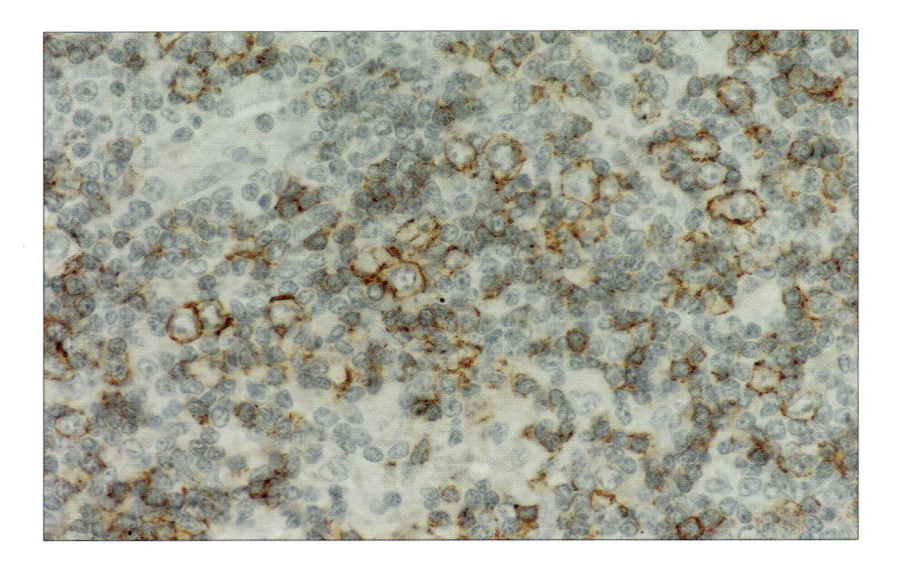

Figure 15.6 *continued*

(d) With antibodies to B cells (L26), the L&H cells and most small lymphocytes are stained. (Immunoperoxidase technique on paraffin sections)

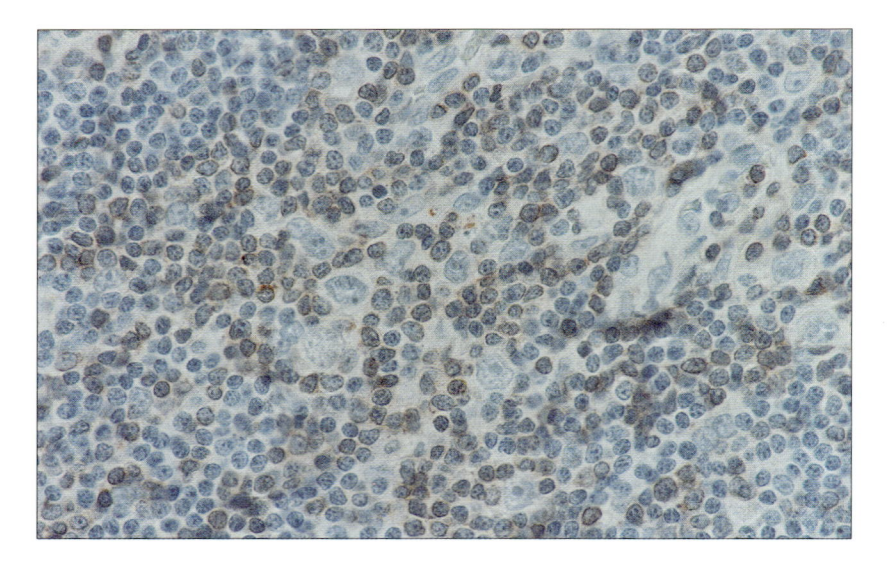

(e) With antibodies to T cells (CD3), there is staining of small lymphocytes surrounding the L&H cells. (Immunoperoxidase technique on paraffin sections)

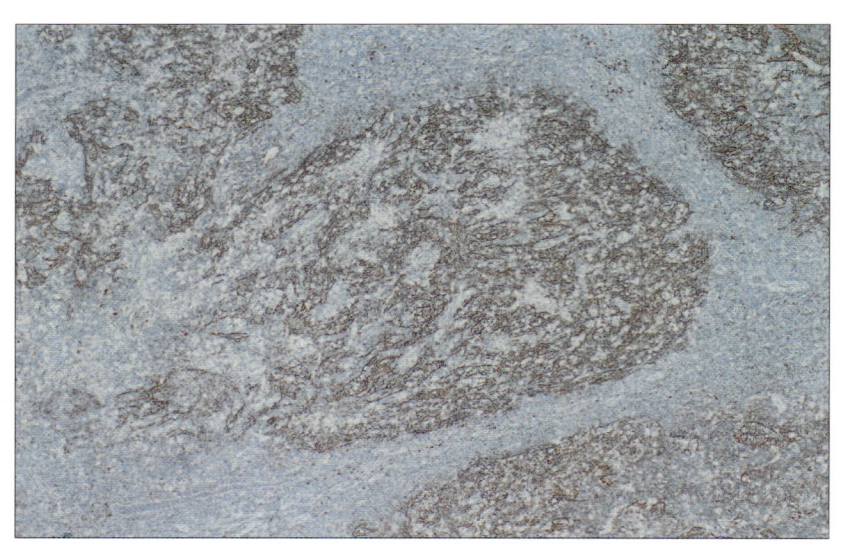

(f) An immunostain for CD21 (follicular dendritic cells) highlights the nodular pattern of the Hodgkin's disease. (Immunoperoxidase technique on paraffin sections)

Lymphocyte-rich classic Hodgkin's disease

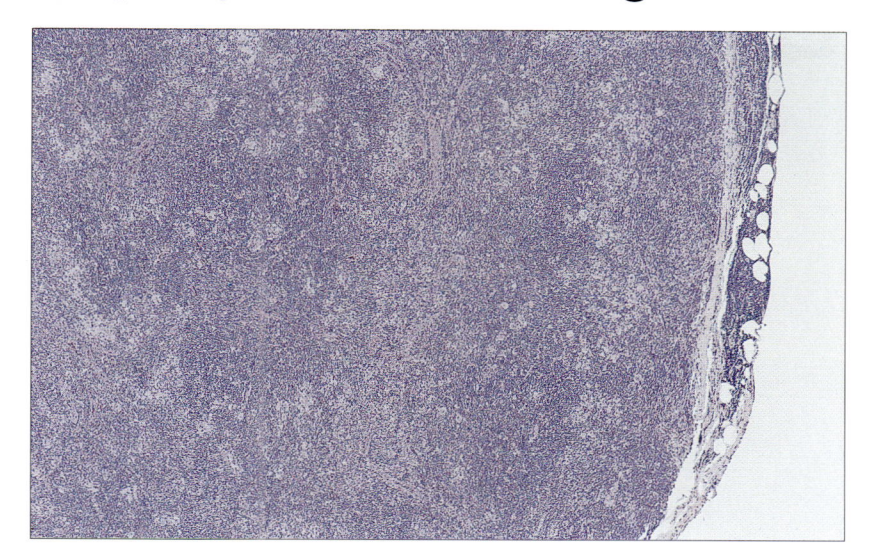

Figure 15.7

Lymphocyte-rich classic Hodgkin's disease:

(a) On low-power examination, the normal architecture of the lymph node is obliterated. (H&E stain)

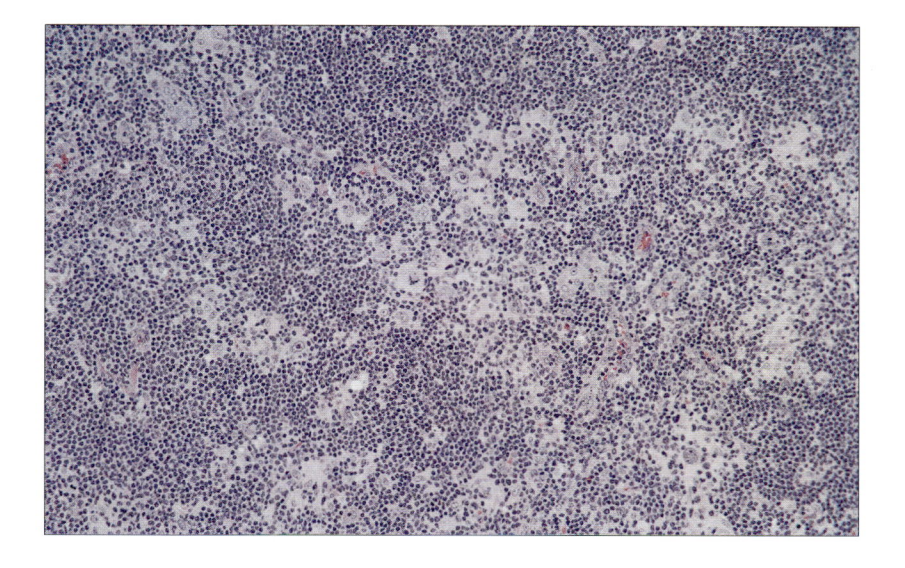

(b) Slightly higher power shows a proliferation with a mottled blue and pink color due to the admixture of lymphocytes and histiocytes. (H&E stain)

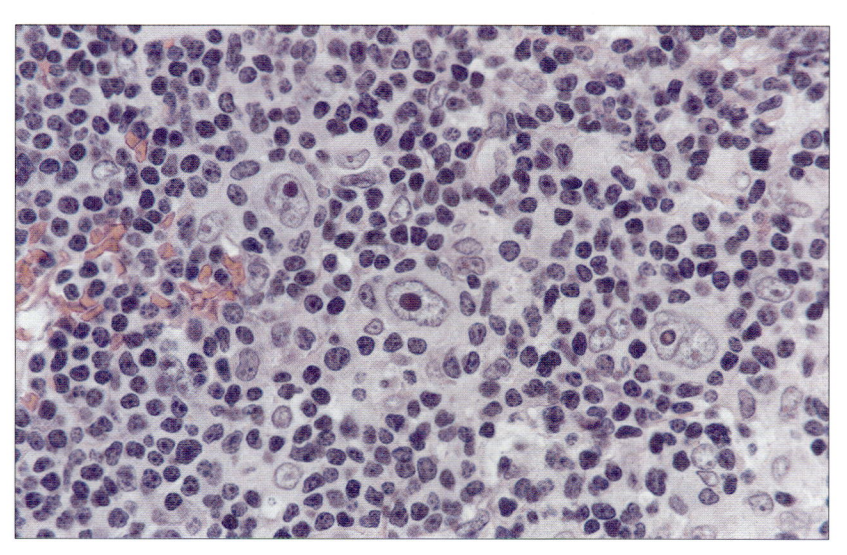

High power shows that the mononuclear Reed–Sternberg variants (c) and diagnostic Reed–Sternberg cells (d) have the morphology expected in classic Hodgkin's disease, rather than resembling the L&H cells of lymphocyte-predominant Hodgkin's disease. (H&E stain)

(c)

Contd

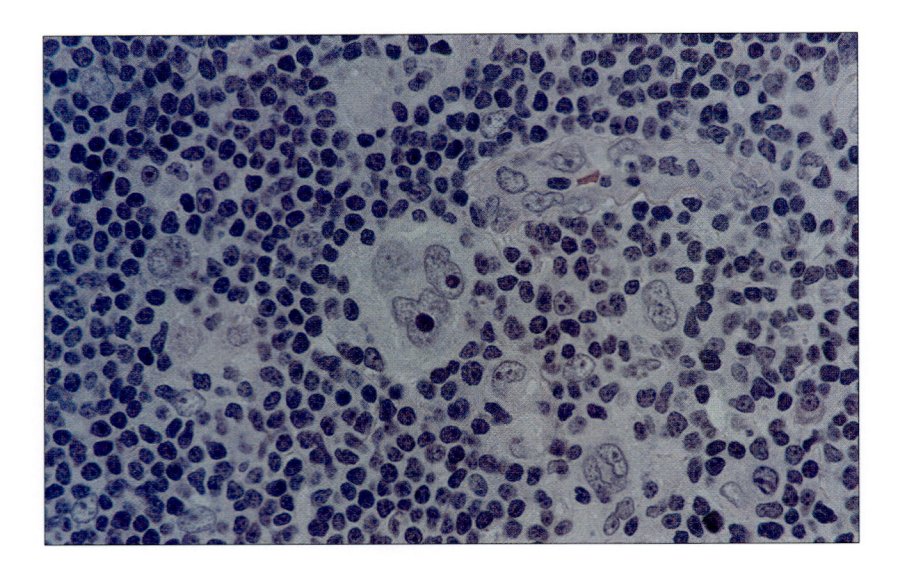

Figure 15.7 *continued*

(d)

Hodgkin's disease in the bone marrow

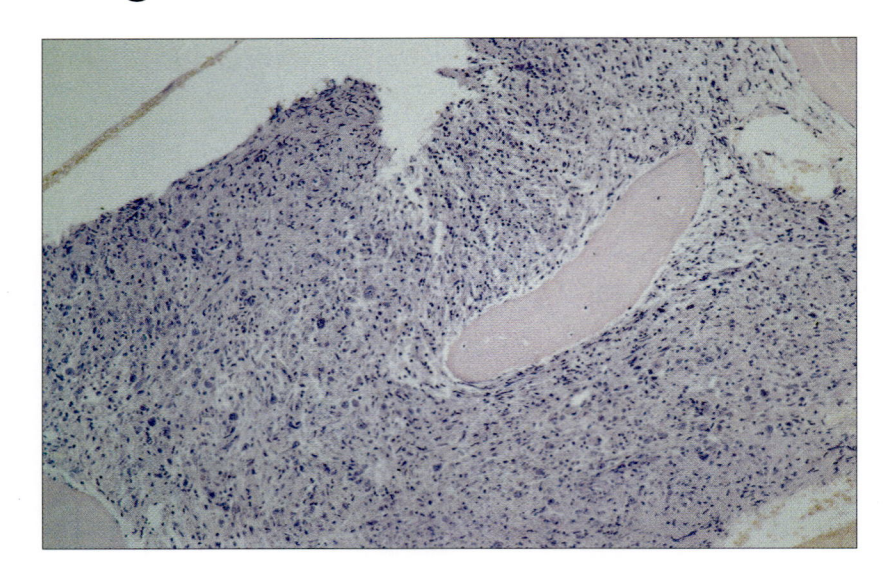

Figure 15.8

Hodgkin's disease in the bone marrow:

The patient was HIV+ and had a diagnosis of mixed-cellularity Hodgkin's disease in a lymph node. This marrow biopsy was obtained during staging.

(a) Low power shows a cellular infiltrate replacing normal marrow elements. (Giemsa stain)

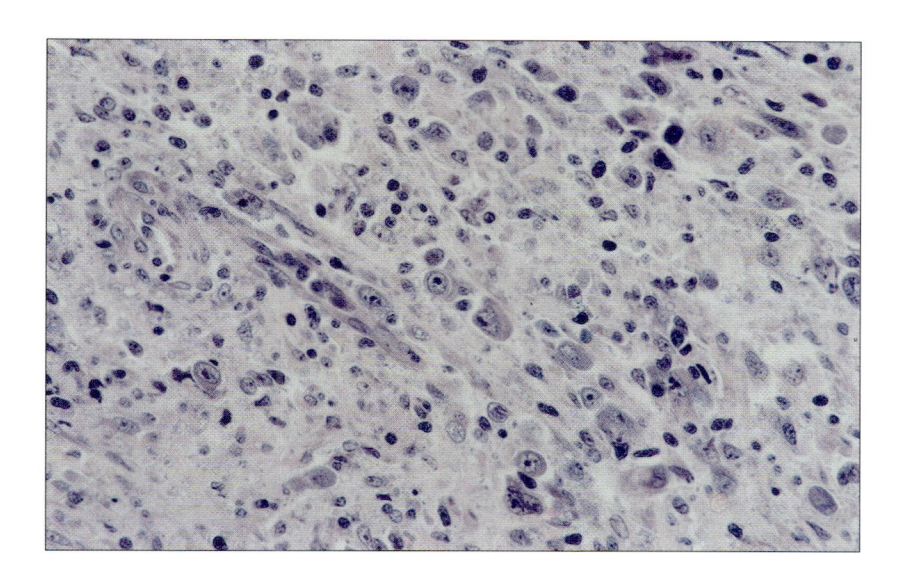

Figure 15.8 *continued*

(**b**) There is a mixture of small lymphocytes, histiocytes and large atypical cells with large nucleoli, consistent with mononuclear variants of Reed–Sternberg cells, in a fibrotic background. (Giemsa stain)

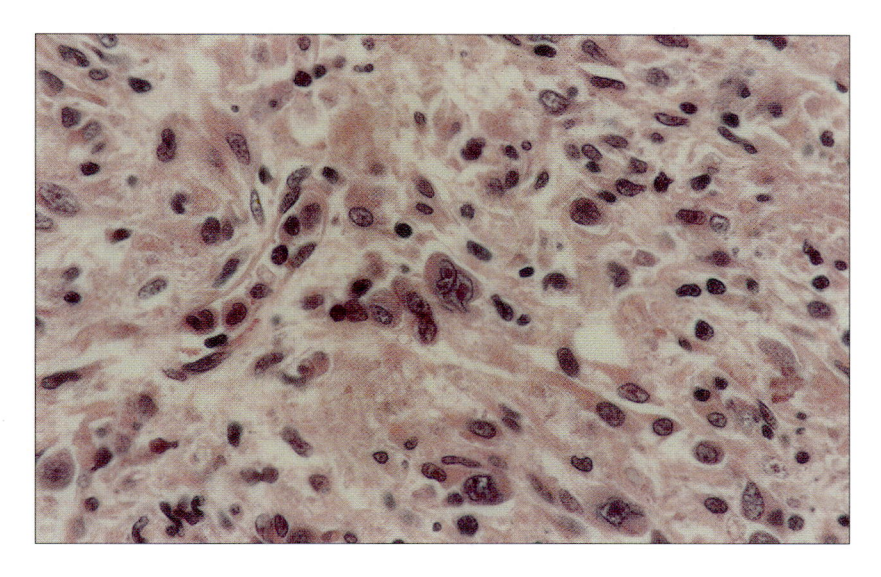

(**c**) Occasional binucleated Reed–Sternberg cells are also seen (center). (H&E stain)

16 Rare subtypes

The subtypes described in this chapter are not an official part of any of the new lymphoma classification schemes. The reasons for the omissions are several. In some cases, the entities are newly described (e.g. body cavity lymphoma). In others, their neoplastic nature is still being discussed (e.g. multicentric Castleman's disease). True histiocytic lymphoma and follicular dendritic cell sarcoma are derived from hematopoietic lineage cells but not lymphocytes, though they probably originate in lymph nodes. Angiotropic lymphoma is not yet an unequivocally distinct entity in that it can be of either B-cell or T-cell lineage and has protean manifestations; furthermore, no single measurable feature identifies it as distinct from other aggressive lymphomas – a defect it shares with T-cell-rich B-cell lymphoma.

The clinical approach to these lesions reflects an old saying: 'When the only tool you have is a hammer, the whole world looks like a nail'. The usual treatment given to patients presenting with these diagnoses is multiagent doxorubicin-containing chemotherapy. However, progress in understanding the causes and underlying biology of these disorders is beginning, and the management approach is bound to be altered by new information.

T-cell-rich B-cell lymphoma

A small percentage of diffuse aggressive-histology lymphomas comprise a mixture of B cells and T cells, with the T cells outnumbering the B cells by at least 2:1. Conventional phenotyping of the cells by flow cytometry reveals the numerical dominance of the T cells, but clonal T-cell receptor gene (*TCR*) rearrangements are not detectable. Instead, the minority B-cell population has a clonal rearrangement of the immunoglobulin genes. In some instances, the malignant B-cell clone is below the threshold of detectability by Southern analysis (<5%); when the percentage of malignant cells is small, diagnosis can be very difficult.

The morphologic picture is that of a mixed cellular infiltrate of small and large cells. The large cells are usually the malignant B cells, which occur singly or in small clusters, and the small cells are reactive polyclonal T cells. The majority of cases of T-cell-rich B-cell lymphoma are misdiagnosed. They are often confused with mixed-cellularity Hodgkin's disease or peripheral T-cell lymphoma. In one large series of peripheral T-cell lymphomas, 10% were actually T-cell-rich B-cell lymphomas. In the Working Formulation, most of these cases have been classified as diffuse mixed lymphoma. No unique features enable this subtype to be distinguished from other B-cell neoplasms. However, it seems likely that the neoplastic B cells produce a T-cell-attracting chemokine. Several candidates exist, but have not yet been assessed. These lymphomas do appear to produce large amounts of interleukin-4 (IL-4), but its relationship to the pathogenesis is unclear.

Patients with T-cell-rich B-cell lymphoma do not have distinctive clinical characteristics. Splenomegaly is present in about one-third; B symptoms are noted in one-half. The median age (53 years), sex distribution (M/F 1.4), and stage distribution are about the same as those of diffuse large B-cell lymphoma. Treatment with regimens used in diffuse large B-cell lymphoma appears to give similar results. In the author's experience (DLL), some of these patients carry a diffuse aggressive lymphoma designation, but they follow a chronic responding and relapsing course more suggestive of follicular lymphoma.

Angiotropic lymphoma

Angiotropic lymphoma has been called 'malignant angioendotheliomatosis', 'intravascular lymphoma' and 'angioendotheliomatosis proliferans systemisata' in various reports. The subtype is a very rare diffuse large B-cell lymphoma that is extranodal in nearly all cases, and has protean manifestations, including skin rash and telangiectasia (often the skin nodules are painful and present on the lower extremity), central nervous system (CNS) symptoms such as dementia and non-localizing functional deficits, respiratory failure from invasion of small lung vessels, adrenal failure, peripheral nerve dysfunction, skeletal muscle masses or myalgia, prostate enlargement, abdominal pain and ischemia from mesenteric vessel involvement, thyroid dysfunction and mass, lytic bone lesions, and others. Older patients are disproportionately affected. Although the tumor usually contains clonally rearranged immunoglobulin genes, occasional patients have tumors with T-cell markers and *TCR* gene rearrangements. The T-cell-derived lesions can show Epstein–Barr virus (EBV) infection. Rare patients have tumors expressing histiocyte markers. Patients often have B symptoms. They may have a history of an antecedent malignant lymphoma. The clinical manifestations of this subtype are so diverse and the disease is so rare that many patients die of progressive multiorgan failure without a definitive diagnosis. Clinicians who aggressively biopsy symptomatic sites or malfunctioning organs often make the diagnosis, and the disease appears to be highly responsive and curable with combination chemotherapy used in other diffuse large B-cell lymphomas. Without combination chemotherapy, the disease runs an aggressive course. The symptoms are generally caused by occlusion of small vessels with tumor cells and fibrin. It seems likely that the expression of a particular adhesion molecule on the tumor cell is responsible for its predilection to stick to endothelial surfaces.

Angiotropic lymphoma cases have been identified all over the world. However, a distinct variant appears to occur exclusively in Asians. Patients present with fever, hepatosplenomegaly and hemophagocytosis. The tumor is a neoplastic B cell, and it involves the bone marrow, liver and spleen, but it is accompanied by a hemophagocytosing histiocytic infiltrate. The disease is rapidly progressive, but spares the skin and CNS. The involvement of the bone marrow, the hemophagocytosis, and the skin-sparing and CNS-sparing distribution may make this disease a distinct variant of angiotropic lymphoma.

Primary effusion (body cavity) lymphoma

Primary effusion lymphoma is a B-cell lymphoma that occurs in effusions without associated tumor masses. This entity was first described in male patients infected with HIV and EBV. The neoplastic cells have a distinctive morphology that appears to be on a continuum between anaplastic large cell lymphoma and diffuse large B-cell lymphoma ('immunoblastic' in the terminology of the Working Formulation). Some cells are binucleate or trinucleate, and mitotic figures are frequent and often abnormal in appearance. Molecular characterization of these lymphomas demonstrated their clonal B-cell nature. All of the cases show infection with Kaposi's sarcoma-associated herpesvirus/human herpesvirus 8 (KSHV/HHV-8). Although coinfection with EBV is common, it is not universal, and the pattern of EBV gene expression is latency I: EBNA is the only viral gene product detected. This result suggests that EBV may be a cofactor in the initiation of the tumor, but that it is not required for its persistence. The tumor cells lack *BCL6* and *p53* gene alterations. They express and appear to respond to the KSHV viral IL-6, a virus-encoded cytokine that binds the IL-6 receptor. Thus an IL-6-based autocrine mechanism is hypothesized to be at work in this tumor. Efforts to use this pathway to treat the tumor have not yet been reported.

The role of HIV infection in the pathogenesis of the tumor is unclear; cases have been reported in HIV-uninfected women. However, KHSV is a universal feature. There are occasionally Burkitt's lymphomas in AIDS patients that manifest early as malignant effusions. However, these tumors all demonstrate c-*MYC* activation and are morphologically distinct from KHSV-associated body cavity lymphoma. Primary effusion lymphoma is also distinct from pyothorax-associated lymphoma. Although the latter also produces malignant pleural effusions and is a diffuse large B-cell lymphoma according to the REAL and WHO classifications, it is pathogenetically distinct from primary effusion lymphoma. Pyothorax-associated lymphoma occurs in a distinctive clinical setting (decades after artificial pneumothorax treatment for tuberculosis); it is nearly always associated with EBV infection in which many EBV genes are expressed (latency III), and it is not associated with KSHV.

The median survival for patients with HIV infection and primary effusion lymphoma is about six months, which is similar to that for other lymphomas occurring in AIDS patients. The disease may spread viscerally late in its course, but it remains confined to a body cavity for much of its natural history. Combination chemotherapy may kill the tumor, but toxicity is too great in patients with underlying immune defects. Therapies aimed either at the IL-6 autocrine loop or at the KHSV virus may be more effective.

Multicentric Castleman's disease

Castleman's disease comes in two clinical forms and two morphologic forms. Clinically, the disease can be localized or multicentric (disseminated or generalized). The two morphologic types are hyaline vascular type and plasma cell type. The hyaline vascular type is always localized; the plasma cell type may be localized or multicentric. The disease is also known as 'angiofollicular lymphoid hyperplasia'; as originally described by Benjamin Castleman and his colleagues, the disease was a rare cause of a mediastinal mass. Subsequently, localized manifestations have been seen in many other sites.

The morphologic features of Castleman's disease are distinctive. In the hyaline vascular type, the involved lymph node retains a follicular pattern, but contains atypical large vessels. The follicles are hyperplastic, and capillary proliferation with endothelial hyperplasia is noted. In the plasma cell type, the altered germinal centers and vascular proliferation are accompanied by a prominent plasma cell infiltration. When Castleman's disease is localized, whether it is hyaline vascular type or plasma cell type in morphology, nearly all patients are curable with surgical resection of the mass. This lesion is fundamentally a hamartoma.

However, when the disease is more widespread, it reflects a systemic illness. Patients present with systemic symptoms in 95% of cases, including malaise, weakness, fever, night sweats, weight loss and anorexia. All patients have lymphadenopathy in multiple sites. About 80% have splenomegaly, 65% have hepatomegaly, 50% have edema or effusions, 37% have skin rashes, and about 25% have neurologic symptoms involving the CNS, peripheral nerves or both. The patients with neurologic symptoms appear to be a distinct subset with another rare systemic syndrome called POEMS: polyneuropathy, organomegaly, endocrinopathy, serum monoclonal M protein (and the clonal plasma cell disorder it implies, usually accompanied by osteosclerosis; the paraprotein nearly always contains λ light chains), and skin changes. Patients with multicentric Castleman's disease often have other autoimmune symptoms such as Raynaud's phenomenon, xerostomia, keratoconjunctivitis sicca and arthritis/arthralgia.

Nearly all patients are anemic at diagnosis. In addition, 20% are neutropenic, 60% are thrombocytopenic, 95% have elevated erythrocyte sedimentation rates, 85% have elevated gammaglobulin levels, all patients are hypoalbuminemic, and many have liver function test abnormalities and proteinuria. The clinical picture is one of a systemic acute-phase reaction. In keeping with that observation, patients often manifest elevated levels of IL-6 and IL-1β, cytokines involved in mediating the acute-phase reaction in response to immune activation.

Multicentric Castleman's disease is often associated with other conditions or tumors, such as lymphomas, Hodgkin's disease, Kaposi's sarcoma or AIDS. The clinical course untreated is progressive, with about three-quarters of patients dying of infection and one-quarter of a malignancy.

The fundamental nature of the disease is still unclear. The plasma cells infiltrating the lymph nodes are usually polyclonal, but occasionally they are monoclonal; the prognosis is apparently unaffected by the clonality of the plasma cell infiltrate. The plasma cells respond to IL-6, which was thought to be produced in this disease by the follicular dendritic cells that are present in the lymphoid follicles and that can be hyperplastic in this disease. However, another potential source is the viral IL-6 molecule encoded by the KSHV virus. All the patients with AIDS who develop Castleman's disease and about 40% of the Castleman's disease patients who do not have AIDS have KSHV sequences in their lesions. Current data are most consistent with the hypothesis that Castleman's disease is a non-neoplastic lymphoproliferative disorder driven by the overproduction of IL-6 from either endogenous or viral sources.

The approach to the therapy of multicentric Castleman's disease is largely determined by the degree to which it is the cause of the patient's morbidity. In patients without AIDS, Castleman's disease is often the most serious and life-threatening condition. Glucocorticoids can alleviate the symptoms, at least temporarily, for patients without neuropathy (i.e. without POEMS), but they are not effective in the long term and do not work at all in POEMS patients. Experience with combination chemotherapy is limited, but the approach appears to be more successful than single-agent glucocorticoids at controlling the disease. Anecdotal evidence that antibody to IL-6 may alleviate the systemic manifestations of multicentric Castleman's disease leads to optimism that a biologic approach aimed at blocking the IL-6 receptor might be of benefit.

True histicytic lymphoma

About 0.5–1% of lymphomas diagnosed as diffuse large cell lymphoma are actually true histiocytic lymphomas, the malignant cells of which are derived from phagocytic histiocytic cells. There are two main types of histiocytes: those that are specialized to present antigens to T and B cells are called dendritic cells, and those that are specialized to phagocytose cellular debris are called phagocytes. Abnormal proliferative disorders of the two lineages can be either benign reactive processes or neoplastic processes. The reactive disorders of phagocytes include the hemophagocytic syndromes, sinus histiocytosis with massive lymphadenopathy (Rosai–Dorfman disease), and histio- cytic necrotizing lymphadenitis (Kikuchi's disease). Neoplasias of phagocytes are very rare, and include malignant histiocytosis and true histicytic lymphoma. The disorders of antigen-presenting cells (dendritic cells) are discussed in the next section.

Malignant histiocytosis (MH) and true histiocytic lymphoma are thought to be derived from distinct types of phagocytes: MH from circulating monocytes or tissue macrophages, and true histiocytic lymphoma from fixed tissue histiocytes. The differences between the cells can be subtle. Lymph nodes in patients with true histiocytic lymphoma show diffuse effacement or a paracortical pattern of infiltration. The malignant cells have abundant eosinophilic cytoplasm and large, indented eccentrically placed nuclei with prominent nucleoli. The cells maintain their immune receptor genes in germline configuration and express CD11c, CD14, CD68 and HLA-DR on their surface. Histochemical staining for non-specific esterase is positive. The cells are negative for CD30 and epithelial membrane antigen – markers that are important in distinguishing true histiocytic lymphoma from sinusoidal anaplastic large cell lymphoma.

The clinical presentation is not readily distinguishable from that of other forms of aggressive lymphoma. Patients have diffuse adenopathy, and may have extranodal sites of disease – especially the skin. Patients with MH are usually sicker; they have systemic symptoms, fever, wasting, hepatosplenomegaly and pancytopenia. Patients with true histiocytic lymphoma are rarely diagnosed accurately before treatment, and they usually receive multiagent doxorubicin-containing chemotherapy, just like other patients with diffuse large cell lymphoma. The experience in any single institution or study is not great enough to allow firm conclusions to be drawn, but it appears that these patients have a similar outcome to patients with diffuse large B-cell lymphoma.

Follicular dendritic cell sarcoma

Reactive proliferative disorders of dendritic cells include dermatopathic lymphadenitis, seen in cutaneous T-cell lymphoma, and Langerhans cell histiocytosis (histiocytosis X), a group of illnesses usually localized to bone that manifest most commonly in childhood. Malignancy of dendritic cells is called 'follicular dendritic cell sarcoma' and is very rare. In a series of 17 patients, the median age of disease onset was 40 years, with a slight female predominance. About half the patients had adenopathy, and 10 had involvement of extranodal sites. Two patients had localized hyaline vascular-type Castleman's disease. Adenopathy was quite large, the median being nearly 7 cm in diameter. The histologic picture features a storiform or fascicular pattern of growth of spindle-shaped or polygonal cells with oval nuclei, vesicular nucleoli and well-defined nucleoli. The tumor cells express CD21, CD35 and epithelial membrane antigen (EMA); half the cases expressed desmoplakin, but no case expressed cytokeratin. Electron microscopy demonstrated the presence of villous processes connecting to other cells by desmosomes. EBV infection was rare. With a median follow-up of three years, only 3 of 13 patients had died. However, the best therapeutic approach to these patients has not been defined.

Bibliography

Beck JT, Hsu SM, Wijdenes J et al, Brief report: alleviation of systemic manifestations of Castleman's disease by monoclonal anti-interleukin-6 antibody. *N Engl J Med* 1994; **330**: 602–5.

Carter DK, Batts KP, deGrouen PC, Kurtin PJ, Angiotropic large cell lymphoma (intravascular lymphomatosis) occurring after follicular small cleaved cell lymphoma. *Mayo Clin Proc* 1996; **71**: 869–73.

Chan JK, Fletcher CD, Nayler SJ, Cooper K, Follicular dendritic cell sarcoma. Clinicopathologic analysis of 17 cases suggesting a malignant potential higher than currently recognized. *Cancer* 1997; **79**: 294–313.

Egeler RM, Schmitz L, Sonneveld P et al, Malignant histiocytosis: a reassessment of cases formerly classified as histiocytic neoplasms and review of the literature. *Med Pediatr Oncol* 1995; **25**: 1–7.

Ferry JA, Harris NL, Picker LJ et al, Intravascular lymphomatosis (malignant angioendotheliomatosis): a B-cell neoplasm expressing surface homing receptors. *Mod Pathol* 1988; **1**: 444–52.

Gherardi RK, Belec L, Fromont G et al, Elevated levels of interleukin-1β (IL-1β) and IL-6 in serum and increased production of IL-1β mRNA in lymph nodes of patients with polyneuropathy, organomegaly, endocrinopathy, M protein, and skin changes (POEMS) syndrome. *Blood* 1994; **83**: 2587–93.

Gonzalez CL, Jaffe ES, The histiocytoses: clinical presentation and differential diagnosis. *Oncology* 1990; **4**: 47–60.

Greer JP, Macon WR, Lamar RE et al, T-cell-rich B-cell lymphomas: diagnosis and response to therapy of 44 patients. *J Clin Oncol* 1995; **13**: 1742–50.

Horenstein MG, Nador RG, Chadburn A et al, Epstein–Barr virus latent gene expression in primary effusion lymphomas containing Kaposi's sarcoma-associated herpesvirus/human herpes virus-8. *Blood* 1997; **90**: 1186–91.

Kamel OM, Gocke CD, Kell DL et al, True histiocytic lymphoma: a study of 12 cases based on current definition. *Leuk Lymphoma* 1995; **18**: 81–6.

Levine EG, Hanson CA, Jaszcz W, Peterson BA, True histiocytic lymphoma. *Semin Oncol* 1991; **18**: 39–49.

McCarty MJ, Vukelja SJ, Banks PM, Weiss RB, Angiofollicular lymph node hyperplasia (Castleman's disease). *Cancer Treat Rev* 1995; **21**: 291–310.

Macon WR, Cousar JB, Waldron JA et al, Interleukin-2 may contribute to the abundant T-cell reaction and paucity of neoplastic B cells in T-cell-rich B-cell lymphoma. *Am J Pathol* 1992; **141**: 1031–6.

Murase T, Nakamura S, Tashiro K et al, Malignant histiocytosis-like B-cell lymphoma, a distinct pathologic variant of intravascular lymphomatosis: a report of five cases and review of the literature. *Br J Haematol* 1997; **99**: 656–64.

Nador RG, Cesarman E, Chadburn A et al, Primary effusion lymphoma: a distinct clinicopathologic entity associated with the Kaposi's sarcoma-associated herpes virus. *Blood* 1996; **88**: 645–56.

Parravinci C, Corbellino M, Paulli M et al, Expression of a virus-derived cytokine, KSHV vIL-6 in HIV-seronegative Castleman's disease. *Am J Pathol* 1997; **151**: 1517–22.

Peterson BA, Frizzera G, Multicentric Castleman's disease. *Semin Oncol* 1993; **20:** 636–47.

Rodriguez J, Pugh WC, Cabanillas F, T-cell-rich B-cell lymphoma. *Blood* 1993; **82:** 1586–9.

Said JW, Tasaka T, Takeuchi S et al, Primary effusion lymphoma in women: report of two cases of Kaposi's sarcoma herpes virus-associated effusion-based lymphoma in human immunodeficiency virus-negative women. *Blood* 1996; **88:** 3124–8.

Sanna P, Bertoni F, Roggero E et al, Angiotropic (intravascular large cell lymphoma): case report and short discussion of the literature. *Tumori* 1997; **83:** 772–5.

Sheibani K, Battifora H, Winberg CD et al, Further evidence that malignant angioendotheliomatosis is an angiotropic large cell lymphoma. *N Engl J Med* 1986; **314:** 943–8.

Soubrier MJ, Dubost JJ, Sauvezie BJ, POEMS syndrome: a study of 25 cases and a review of the literature. *Am J Med* 1994; **97:** 543–53.

Soulier J, Grollet L, Oksenhendler E et al, Molecular analysis of clonality in Castleman's disease. *Blood* 1995; **86:** 1131–8.

Soulier J, Grollet L, Oksenhendler E et al, Kaposi's sarcoma-associated herpesvirus-like DNA sequences in multicentric Castleman's disease. *Blood* 1995; **86:** 1276–80.

Stroup RM, Sheibani K, Moncada A et al, Angiotropic (intravascular) large cell lymphoma. A clinicopathologic study of seven cases with unique clinical presentations. *Cancer* 1990; **66:** 1781–8.

Szekely L, Chen F, Teramoto N et al, Restricted expression of Epstein–Barr virus (EBV)-encoded, growth transformation-associated antigens in an EBV- and human herpesvirus type 8-carrying body cavity lymphoma line. *J Gen Virol* 1998; **79:** 1445–52.

Tanier P, Manai A, Charpentier R et al, Pyothorax-associated lymphoma: relationship with Epstein–Barr virus, human herpes virus-8 and body cavity-based high grade lymphomas. *Eur Respir J* 1998; **11:** 779–83.

T-cell-rich B-cell lymphoma

Figure 16.1

T-cell-rich B-cell lymphoma:

This lymphoma involves perisplenic lymph nodes (**a**), and has also formed large nodules in the spleen (**b**). (H&E stain)

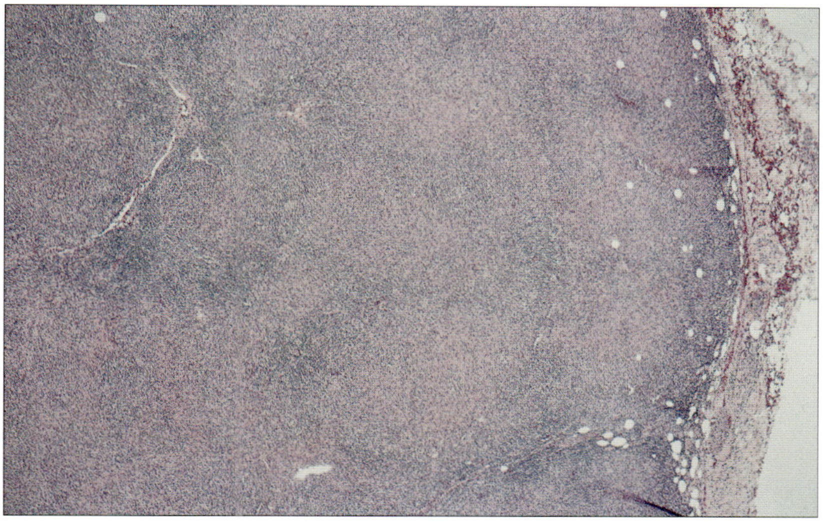

(a)

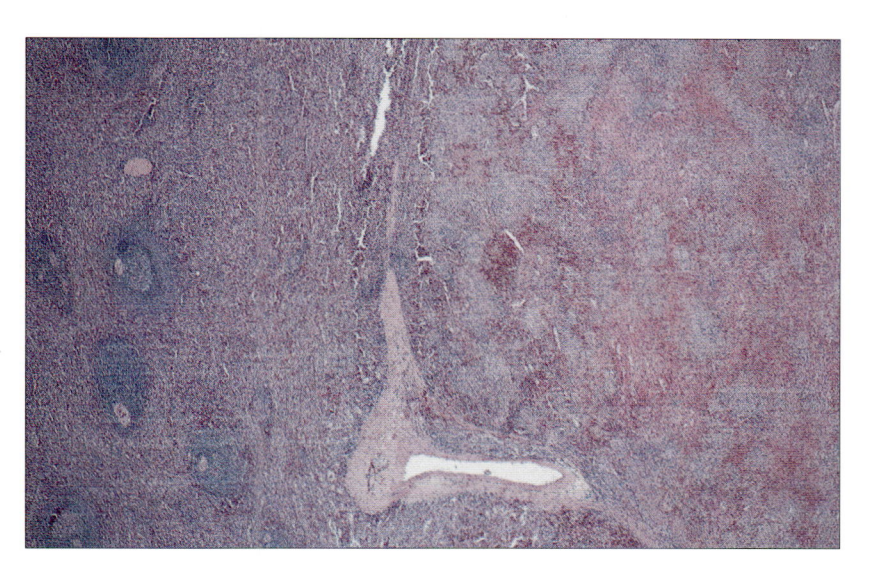

(b)

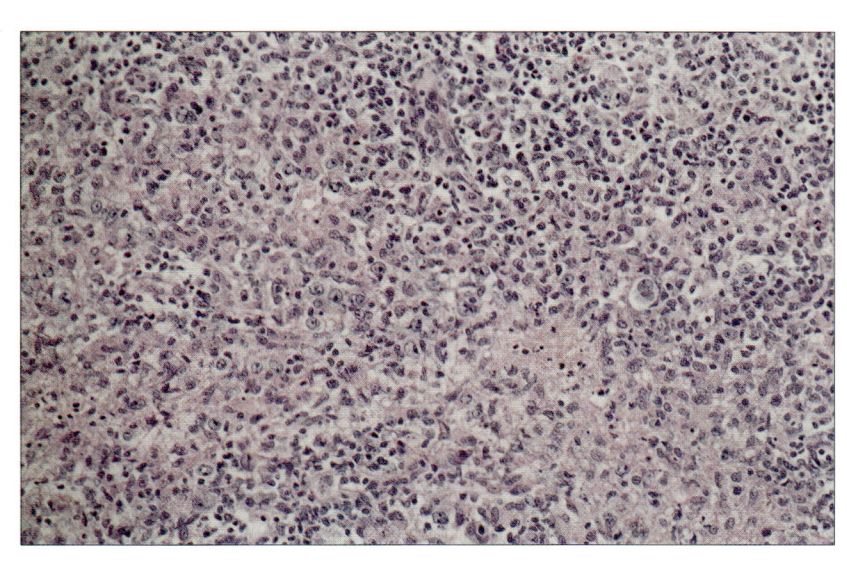

(c) Most cells present are lymphocytes and histiocytes. (H&E stain)

Contd

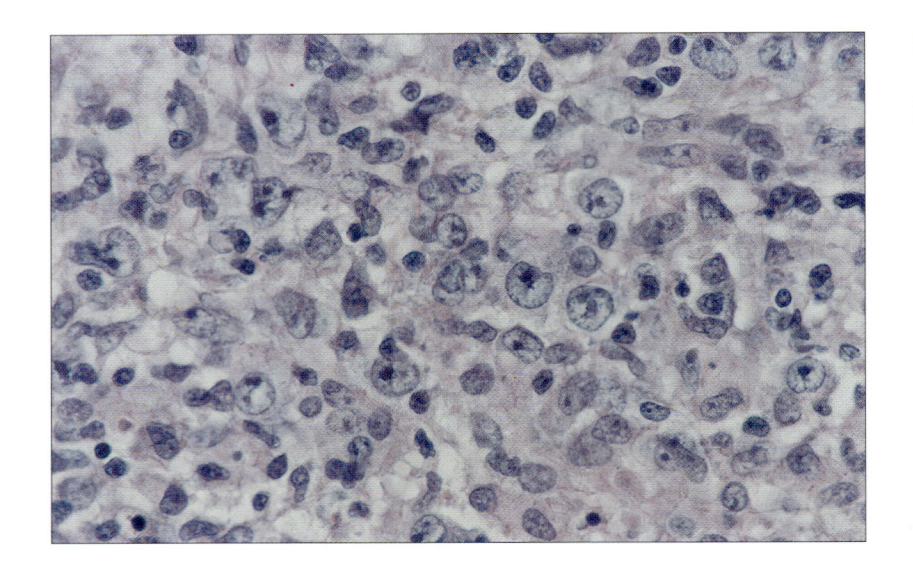

Figure 16.1 *continued*

(d) Scattered among the reactive cells are occasional large lymphoid cells, many of which resemble immunoblasts. (H&E stain)

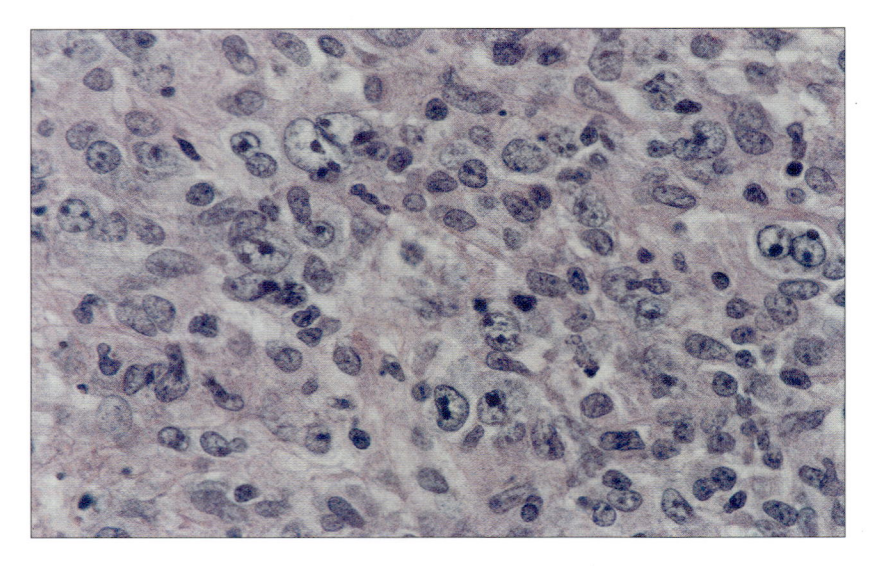

(e) A few binucleated neoplastic cells are seen (H&E stain)

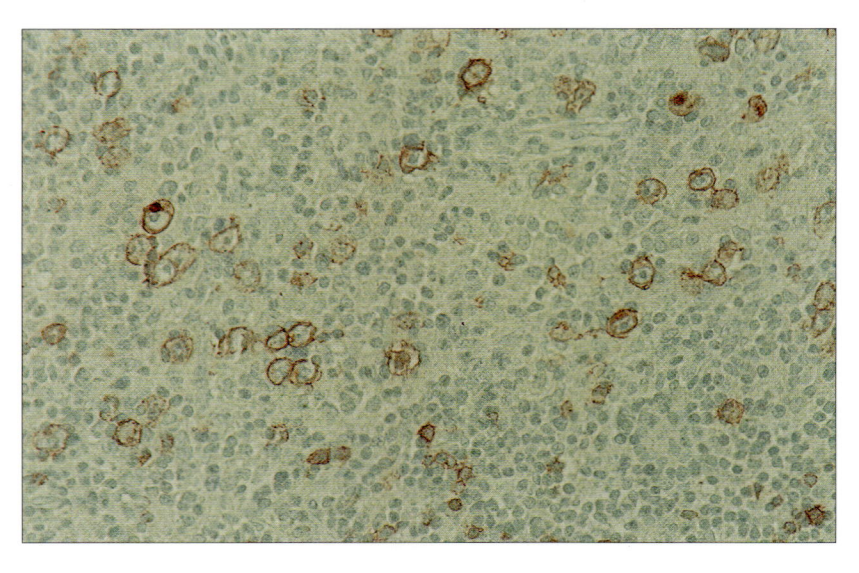

Large cells are CD20$^+$ (f) and CD15$^-$ (g), consistent with B cells. (Immunoperoxidase technique on paraffin sections)

(f)

Rare subtypes

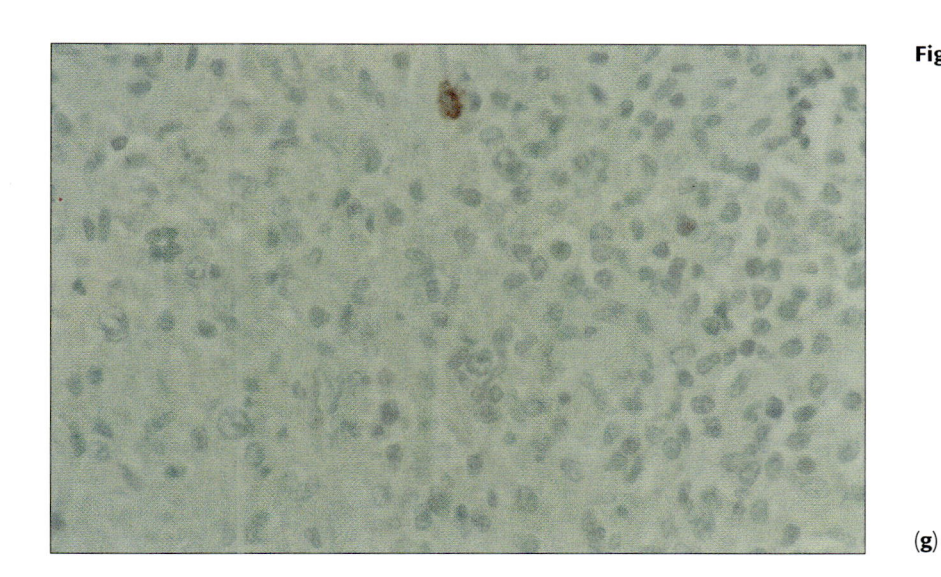

Figure 16.1 *continued*

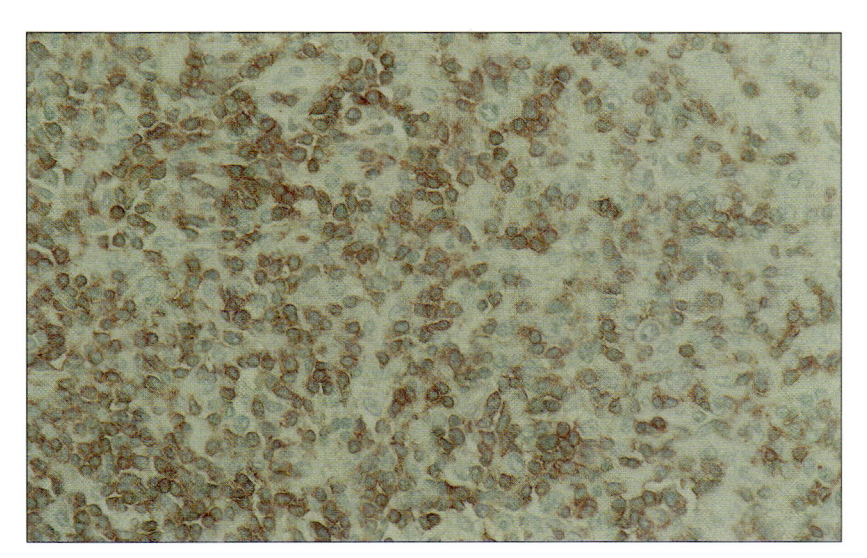

(g)

(h) The majority of cells present, however, are small cells of T lineage (CD3⁺). (Immunoperoxidase technique on paraffin sections)

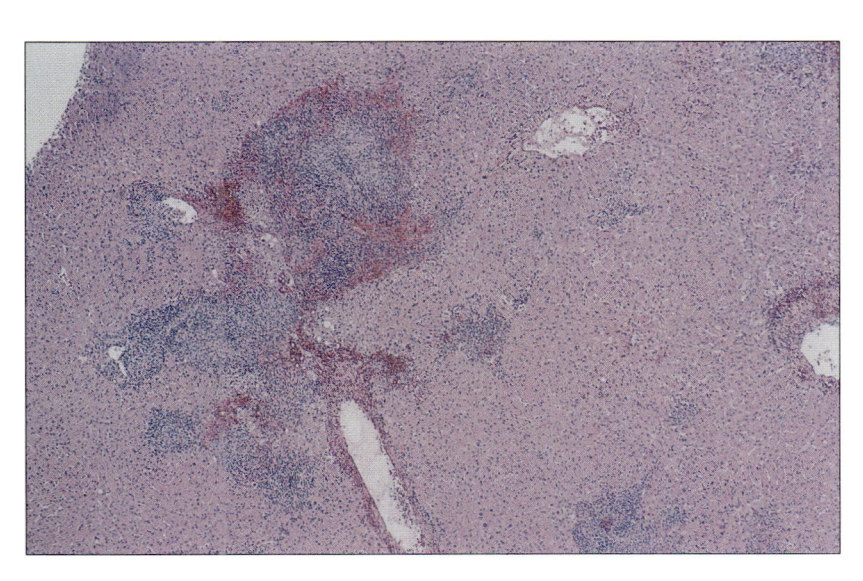

The liver is also involved by lymphoma. Low power (i) shows irregular aggregates of lymphoid cells. Medium power (j) shows a mixture of lymphocytes and histiocytes, similar to that seen in the spleen and lymph node. High power (k) shows a few large atypical lymphoid cells in a background of small lymphocytes. (H&E stain)

(i)

Contd

Figure 16.1 *continued*

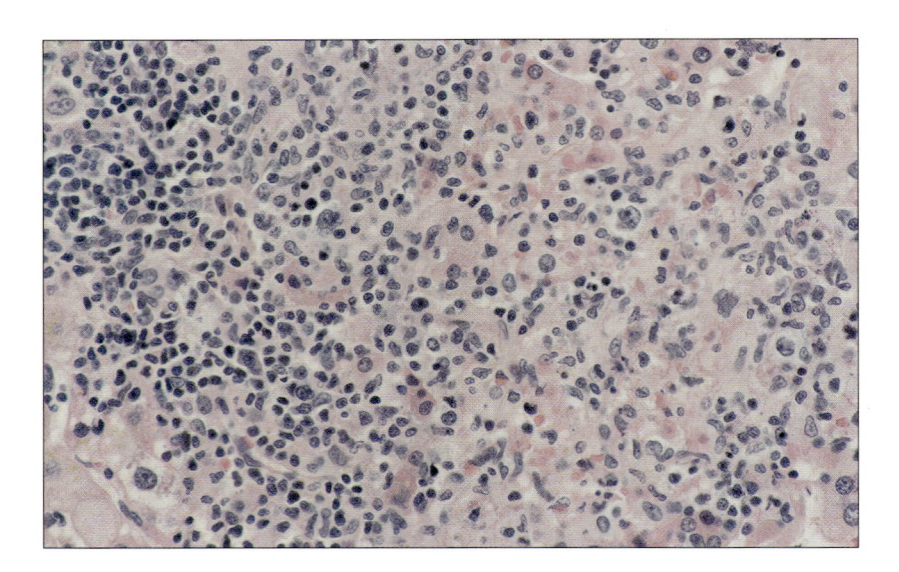

(j)

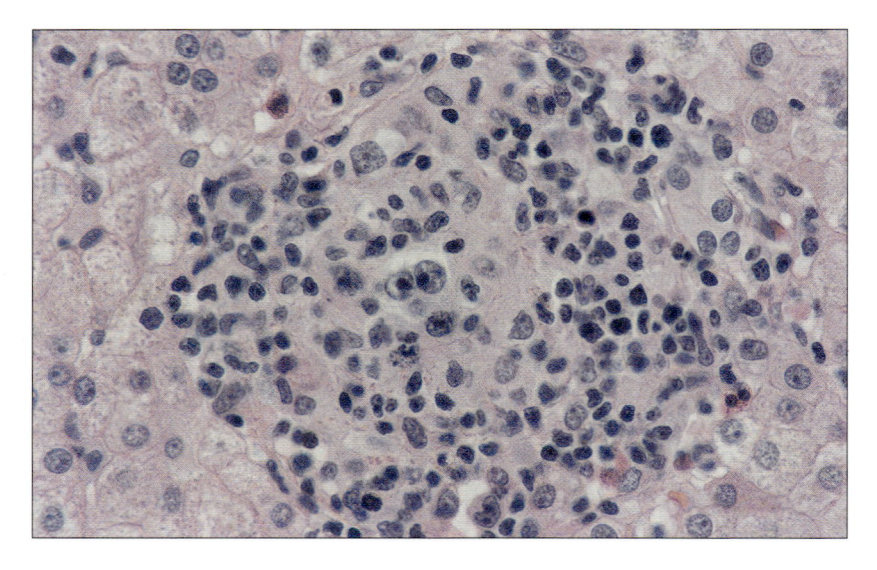

(k)

Angiotrophic lymphoma

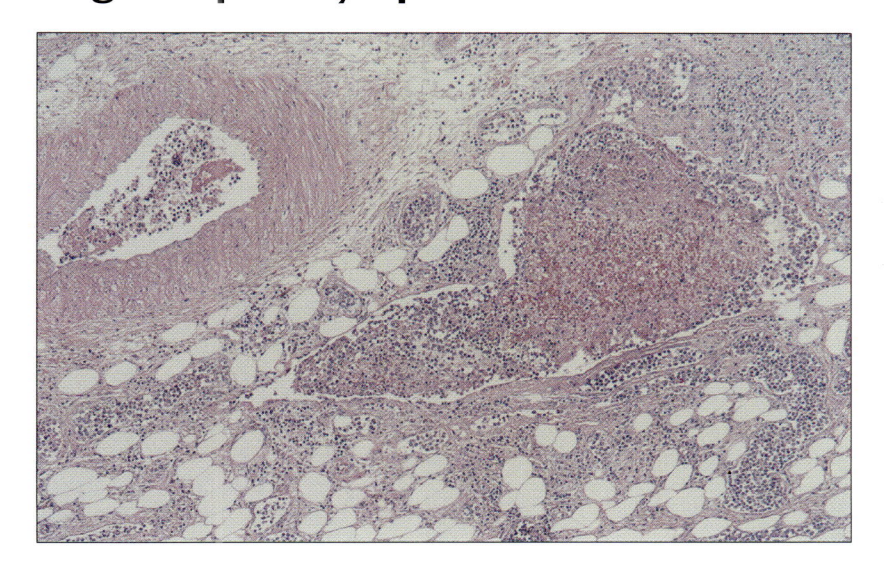

Figure 16.2

Angiotropic lymphoma:

(a) This case is associated with venous thrombosis. (H&E stain)

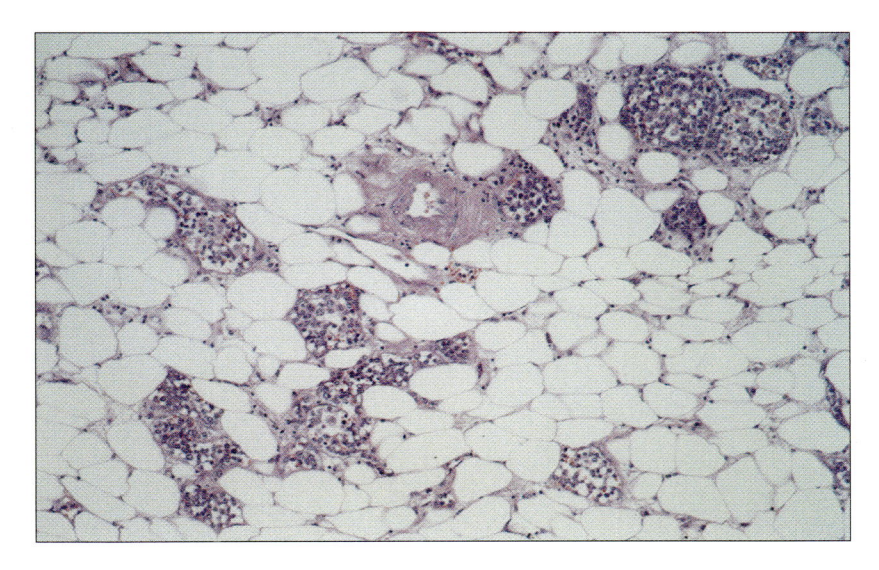

(b) Multiple small blood vessels contain atypical lymphoid cells. (H&E stain)

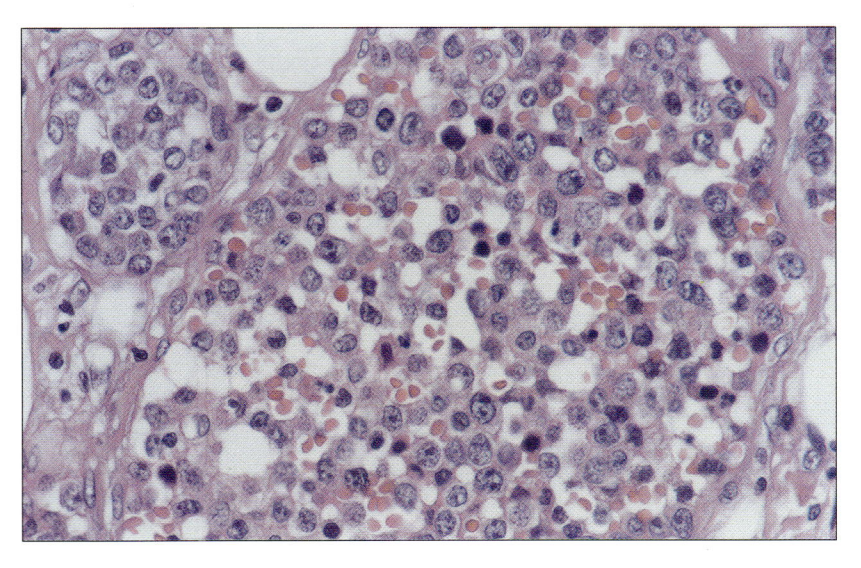

(c) High power shows large lymphoid cells with a moderate amount of pink cytoplasm. (H&E stain)

Contd

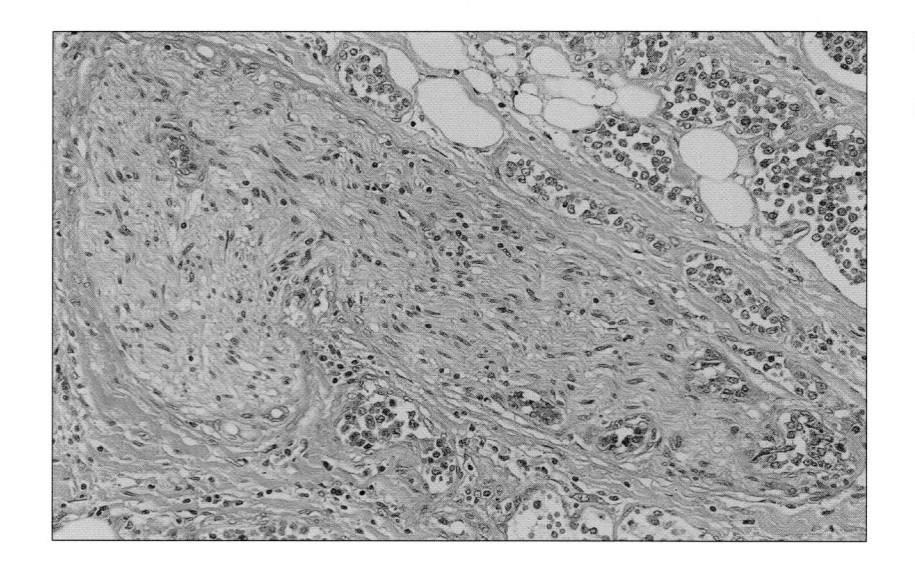

Figure 16.2 continued

(d) In this case, small blood vessels in and around nerves contain neoplastic cells. (H&E stain)

Primary effusion (body cavity) lymphoma

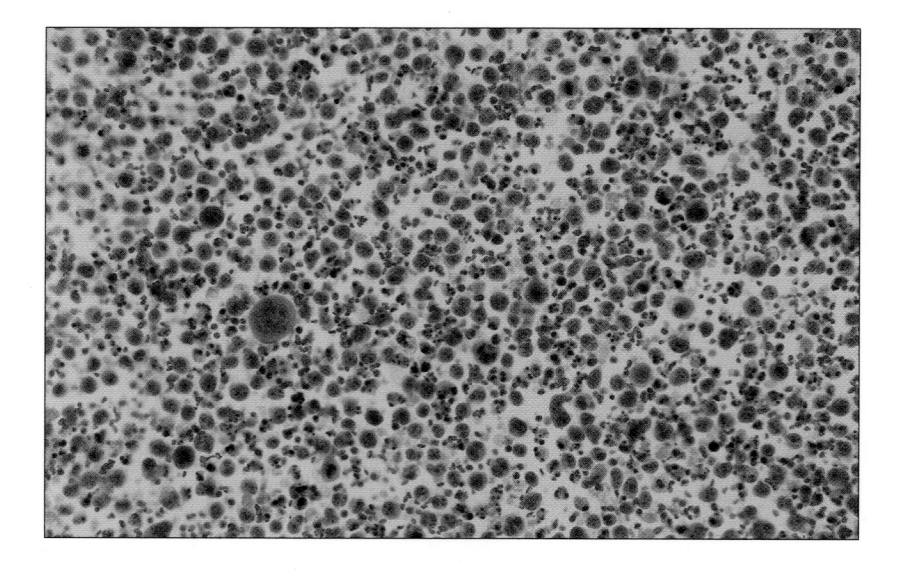

Figure 16.3

Primary effusion (body cavity) lymphoma:

(a) This pleural effusion is extremely cellular. (Papanicolaou stain)

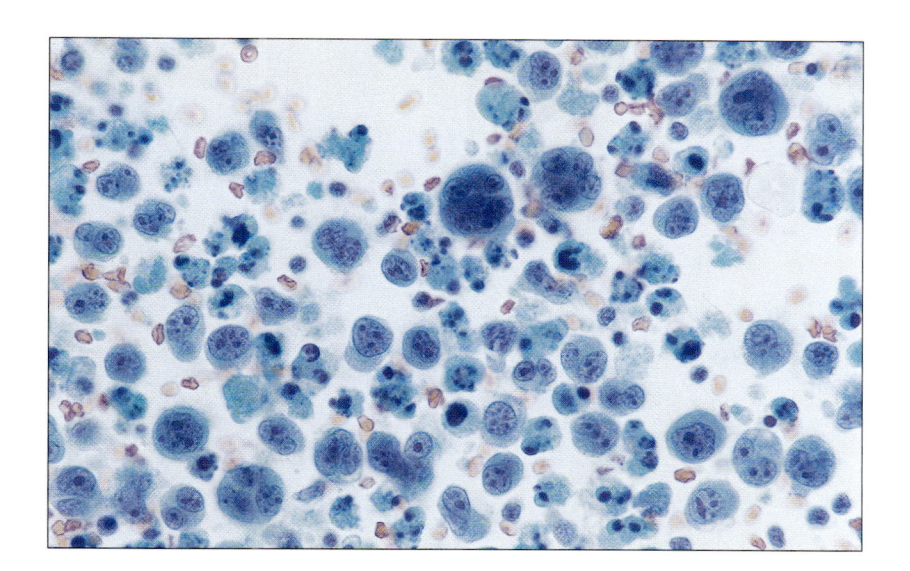

Figure 16.3 *continued*

(**b**) Higher power shows large atypical lymphoid cells, some of which are bi- or multinucleated. (Papanicolaou stain)

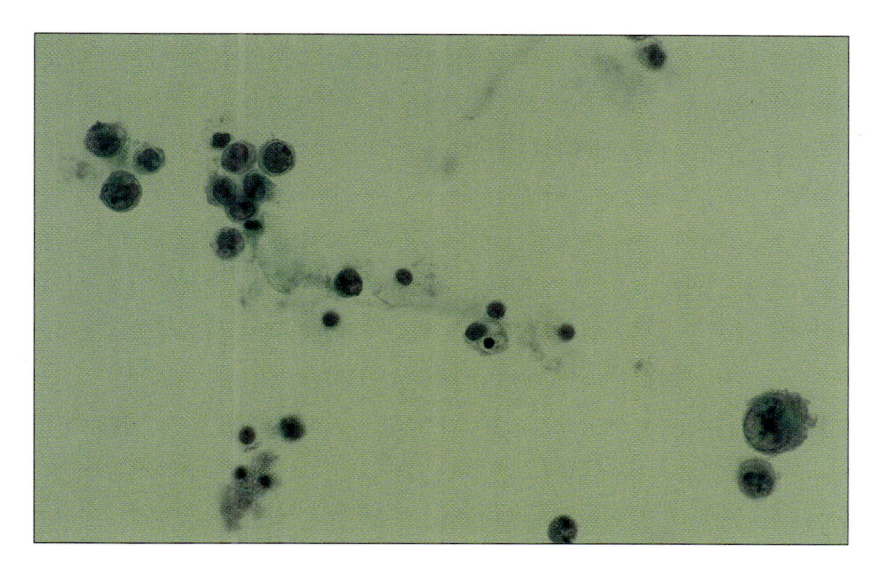

(**c**) In an example from another patient, the cytologic appearance is similar. (Papanicolaou stain)

Multicentric Castleman's disease, mixed type

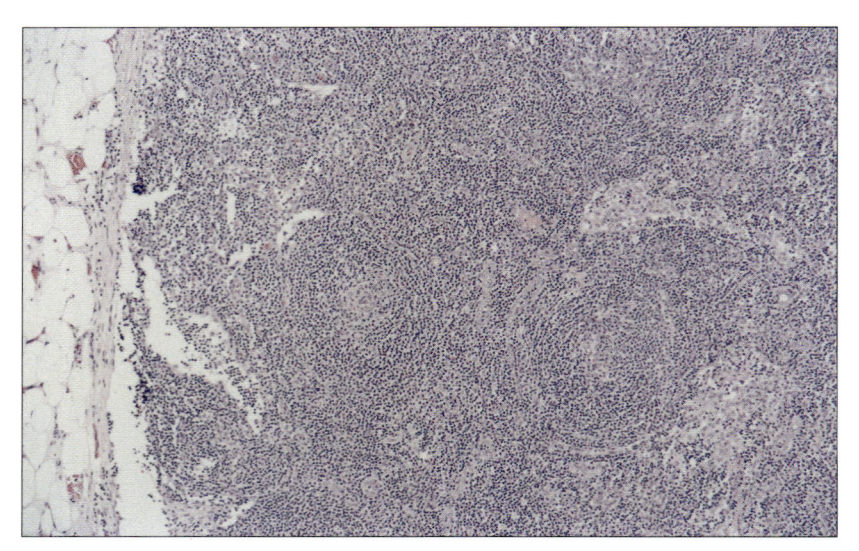

Figure 16.4

Multicentric Castleman's disease, mixed type (combination of hyaline vascular and plasma cell types):

(a) Lymph node showing distortion of the normal architecture by a proliferation of follicles with prominent mantle zones. Some sinuses remain patent. (H&E stain)

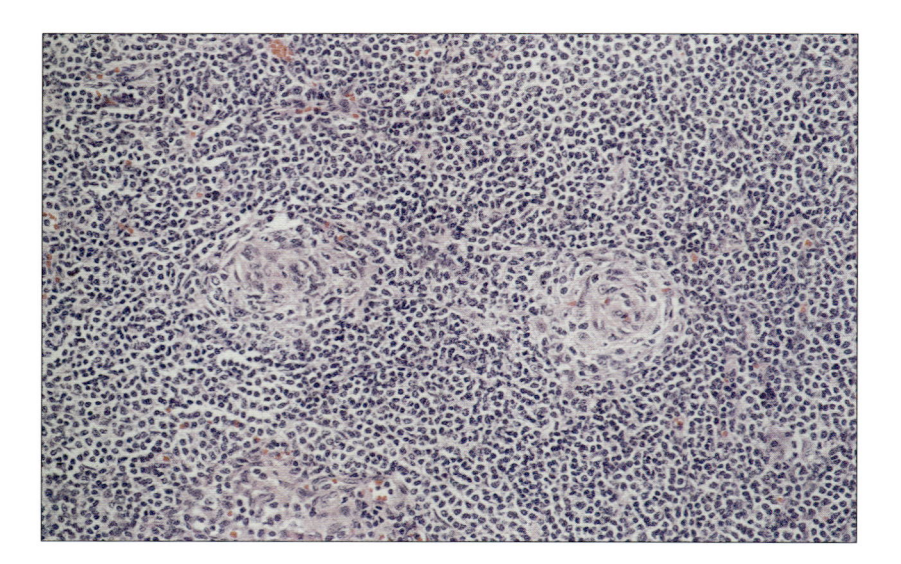

(b) The follicles have small, pink, sclerotic centers and broad mantles.

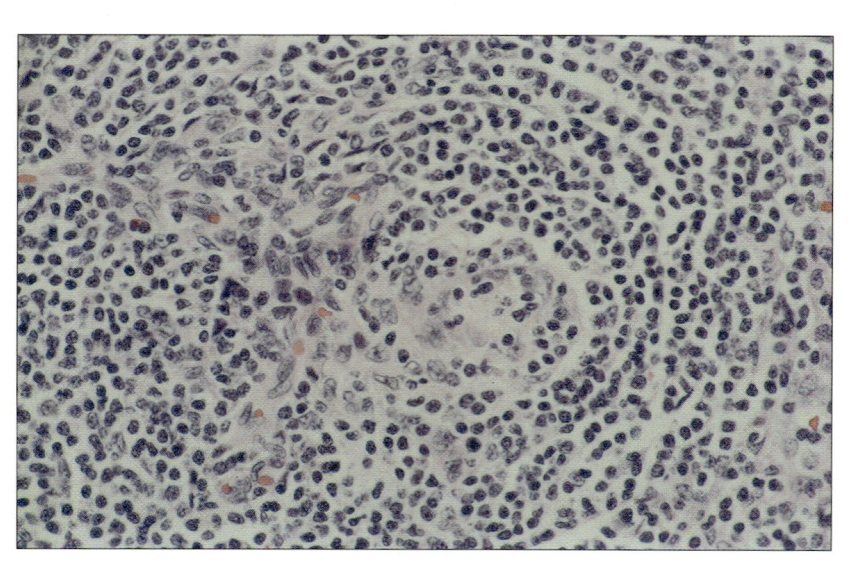

(c) The follicular centers contain a high proportion of follicular dendritic cells with pale nuclei, and relatively few lymphoid cells. The mantle-zone lymphocytes are arrayed in concentric rings. (H&E stain)

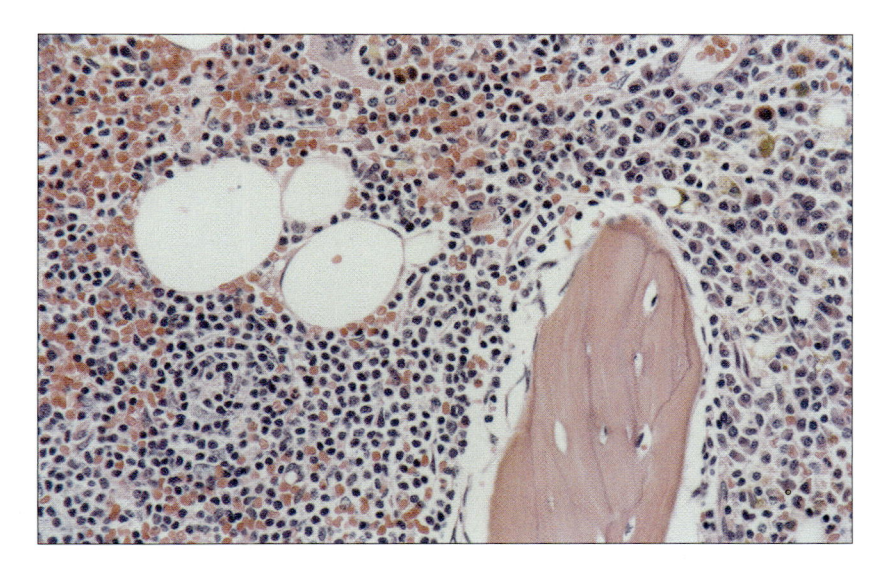

Figure 16.4 *continued*

(**d**) The marrow is also involved by Castleman's disease in this case. A lymphoid aggregate forming an ill-defined follicle is present on one side of the bony trabecula; a cluster of plasma cells is found on the opposite side. (H&E stain)

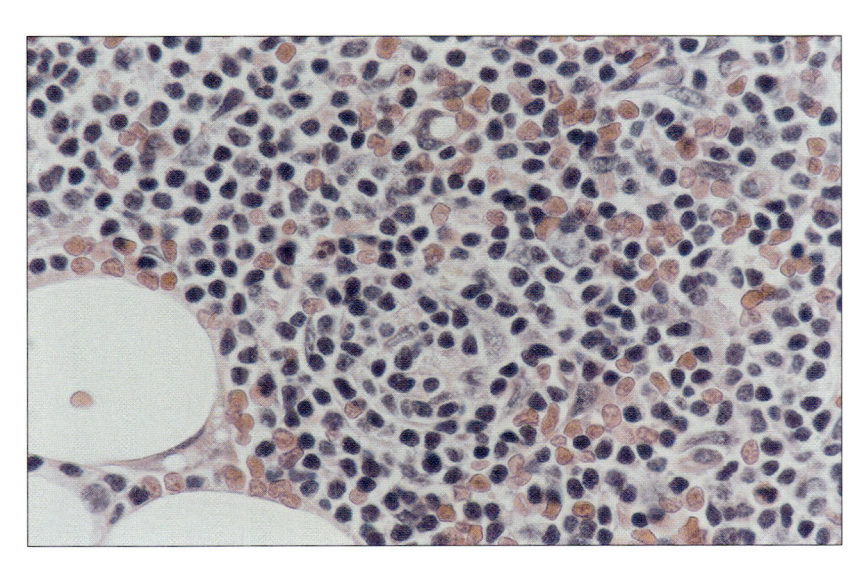

(**e**) Higher power shows the follicle with its inconspicuous follicular center and focal lining-up of lymphocytes along the processes of follicular dendritic cells. (H&E stain)

True histiocytic lymphoma

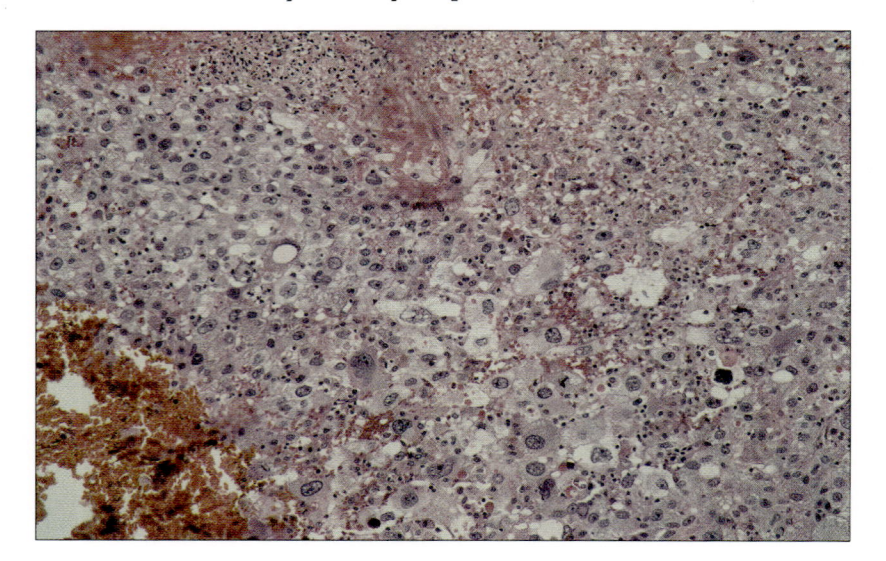

Figure 16.5

A possible case of true histiocytic lymphoma:

Low power shows a cellular tumor with areas of hemorrhage (**a**) and necrosis (**b**). (H&E stain)

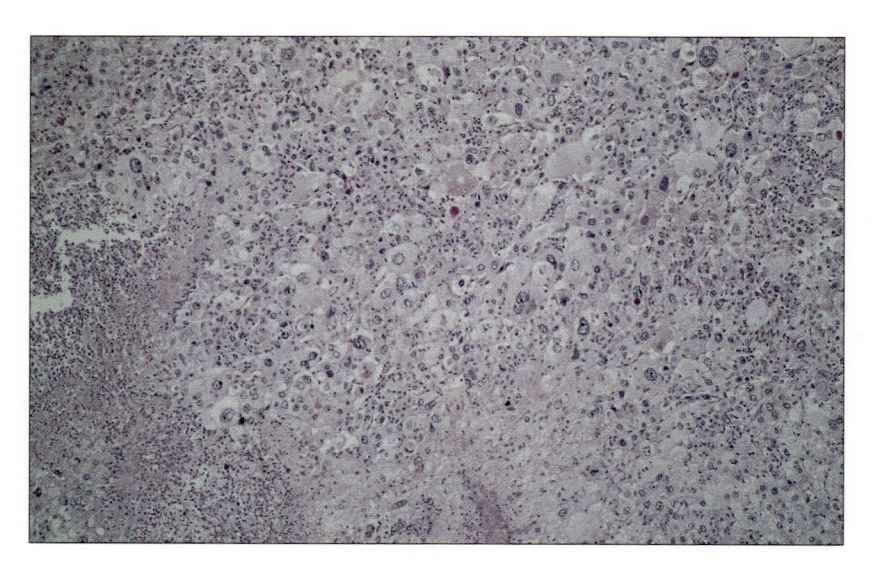

(a)

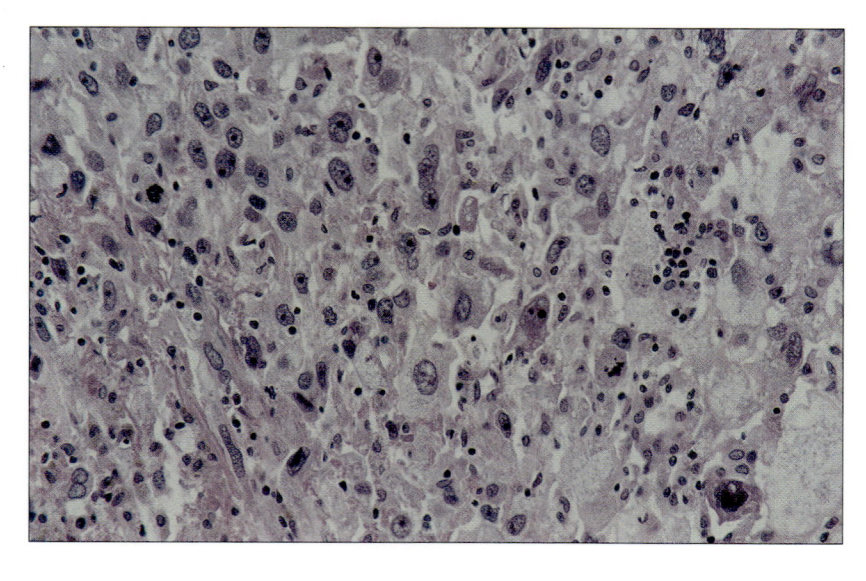

(b)

Medium- and high-power views (**c–f**) show an extremely pleomorphic neoplasm composed of very large, polygonal cells with bizarre nuclei and abundant pale cytoplasm. (H&E stain)

(c)

Figure 16.5 *continued*

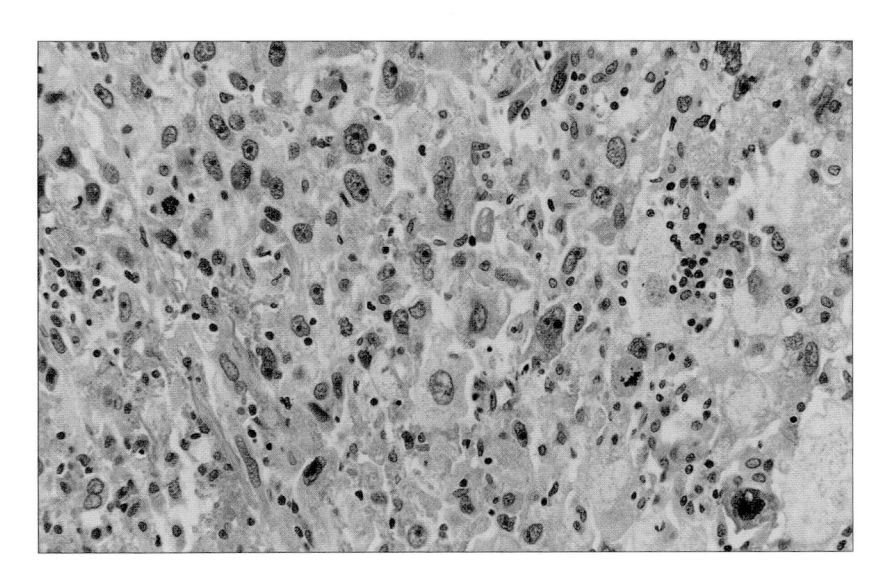

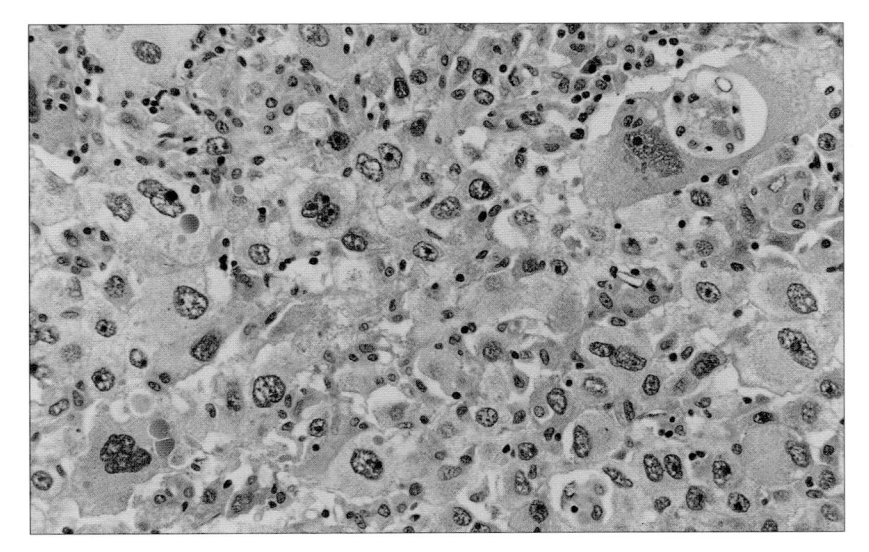

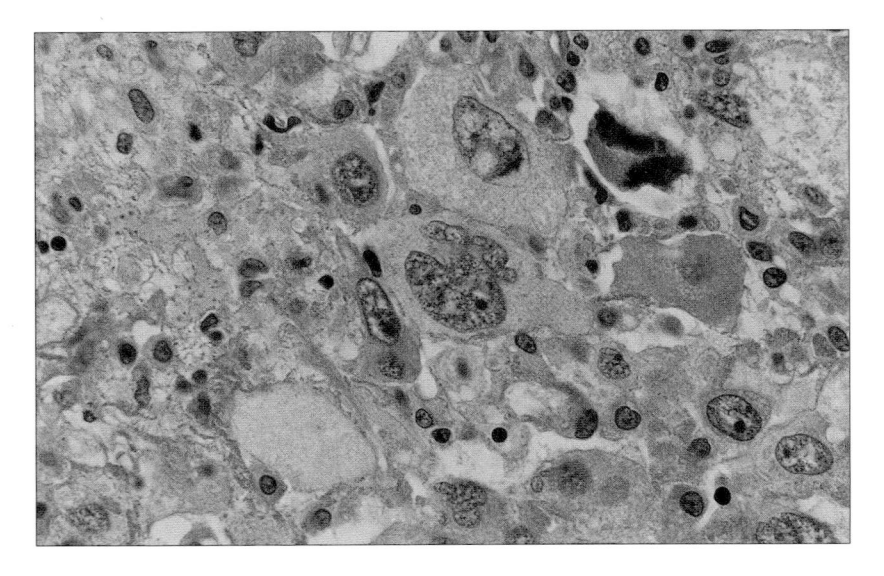

Follicular dendritic cell sarcoma

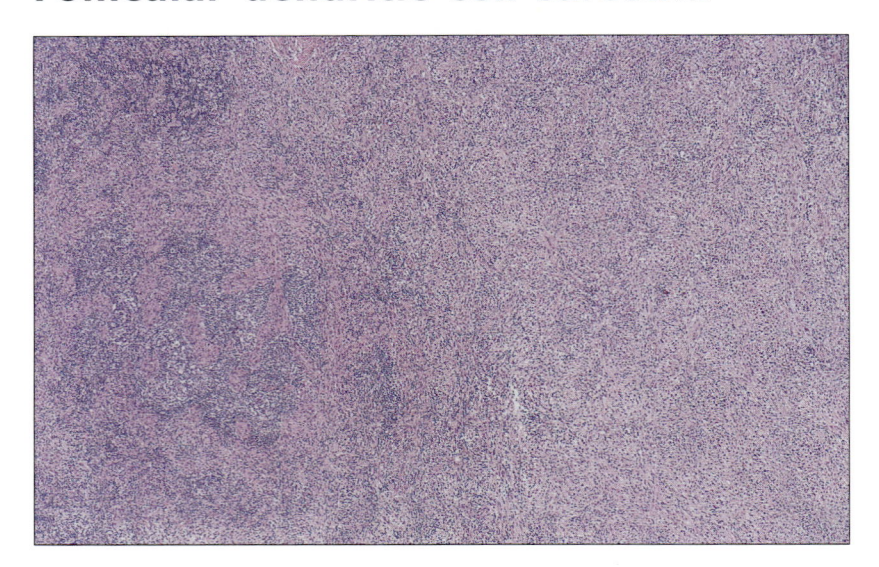

Figure 16.6

Follicular dendritic cell sarcoma:

(a) In areas, the normal architecture of the lymph node is almost entirely obliterated by the neoplasm. (H&E stain)

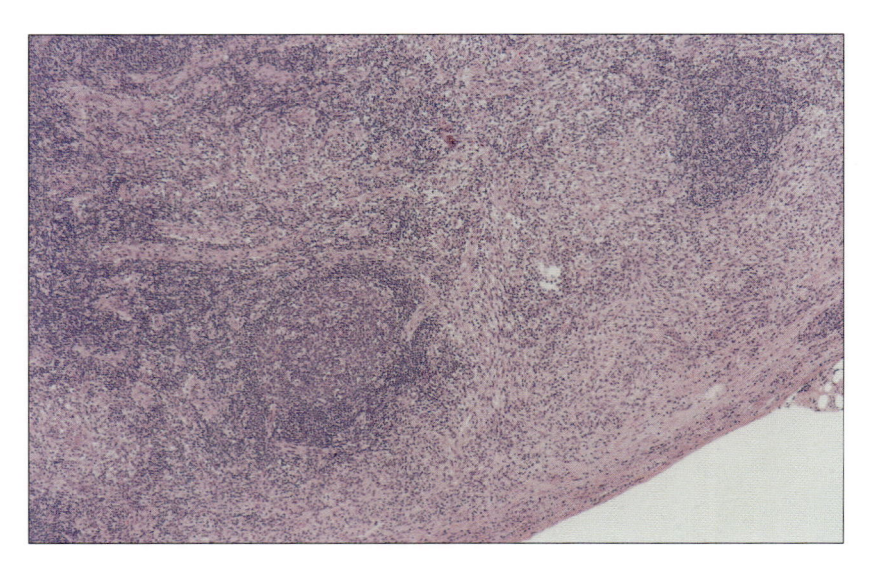

In other areas, there is sparing of follicles (**b,c**). (H&E stain)

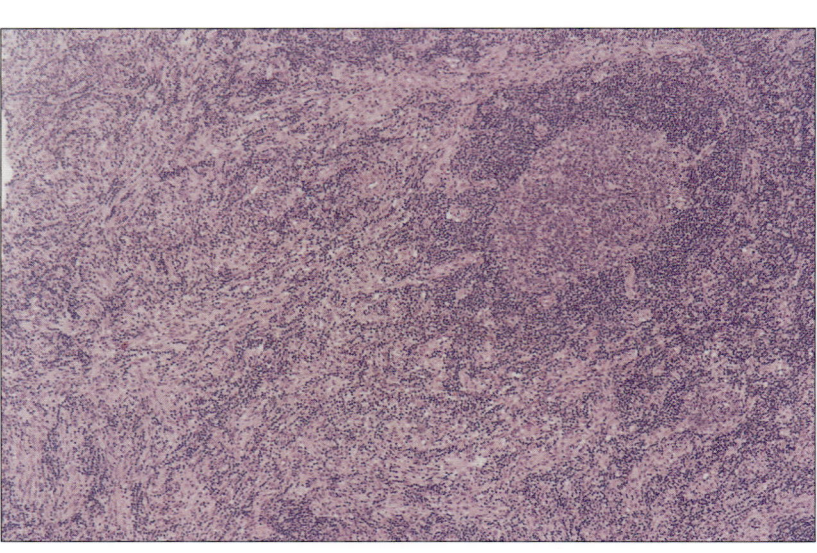

(b)

(c)

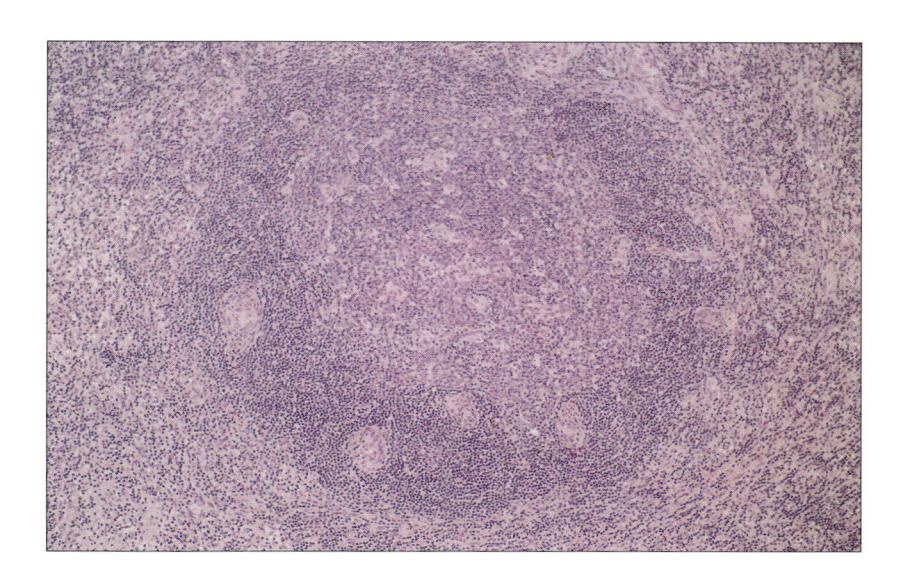

Figure 16.6 *continued*

(**d**) Closer examination reveals clusters of pale cells in the mantles of one of the follicles. (H&E stain)

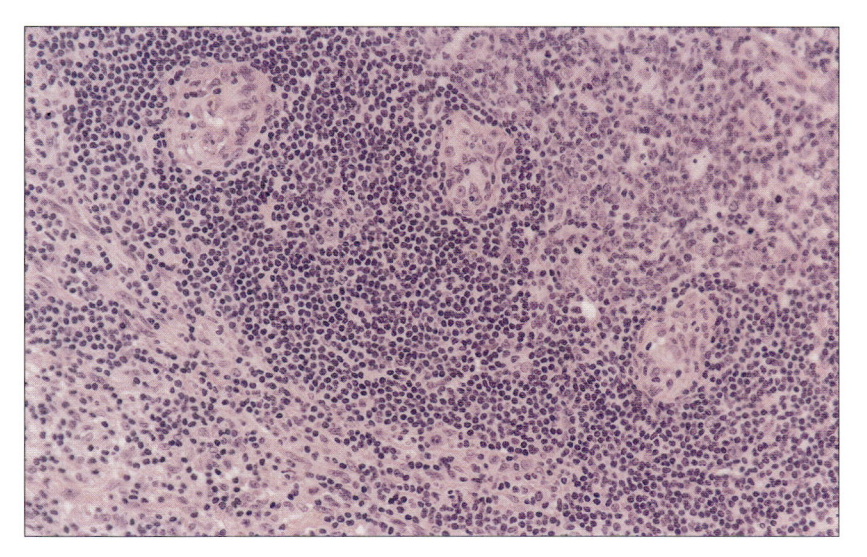

(**e**) The pale cells are clusters of follicular dendritic cells. (H&E stain)

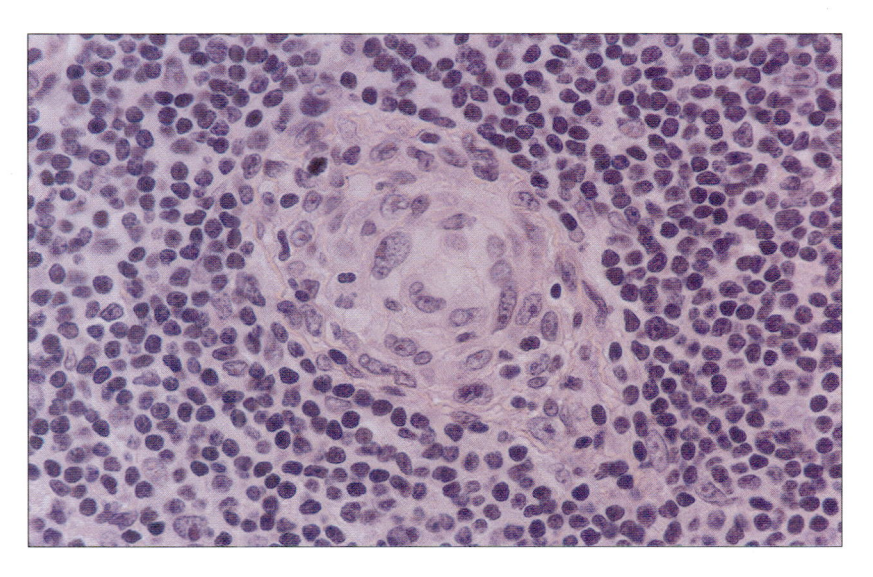

(**f**) High-power examination of one of these clusters shows an aggregate of follicular dendritic cells with pale, oval to slightly elongate and irregular nuclei. The appearance in this field by itself is reminiscent of the hyaline vascular follicles of Castleman's disease. (H&E stain)

Note: The changes shown in the follicles (**d–f**) are unusual, and are not found in the majority of follicular dendritic cell sarcomas. It is possible that they represent some sort of precursor lesion to the follicular dendritic cell sarcoma.

Contd

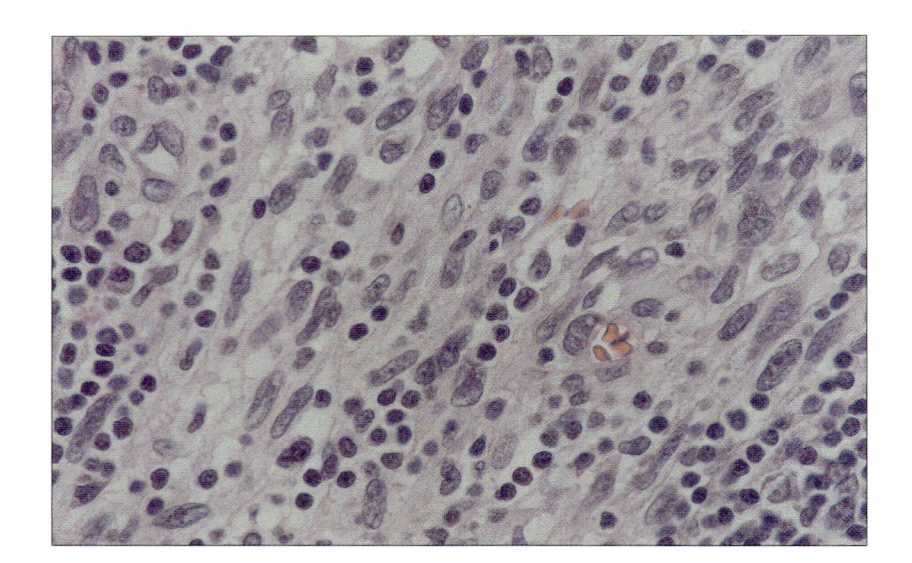

Figure 16.6 *continued*

(g) Away from the follicles, the tumor cells are elongated and spindled, with abundant pink cytoplasm and ill-defined cell borders. Some cells have prominent red nucleoli. There are many interspersed small lymphocytes. (H&E stain)

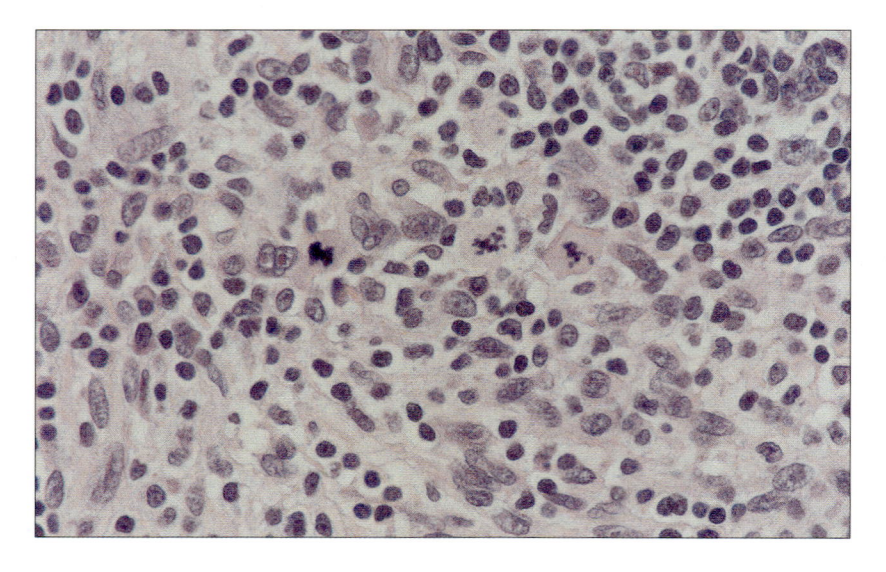

(h) In areas, mitotic figures are numerous. (H&E stain)

17 Summary

A comparison of the features of the major subtypes of non-Hodgkin's lymphoma is shown in Table 17.1. By combining histological, biological and clinical observations, it is possible to identify 'real' clinical/pathological entities. Oncologists who care for patients with lymphoma need to be acquainted with the major groups of lymphomas. Pathologists need both to acknowledge the diagnostic criteria and to be experienced in their application in the diagnosis of lymphomas.

What pathologists need to know

The diagnosis of non-Hodgkin's lymphoma and Hodgkin's disease and the identification of a specific subtype should always be made by a pathologist who has taken the time to become an expert in this area. This is one of the most difficult diagnoses pathologists are called upon to make, and, since treatments vary, accurate diagnosis is important. Pathologists need to work from clear and widely accepted definitions and to have made the commitment to spend the time necessary to make themselves experts.

Pathologists must have adequate tissue with which to work. Needle aspirates can be useful in confirming relapse in a patient with a known type of lymphoma, but should very rarely be the basis for initial diagnosis. Cutting needle biopsies provide more tissue, but in general it would be better to have an excisional biopsy and a generous amount of tissue. A pathologist needs to have access to immunostaining and genetic studies to resolve difficult cases.

Finally, for the pathologist to make the best possible diagnosis, it is necessary that they communicate with the clinician seeing the patient. Mediastinal large B-cell lymphoma cannot be diagnosed without knowing there is a mediastinal mass. Distinction between lymphomatoid papulosis and anaplastic large T/null cell lymphoma in the skin is only possible when the pathologist and the clinician communicate. They must act as a team for the patient to have the best chance for a good outcome.

What clinicians need to know

Since the therapy of non-Hodgkin's lymphomas continues to be based on the diagnosis of a specific subtype, clinicians should not undertake therapy until the slides have been reviewed by a pathologist with special skills in this area. The clinician and the pathologist must communicate to give the pathologist the best opportunity to reach an accurate diagnosis. The clinician also must support the pathologist in the latter's need for adequate tissue. It is better for the patient to undergo a second biopsy than for treatment to be based on a diagnosis reached on inadequate tissue.

Clinicians must be acquainted with the clinical characteristics of the most common subtypes of

Table 17.1
Comparison of the major subtypes of non-Hodgkin's lymphoma

Lymphoma subtype	Median age (years)	Male (%)	Stage III/IV (%)	B symptoms (%)	Elevated LDH (%)	Tumor mass ≥10 cm (%)	Bone marrow involved (%)	IPI score 0/1 (%)	IPI score 4/5 (%)	5-year FFS (%)	5-year OS (%)
Small lymphocytic	65	53	91	33	41	13	72	23	13	25	51
Lymphoplasmacytic	63	53	80	13	15	25	73	16	15	25	59
Follicular	59	42	67	28	30	28	42	45	7	40	72
Marginal-zone, nodal	58	42	74	37	40	0	32	60	13	29	57
Marginal-zone, MALT	60	48	33	19	27	8	14	44	8	60	74
Mantle-cell	63	74	80	28	40	25	64	23	23	11	27
Diffuse large B-cell	64	55	46	33	53	30	16	35	19	41	46
Primary mediastinal large B-cell	37	34	34	38	81	52	43	52	11	48	50
Burkitt-like	57	59	48	39	61	42	21	30	22	43	47
Burkitt's	31	89	38	22	75	22	33	57	14	44	44
Peripheral T-cell	61	55	80	50	64	12	36	17	31	18	25
Anaplastic large T/null cell	34	69	49	53	45	17	13	61	21	58	77
Lymphoblastic	28	64	89	32	70	32	50	33	26	24	26

LDH, lactate dehydrogenase; IPI, International Prognostic Index; FFS, failure-free survival; OS, overall survival.

non-Hodgkin's lymphoma. At a minimum, this should include those described in this volume. The best treatment plan for an individual patient should be reached when an accurate diagnosis is combined with the information from a careful clinical evaluation. The patient's score in the International Prognostic Index (IPI) will help determine therapy, and is necessary to impart an accurate prognosis to the patient.

It is also necessary for clinicians to be aware of the more subtle, unique characteristics of specific subtypes of lymphoma or unusual clinical presentations. For example, patients who present with diffuse large B-cell lymphoma and sinus involvement, epidural involvement or testicular involvement should receive central nervous system prophylactic therapy because of a high chance of meningeal relapse in the absence of such therapy. Patients who present with lymphomas involving Waldeyer's ring need to have their distal gastrointestinal tract evaluated to rule out involvement at that site. Conversely, patients who present with distal gastrointestinal-tract involvement should have a careful evaluation of Waldeyer's ring before therapy is initiated, because of the high likelihood of involvement. Patients with lymphoblastic and Burkitt's lymphoma should always receive central nervous system prophylactic therapy because of the high likelihood of meningeal dissemination. These and numerous other, similar facts need to be taken into account in planning a patient's management.

Clinicians need to be expert in the administration of the therapies used to treat patients with non-Hodgkin's lymphoma. There is a widespread tendency to believe that surgeons should not treat patients unless they have become expert in the particular operation involved, and radiotherapists should have experience in treating a particular disease before they manage a patient. However, there is an equally widespread feeling that any clinician who sees patients with cancer can look up a chemotherapy regimen in a book and administer it. There are as many mistakes to be made in the administration of chemotherapy as there are to be made in performing surgery, and these mistakes can have equally devastating consequences. It is important that individuals who treat patients with lymphoma using chemotherapy be experienced in the use of the particular regimen being administered.

The future

The classification system for non-Hodgkin's lymphomas is not in its last iteration, and new insights into biology of the immune system will undoubtedly lead to the identification of new subtypes of non-Hodgkin's lymphoma. It is also possible that advances in lymphoma therapy will alter lymphoma classification. Pneumococcal pneumonia was once subdivided into multiple categories based on identification of specific subtypes of the organism. The importance of this complicated system disappeared with the advent of penicillin. It is possible that the discovery of an effective new therapy for lymphoma will diminish the need for a precise system of classification. We should all like to see the discovery of a 'penicillin' for lymphoma. Unfortunately, this is not likely in the near future.

It is possible that increased understanding of the genetic abnormalities found in lymphomas will lead to a classification system based on gene expression. The advent of chip technology that allows rapid identification of gene expression in a particular neoplasm might become the standard approach to the diagnosis and categorization of lymphomas. However, previous experience and understanding the genetics of lymphomas might suggest that this will complicate rather than simplify the process, and histologic and clinical findings might remain important.

Lymphomas have taught us much about malignancy and its management. They are almost certainly going to continue to do so in the future.

Bibliography

Cabanillas F, Armitage J, Pugh WC et al, Lymphomatoid papulosis: a T-cell dyscrasia with a propensity to transform into malignant lymphoma. *Ann Int Med* 1995; **122:** 210–17.

International Non-Hodgkin's Lymphoma Prognostic Factors Project, A predictive model for aggressive non-Hodgkin's lymphoma. *N Engl J Med* 1993; **329:** 987–94.

Index

Note: Page references in *italic* refer to tables and those in **bold** refer to figures. The abbreviation CLL used in subheadings stands for chronic lymphocytic leukemia.

Abdominal lymph node, hairy cell leukemia, **54**
ABVD regimen, Hodgkin's disease, 159
Adriamycin *see* Doxorubicin
Adult T-cell leukemia/lymphoma (ATL), **41–3**
　classification, *2*, 29, 33–4
　clinical characteristics, 34–5
　definition, 33–4
　diagnostic criteria, *35*
　flower cells, 35, **43**
　frequency, 30, 34
　genetics, 34
　histology, 34
　HTLV, 33, 34, 35
　immunophenotype, 34, **41**
　prognosis, 35
　treatment, 35
AIDS-associated lymphomas
　Burkitt's, 84, 87–8, 179
　Castleman's disease, 180
　primary central nervous system, 139
Alkylating agents
　CLL/small lymphocytic lymphoma, 48
　marginal-zone B-cell lymphoma, 126
　see also Chlorambucil; Cyclophosphamide
Allogenic stem cell transplantation, 48, 110
Amyloid deposition, MALT lymphoma, **81**
Anaplastic carcinomas, 91, 92, 93
Anaplastic large T/null cell lymphoma, **95–6**
　classification, 29, 91
　clinical characteristics, 92–3, *93*
　definition, 91
　frequency, 91
　genetics, 91, 92, *92*
　histology, 91–2, *91*
　Hodgkin-like, 92, **97–8**
　immunophenotypes, 91, 92, *92*, **96**
　other lymphomas compared, *198*
　prognosis, 91, 93–4, **93**
　treatment, 31, 93–4
　and true histiocytic lymphoma, 180
Angiocentric T/NK-cell lymphomas, 29, 30, 31, 141, **147–9**
Angioendotheliomatosis proliferans systemisata (angiotropic lymphoma), *138*, 177, 178, **187–8**
Angiofollicular lymphoid hyperplasia (Castleman's disease), 179–80, **190–1**
Angioimmunoblastic lymphadenopathy with dysproteinemia (AILD), 32, 33
Angioimmunoblastic T-cell lymphomas, **39–40**
　classification, 29, 32
　clinical characteristics, 33
　definition, 32
　frequency, 30, 32
　genetics, 33
　histology, 32–3
　immunophenotype, 33, **40**
　treatment, 33
Angiotropic lymphoma, *138*, 177, 178, **187–8**

Antibiotics, 72–3, *73*, 136, 139
Anti-CD20 antibody, 19
Anti-CD20 (Rituximab), 19, 64
Asparaginase, BFM 86 protocol, 86, *86*, **109**, 110
Autoimmune phenomena, CLL/small lymphocytic lymphoma, 47
Autologous stem cell transplantation
　anaplastic large T/null cell lymphoma, 94
　Burkitt's lymphoma/leukemia, 87
　CLL/small lymphocytic lymphoma, 48
　diffuse large B-cell lymphoma, 9
　follicular lymphoma, 18, 20
　Hodgkin's disease, 160
　lymphoblastic lymphoma, 110
　mantle-cell lymphoma, 64
　primary mediastinal large B-cell lymphoma, 101, 102
　unspecified peripheral T-cell lymphoma, 32

B-cell acute lymphoblastic leukemia *see* Burkitt's leukemia
B-cell chronic lymphocytic leukemia (CLL)/small lymphocytic lymphoma, **51–2**
　classification, *2*, 45
　clinical characteristics, 46–7
　definition, 45
　frequency, 45
　genetics, 46
　histology, 45–6
　immunophenotype, 45, 46
　staging systems, 47, *47*
　treatment, 47–8

B-cell lymphoblastic lymphoma, 2, 105, 106, 108, **114–15**
B-cell lymphomas, 2
  major features compared, *198*
  T-cell-rich, 6, *6*, 177–8, **183–6**
  see also B-cell chronic lymphocytic leukemia; B-cell lymphoblastic lymphoma; Burkitt-like lymphoma; Burkitt's lymphoma; Diffuse large B-cell lymphoma; Extranodal lymphomas; Follicular lymphoma; Lymphoplasmacytic lymphoma; MALT lymphomas; Mantle-cell lymphoma; Nodal marginal-zone B-cell (monocytoid) lymphoma; Primary mediastinal large B-cell lymphoma; Small lymphocytic lymphomas; Splenic marginal-zone B-cell lymphoma
B-cell prolymphocytic leukemia, 48–9
BEACOPP regimen, Hodgkin's disease, 159
BFM 86 protocol
  Burkitt's lymphoma/leukemia, 86, *86*
  lymphoblastic lymphoma, **109**, 110
Binet clinical staging system, 47, *47*
Biopsies, 197
Blackledge staging system, 135, *135*
Bleomycin, Hodgkin's disease, 159
Body cavity lymphomas, 141, 178–9, **188–9**
Bone
  Burkitt's lymphoma, 85
  extranodal lymphomas, **76–8**, 134, *134*
  lymphoblastic lymphoma, 107–8
  MALT lymphomas, **76–8**
Bone marrow
  anaplastic large T/null cell lymphoma, 92
  Burkitt's lymphoma/leukemia, 85, 87, **87**
  Castleman's disease, **191**
  diffuse large B-cell lymphoma, 7, 8
  extranodal lymphomas, *72*, 135, 136–7, 141, **152**
  follicular lymphoma, 16, **27**
  hairy cell leukemia, **55**
  hepatosplenic lymphoma, **152**
  Hodgkin's disease, **174–5**
  lymphoblastic lymphoma, 105, 107–8, **107**
  lymphoplasmacytic lymphoma, 117, 118
  major lymphomas compared, *198*
  mantle-cell lymphoma, 62, *63*, 64, **66–7**
  nodal marginal-zone B-cell (monocytoid) lymphoma, 125
  splenic marginal-zone B-cell lymphoma, 126
Borrelia burgdorferi, 139
Brain
  diffuse large B-cell lymphoma, 9
  primary lymphoma, 139–40
Burkitt-like lymphoma, **90**
  classification, *2*, 83
  genetics, 83, 85
  other lymphomas compared, *198*
Burkitt's leukemia, 85, 86–7, **87**
Burkitt's lymphoma, **89**
  classification, *2*, 83
  clinical characteristics, 85–6, *85*, 179
  definition, 83
  frequency, 83–4
  genetics, 84–5
  histology, 84
  immunophenotypes, 84
  other lymphomas compared, *198*
  prognosis, 86–8, *86*
  staging, 85–6, *85*
  starry sky appearance, 84, **89**, **111**
  treatment, 86–8, *87*, *198*

Carcinomas, anaplastic, 91, 92, 93
Castleman's disease, 179–80, **190–1**
Celiac disease, 134, 136
Central nervous system
  adult T-cell leukemia/lymphoma, 35
  Burkitt's lymphoma, 85, 198
  Castleman's disease, 179, 180
  diffuse large B-cell lymphoma, 5, 9, 198
  lymphoblastic lymphoma, 108, 198
  primary lymphomas, 133, 134, *134*, 139–40
Centrocytic lymphoma *see* Mantle-cell lymphoma
Chemotherapy, 198–9
  anaplastic large T/null cell lymphoma, 93–4
  angioimmunoblastic T-cell lymphoma, 33
  angiotropic lymphoma, 178
  Burkitt's lymphoma/leukemia, 86–7, **87**
  Castleman's disease, 180
  CLL/small lymphocytic lymphoma, 48
  diffuse large B-cell lymphoma, 8–9, *8*
  extranodal lymphomas, 73, 125, 135–6, 137, 139, 140
  follicular lymphoma, 16, 18–19, 20
  Hodgkin's disease, 158, 159–60
  lymphoblastic lymphoma, 108, **109**, 110
  lymphoplasmacytic lymphoma, 119
  MALT lymphomas, 73, 125
  mantle-cell lymphoma, 63–4
  nodal marginal-zone B-cell (monocytoid) lymphoma, 125
  primary effusion lymphoma, 179
  primary lymphoma of brain, 140
  primary mediastinal large B-cell lymphoma, 101
  splenic marginal-zone B-cell lymphoma, 126
  unspecified peripheral T-cell lymphoma, 32
Chlorambucil
  lymphoplasmacytic lymphoma, 119
  mantle-cell lymphoma, 64
CHOP regimen
  diffuse large B-cell lymphoma, 8, *8*
  mantle-cell lymphoma, 64
  nodal marginal-zone B-cell (monocytoid) lymphoma, 125
  primary mediastinal large B-cell lymphoma, 101
Chronic lymphocytic leukemia (CLL)
  B-cell derived, 2, 45–8, **51–2**
  T-cell derived, 45, 49, **56**
CHVP regimen, follicular lymphoma, 18
Cladribine
  CLL/small lymphocytic lymphoma, 48
  lymphoplasmacytic lymphoma, 119
Classification of lymphomas, 1–3, 199
  rare subtypes, 177
  see also classification *under specific lymphomas*
Clinicians, 197–9
CODOX-M regimen, Burkitt's lymphoma/leukemia, 86–7, *86*

COP-BLAM III, follicular lymphoma, 20
Cutaneous lymphomas *see* Skin
CVP regimen, mantle-cell lymphoma, 64
Cyclophosphamide
  Burkitt's lymphoma/leukemia, **87**
  follicular lymphoma, 18
  Hodgkin's disease, 159
  mantle-cell lymphoma, 64
  unspecified peripheral T-cell lymphoma, 32
  see also BFM 86 protocol; CHOP regimen
Cyclosporine, angioimmunoblastic T-cell lymphoma, 33
Cytarabine, BFM 86 protocol, 86, *86*, **109**, 110
Cytogenetics *see* genetics *under specific lymphomas*
Cytosine arabinoside
  Burkitt's lymphoma/leukemia, **87**
  CLL/small lymphocytic lymphoma, 48

Dacarbazine, Hodgkin's disease, 159
Dendritic cells, follicular dendritic cell sarcoma, 177, 181, **194–6**
Dexamethasone
  BFM 86 protocol, 86, *86*, **109**, 110
  follicular lymphoma, 19
Diffuse histiocytic lymphoma *see* Diffuse large B-cell lymphoma
Diffuse large B-cell lymphoma
  anaplastic appearance, 92
  angiotropic lymphoma, *138*, 178
  Burkitt-like lymphoma, 83, 85
  classification, 2, 5, **11–12**
  clinical characteristics, 7–8, *7*
  definition, 5
  extranodal, 134
  and follicular lymphoma, 14, 15, 22, 46
  frequency, 5–6
  genetics, *6*, 7
  histology, 6, *6*
  immunophenotype, 6, *6*
  legs, 137, *138*, 139
  other lymphomas compared, *99*, 101, *198*
  predisposing factors, 6
  prognosis, **8**, 9, **9**
  pyothorax-associated, 179

  skin, 5, 9, 137, *138*, 139
  and small lymphocytic lymphoma, 46, 48
  treatment, 8–9, *8*, 198
  and true histiocytic lymphoma, 180–1
Diffuse large cell lymphomas *see* Diffuse large B-cell lymphoma; Peripheral T-cell lymphomas
Diffuse mixed lymphoma *see* Peripheral T-cell lymphomas
Diffuse small cleaved cell lymphoma *see* Lymphoblastic lymphoma
Doxorubicin
  BFM 86 protocol, 86, *86*, **109**, 110
  Burkitt's lymphoma/leukemia, 86, *86*, **87**
  follicular lymphoma, 18
  Hodgkin's disease, 159
  lymphoblastic lymphoma, **109**, 110
  mantle-cell lymphoma, 64
  unspecified peripheral T-cell lymphoma, 32
  see also CHOP regimen

Effusion lymphoma, 141, 178–9, **188–9**
Enteropathy-associated T-cell lymphoma (EATCL), 134, *135*, 136
EORTC Cutaneous Lymphoma Study Group, 137, *138*, 139
Epididymis, diffuse large B-cell lymphoma, **11**
Epidural tissue, diffuse large B-cell lymphoma, 5, 9, 198
Epstein–Barr virus
  angiotropic lymphoma, 178
  Burkitt's lymphoma, 85
  extranodal lymphomas, 141, 178–9
  Hodgkin's disease, 154, 155, **166**
  primary effusion lymphoma, 178–9
  pyothorax-associated lymphoma, 179
Etoposide
  Hodgkin's disease, 159
  peripheral T-cell lymphoma, 32
Extradural lymphoma, primary, 140
Extranodal lymphomas, 133
  angiocentric T/NK-cell, 29, 30, 31, 141, **147–9**
  angiotropic, *138*, 177, 178, **187–8**
  body-cavity-based, 141, 178–9, **188–9**

  central nervous system, 133, 134, *134*, 139–40
  classification, 133, 134–5, *135*, 137–9
  clinical characteristics, 133–4, 135, 136, 137, 139–40
  cutaneous, 133, 134, *134*, 137–9, **145–6**
  definition, 133, 134–5, 137
  frequency, 133, 134, 136, 137, *138*, 139
  gastrointestinal, 133, 134–7, *134*, **143–4**
  hepatosplenic, 30, 141, **150–2**
  marginal-zone B-cell *see* MALT lymphomas
  prognosis, 134, *134*, 135–6, 137, *138*, 139, 140
  treatment, 135–6
Eye
  Burkitt's lymphoma, 85
  diffuse large B-cell lymphoma, **12**
  MALT lymphoma, **76–8**
  primary lymphoma of brain, 139–40
  primary ocular lymphoma, 140

F-MACHOP
  follicular lymphoma, 20
  primary mediastinal large B-cell lymphoma, 101
Flower cells, 35, **43**
Fludarabine
  CLL/small lymphocytic lymphoma, 48
  follicular lymphoma, 19
  lymphoplasmacytic lymphoma, 119
  mantle-cell lymphoma, 64
FND regimen, follicular lymphoma, 19
Follicle-center cell lymphoma, 137, *138*
Follicular dendritic cell sarcoma, 177, 181, **194–6**
Follicular hyperplasia, **25–6**
Follicular large cell lymphoma *see* Follicular lymphoma, grade III
Follicular lymphoma
  bone marrow, 16, **27**
  classification, *2*, 13, 14, 22
  clinical characteristics, 15–17
  definition, 13
  and diffuse large B-cell lymphoma, 14, 15, 22, 46
  frequency, 13

Follicular lymphoma – *continued*
  genetics, 15
  grade I, 14, 17–19, **22**
  grade II, 14, 17–19, **23**
  grade III, 14, 19–20, 22, **24**
  histology, 13–14, *14*
  immunohistology, 14–15, **25–6**
  immunophenotype, 14–15, 124
  and mantle-cell lymphoma, 62, *62*
  and nodal marginal-zone B-cell
    (monocytoid) lymphoma, 124
  other lymphomas compared, *198*
  prognosis, 16–17, *16*, **17**, 18, 19, 20
  skin, 137, *138*
  staging procedures, 16, *16*
  treatment, 16, 17–20
Follicular mixed lymphoma *see*
  Follicular lymphoma, grade II
Follicular small cleaved lymphoma *see*
  Follicular lymphoma, grade I

Gastrointestinal system
  adult T-cell leukemia/lymphoma, 35
  anaplastic large T/null cell
    lymphoma, 92
  Burkitt's lymphoma, 85, 86
  extranodal lymphomas, 69, 70–3,
    133, 134–7, *134*, **143–4**
  MALT lymphomas, 69, 70–3
  mantle-cell lymphoma, 62–3, *63*,
    136
  nodal marginal-zone B-cell
    (monocytoid) lymphoma, **128**
  and Waldeyer's ring, 198
Genetics *see* genetics *under specific
  lymphomas*
Glucorticoids
  Castleman's disease, 180
  and nucleosides, 48

Hairy cell leukemia, 49, **53–5**, 62, 124
α-Heavy chain disease (IPSID), *135*,
  136
Helicobacter pylori, 70, 72–3, *73*
Hepatosplenic lymphoma, 30, 141,
  150–2
Herpes virus, 141, 178–9, 180
High-grade B-cell lymphoma, Burkitt-
  like, 83
HIV infected patients
  Burkitt's lymphoma, 84, 87

Castleman's disease, 180
  diffuse large B-cell lymphoma, 5, 6
  Hodgkin's disease, **174–5**
  primary effusion lymphoma, 141,
    178–9
Hodgkin-like anaplastic large T/null
  cell lymphoma, 92, **97–8**
Hodgkin's disease
  bone marrow, **174–5**
  classification, 153
  clinical characteristics, 156–7, *157*
  definition, 153
  frequency, 153
  genetics, 155
  histology, 153–4
  immunophenotypes, 154–5, *155*
  lymphocyte-depleted, 154, 155, *155*,
    167–70
  lymphocyte-predominant, 154, 155,
    155, 156–7, 160, **171–2**
  lymphocyte-rich, 154, **173–4**
  mixed-cellularity, 154, 155, *155*,
    164–6
  nodular-sclerosis, 153–4, 155, *155*,
    156, **162–3**
  prognosis, 156–7, 158–9, 160
  staging, 156–7, *157*, 158
  treatment, 157–60
Human T-lymphotropic virus (HTLV),
  33, 34, 35
Hydrocortisone, **87**
Hypogammaglobulinemia, 47

IL-6
  Castleman's disease, 179, 180
  primary effusion lymphoma, 178–9
Immunoblastic lymphomas *see* Diffuse
  large B-cell lymphoma; Peripheral
  T-cell lymphomas
Immunocytomas, 117
  cutaneous, 137–9, *138*
Immunophenotypes *see*
  immunophenotypes *under
  specific lymphomas*
Immunoproliferative small intestinal
  disease (IPSID), *135*, 136
Interferon
  angioimmunoblastic T-cell
    lymphoma, 33
  cutaneous lymphomas, 139
  follicular lymphoma, 18
  hairy cell leukemia, 49

International Lymphoma Study Group,
  2
International Prognostic Index, *3*, 16
  major lymphomas compared, *198*
Intestinal involvement *see*
  Gastrointestinal system
Intestinal T-cell lymphoma, 29, 30,
  134, *135*, 136, **143–4**
Intravascular (angiotropic) lymphoma,
  138, 178, **187–8**
IVAC regimen, 86–7, *86*

Jaw, Burkitt's lymphoma, 83, 85

Kaposi's sarcoma-associated
  herpesvirus, 141, 178–9, 180
Kiel classification, 1
  lymphoplasmacytic lymphoma, 117
  mantle-cell lymphoma, 61
  nodal marginal-zone B-cell
    (monocytoid) lymphoma, 124
  peripheral T-cell lymphomas, 29
  primary cutaneous lymphomas, 137,
    138

Large B-cell lymphoma, primary medi-
  astinal, *2*, 99–102, **103–4**, *198*
Large granular lymphocytic leukemia,
  29, 49, **57–9**
Large transformed cell lymphoma *see*
  Diffuse large B-cell lymphoma
Lennert's lymphoma, 30
Leptomeningeal lymphoma, primary,
  140
Liver
  hepatosplenic lymphoma, 141, **151**
  primary lymphoma, 134
  splenic marginal-zone B-cell
    lymphoma, **131**
  T-cell-rich B-cell lymphoma, **185–6**
LMB 86 protocol, Burkitt's
  lymphoma/leukemia, 86, *86*, **87**
LMT 81 protocol, lymphoblastic
  lymphoma, 110
LNH84 protocol, 101
LNH87 protocol
  follicular lymphoma, 20
  peripheral T-cell lymphoma, 31
  primary mediastinal large B-cell
    lymphoma, 101

LSA$_2$-L$_2$ regimen, 108, 110
Lung, extranodal lymphomas, **75–6**, 134, *134*
Lymphoblastic lymphoma
    B-cell, 105, 106, 108, **114–15**
    classification, *2*, 105
    clinical characteristics, 107–8
    definition, 105
    frequency, 105–6
    genetics, 106, *108*
    histology, 106
    immunophenotypes, 106, **107**, 112
    lymph node, **111–12**
    and mantle-cell lymphoma, 106
    other lymphomas compared, *198*
    prognosis, 108, 110
    soft tissue, **113**
    T-cell, 105, 106, 107–8, **107**, **108**, **111–13**
    treatment, 108–10, **109**, 198
Lymphocyte-depleted Hodgkin's disease (LD), 154, 155, *155*, **167–70**
Lymphocyte-predominant Hodgkin's disease (LP), 154, 155, *155*, 156–7, 160, **171–2**
Lymphocyte-rich Hodgkin's disease, 154, **173–4**
Lymphoid leukemias, acute, 105
    see also Lymphoblastic lymphoma
Lymphomatoid papulosis, 92–3, *138*
Lymphomatous polyposis, 62, *135*, 136–7
Lymphoplasmacytic lymphoma, **121–2**
    classification, *2*, 117
    clinical characteristics, 118, *118*
    definition, 117
    frequency, 117
    genetics, 118, *118*
    histology, 117, *117*
    immunophenotypes, 118, *118*, **122**
    other lymphomas compared, *198*
    prognosis, 118–19, **119**
    treatment, 118–19

MACOP-B
    follicular lymphoma, 20
    primary mediastinal large B-cell lymphoma, 101
Malignant angioendotheliomatosis (angiotropic lymphoma), *138*, 178, **187–8**

Malignant histiocytosis, 91, 180
MALT (extranodal marginal-zone B-cell) lymphomas
    amyloid deposition, **81**
    classification, *2*, 69–70, 125
    clinical characteristics, 71–2, *72*
    cutaneous immunocytoma, 137–9
    definition, 69–70
    frequency, 70, 124
    genetics, 7, *69*
    Helicobacter pylori, 70, 72–3, *73*
    histology, *69*, 70–1, 124
    immunophenotypes, *69*, 71, **77–8**, **82**
    immunoproliferative small intestinal disease, 136
    lung, **75–6**
    nasolacrimal duct region, **80–2**
    orbit, **76–8**
    other lymphomas compared, *198*
    parotid, **79–80**
    predisposing factors, 70
    prognosis, 71–2, 73, 125
    treatment, 72–3, *73*, 125
Mantle-cell lymphoma (MCL), **66–7**
    blastoid variant, 62, 106
    classification, *2*, 61
    clinical characteristics, 62–3, *63*
    definition, 61
    frequency, 61
    genetics, 62, **67**
    histology, 61–2
    immunophenotypes, 62, *62*, 106
    and lymphoblastic lymphoma, 106
    lymphomatous polyposis, 62, *135*, 136
    other lymphomas compared, *198*
    prognosis, 63–4, *63*
    treatment, 63–4, *63*
Marginal-zone B-cell lymphomas, 123–4
    other lymphomas compared, *198*
    see also MALT lymphomas; Nodal marginal-zone B-cell (monocytoid) lymphoma; Splenic marginal-zone B-cell lymphoma
Mediastinum
    Castleman's disease, 179
    Hodgkin's disease, 156, 160
    lymphoblastic lymphoma, 105, 107, 108, 110
    primary large B-cell lymphoma,

    99–102, *99*, **103–4**, *198*
Mercaptopurine, BFM 86 protocol, 86, *86*, **109**, 110
Methotrexate
    Burkitt's lymphoma/leukemia, 86, *86*, **87**
    lymphoblastic lymphoma, **109**, 110
Mitoxantrone, follicular lymphoma, 19
Mixed-cellularity Hodgkin's disease (MC), 154, 155, *155*, **164–6**
Monoclonal antibody treatment
    follicular lymphoma, 19
    mantle-cell lymphoma, 64
Monocytoid lymphoma *see* Nodal marginal-zone B-cell (monocytoid) lymphoma
MOPP regimen, Hodgkin's disease, 159
    see also PRoMACE–MOPP flexitherapy
Mucosa-associated lymphoid tissue lymphomas *see* MALT lymphomas
Multicentric Castleman's disease, 179–80, **190–1**
Multiple lymphomatous polyposis, 62, *135*, 136–7
Mycosis fungoides, *2*, 137, *138*, **145**

Nasal-type T/NK-cell lymphoma, 141, **147–9**
Nasolacrimal duct region, MALT lymphoma, **80–2**
Natural killer (NK) cell-type large granular lymphocytic leukemia, 49, **58–9**
Nitrogen mustard, 159
Nodal marginal-zone B-cell (monocytoid) lymphoma, **128–30**
    classification, *2*, 69, 123–4, 125
    clinical characteristics, 125
    definition, 123–4
    genetics, *123*, 125
    and hairy cell leukemia, 124
    histology, *123*, 124
    immunophenotypes, *123*, 124
    other lymphomas compared, *198*
    prognosis, 125
    treatment, 125
Nodular-sclerosis Hodgkin's disease (NS), 153–4, 155, *155*, 156, **162–3**
Non-Burkitt's type lymphoma, 83

Non-Hodgkin's lymphoma, 1–3
  B-cell *see* B-cell chronic
      lymphocytic leukemia; B-cell
      lymphoblastic lymphoma;
      Burkitt-like lymphoma; Burkitt's
      lymphoma; Diffuse large B-cell
      lymphoma; Extranodal
      lymphomas; Follicular
      lymphoma; Lymphoblastic
      lymphoma; Lymphoplasmacytic
      lymphoma; MALT lymphomas;
      Mantle-cell lymphoma; Nodal
      marginal-zone B-cell
      (monocytoid) lymphoma;
      Primary mediastinal large B-cell
      lymphoma; Small lymphocytic
      lymphomas; Splenic marginal-
      zone B-cell lymphoma
  clinicians' role, 197–9
  major features compared, *198*
  pathologists' role, 197
  T-cell *see* Adult T-cell
      leukemia/lymphoma; Adult T-
      cell leukemia/lymphoma (ATL);
      Anaplastic large T/null cell
      lymphoma; Enteropathy-
      associated T-cell lymphoma;
      Lymphoblastic lymphoma;
      Mycosis fungoides; Peripheral
      T-cell lymphomas; Sézary
      syndrome; T-cell
      prolymphocytic leukemia
Nucleosides
  follicular lymphoma, 19
  lymphoplasmacytic lymphoma, 119
  mantle-cell lymphoma, 64
  peripheral T-cell lymphomas, 31–2
  small lymphocytic lymphomas, 48,
      49
Null cell lymphoma *see* Anaplastic
    large T/null cell lymphoma

Orbit
  Burkitt's lymphoma, 85
  MALT lymphomas, **76–8**
  primary lymphoma, 140
Outcomes, 3
  see also prognosis *under specific
      lymphomas*

Parotid
  MALT lymphoma, **79–80**
  monocytoid lymphoma, 125

Pathologists, 197
Pentostatin, 48
Peripheral T-cell lymphomas, *2*, 29
  adult T-cell leukemia/lymphoma,
      29, 30, 33–5, *35*, **41–3**
  anaplastic large/null cell, 29, 31,
      91–4, *91*, *92*, *93*, **96–8**
  angiocentric T/NK-cell, 29, 30, 31,
      141, **147–9**
  angioimmunoblastic, 29, 30, 32–3,
      39–40
  chronic lymphocytic leukemia, 29,
      45, 49, **56**
  hepatosplenic, 30, 141, **150–2**
  intestinal, 29, 30, 134, *135*, 136,
      143–4
  large granular lymphocytic
      leukemia, 29, 49, **57–9**
  mycosis fungoides, *2*, 29, 137, *138*,
      145
  other lymphomas compared, *198*
  subcutaneous panniculitic, *138*, 139,
      146
  T-cell-rich B-cell lymphoma, 177
  unspecified, 29–32, **37–8**
Plasmacytoma, *138*
Plasmapheresis, 119
POEMS, 179, 180
Prednisone
  angioimmunoblastic T-cell
      lymphoma, 33
  BFM 86 protocol, 86, *86*, **109**, 110
  Burkitt's lymphoma/leukemia, 86,
      86, **87**
  follicular lymphoma, 18
  Hodgkin's disease, 159
  lymphoblastic lymphoma, **109**, 110
  mantle-cell lymphoma, 64
  unspecified peripheral T-cell
      lymphoma, 32
  see also CHOP regimen
Primary effusion lymphoma, 141,
    178–9, **188–9**
Primary extranodal lymphomas *see*
    Extranodal lymphomas
Primary mediastinal large B-cell
    lymphoma, **103–4**
  classification, *2*, 99
  clinical characteristics, 100–1
  definition, 99
  frequency, 99
  genetics, *99*, 100
  histology, 99–100, *99*

  immunophenotypes, *99*, 100
  other lymphomas compared, *99*,
      101, *198*
  prognosis, 100–1, 102
  treatment, 101–2
Procarbazine, Hodgkin's disease, 159
Prognosis, 3, 16
  major lymphomas compared, *198*
  see also specific lymphomas
Prolymphocytic leukemia, 45, 48–9,
    56
ProMACE–CytaBOM, 20
ProMACE–MOPP flexitherapy, 18–19
Pulmonary extranodal lymphomas,
    75–6, 134, *134*
Pyothorax-associated lymphoma, 141,
    179

Radiotherapy
  anaplastic large T/null cell
      lymphoma, 94
  Burkitt's lymphoma/leukemia, 86,
      87
  CLL/small lymphocytic lymphoma,
      48
  extranodal lymphomas, 73, 136,
      137, 139, 140
  follicular lymphoma, 16, 17–19, 20
  Hodgkin's disease, 158–9, 160
  lymphoblastic lymphoma, 110
  MALT lymphomas, 73
  mantle-cell lymphoma, 64
  primary lymphoma of brain, 140
  primary mediastinal large B-cell
      lymphoma, 101–2
RAI clinical staging system, 47, *47*
Rappaport classification, 1
  Burkitt's lymphoma, 83
  lymphoblastic lymphoma, *2*, 105
  small lymphocytic lymphoma, 45
REAL classification, 2, 3
  Burkitt-like lymphoma, *2*, 83
  Burkitt's lymphoma, *2*, 83
  extranodal lymphomas, *2*, 69, 125,
      133, *138*
  follicular lymphoma, *2*, 14
  MALT lymphomas, *2*, 69, 125
  mantle-cell lymphoma, *2*, 61
  nodal marginal-zone B-cell
      (monocytoid) lymphoma, *2*,
      123–4, 125
  peripheral T-cell lymphomas, *2*, 29,
      32, 33, 91

primary mediastinal large B-cell lymphoma, 2, 99
splenic marginal-zone B-cell lymphoma, 2, 124, 125
Reed–Sternberg cell, 153, 154–5, 156, **163–8**, **170**, **173–5**
Richter's syndrome, 46, 48
Rituximab, 19, 64

St Jude staging system, 85, 86
Salivary gland
  nodal marginal-zone B-cell (monocytoid) lymphoma, 125
  primary lymphomas, 134
Sézary syndrome, 2, 49, 137, *138*, **145**
Sinuses, diffuse large B-cell lymphoma, 5, 9, 198
Skin
  anaplastic large T/null cell lymphoma, 92–3
  diffuse large B-cell lymphoma, 5, 9, 137, *138*
  lymphoblastic lymphoma, 108
  primary lymphomas, 133, 134, *134*, 137–9, **145–6**
Skin-associated lymphoid tissue, 139
Small lymphocytic lymphomas
  B-prolymphocytic leukemia, 48–9
  chronic lymphocytic leukemia, 2, 45–8, **51–2**
  hairy cell leukemia, 49, **53–5**, 62, 124
  large granular lymphocytic leukemia, 49, **57–9**
  and mantle-cell lymphoma, 62, *62*
  other lymphomas compared, *198*
  T-chronic lymphocytic leukemia, 45, 49, **56**
  T-prolymphocytic leukemia, 45, 49, **56**
Spleen
  CLL/small lymphocytic lymphoma, 47
  hairy cell leukemia, **53**
  hepatosplenic lymphoma, 141, **150**
  Hodgkin's disease, 156, 158, 159, **167–9**
  lymphomatous polyposis, 136–7
  T-cell-rich B-cell lymphoma, **183**

see also Splenic marginal-zone B-cell lymphoma
Splenic marginal-zone B-cell lymphoma
  classification, *2*, 69, 124, 125
  clinical characteristics, 126
  frequency, 124
  genetics, *123*, 126
  histology, *123*, 126
  immunophenotypes, *123*, 126
  liver, **131**
  peripheral blood, **130**
  periportal lymph node, **130–1**
  prognosis, 126
  spleen, **130**
  treatment, 126
Stanford V regimen, 159
Subcutaneous panniculitic T-cell lymphoma, *138*, 139, **146**
Surgery
  extranodal lymphomas, 73, 136, 140
  Hodgkin's disease, 158, 159
  MALT lymphomas, 73
  primary lymphoma of brain, 140
  splenic marginal-zone B-cell lymphoma, 126
Survival rates, 3
  see also prognosis *under specific lymphomas*

T-cell chronic lymphocytic leukemia, 45, 49, **56**
T-cell lymphoblastic lymphoma, 105, 106, 107–8, **107**, **108**, **111–13**
T-cell lymphomas, 2
  major features compared, *198*
  see also Adult T-cell leukemia/lymphoma (ATL); Anaplastic large T/null cell lymphoma; Peripheral T-cell lymphomas; Sézary syndrome; T-cell lymphoblastic lymphoma; T-cell prolymphocytic leukemia
T-cell prolymphocytic leukemia, 45, 49, **56**
T-cell-rich B-cell lymphoma, 6, *6*, 177–8, **183–6**
Teniposide, follicular lymphoma, 18

Testes
  Burkitt's lymphoma, 85
  diffuse large B-cell lymphoma, 5, 9, 198
  lymphoblastic lymphoma, 108
  primary lymphomas, 134
Thioguanine, BFM 86 protocol, 86, *86*, **109**, 110
Thymus
  lymphoblastic lymphoma, 105, 106, **107**
  primary mediastinal large B-cell lymphoma, 99, 100
Thyroid lymphomas, 134
True histiocytic lymphoma, 177, 180–1, **192–3**

Uganda Cancer Institute staging system, 85, 86

VACOP-B, 20, 101
VACPE regimen, 32
Vinblastine, Hodgkin's disease, 159
Vincristine
  BFM 86 protocol, 86, *86*, **109**, 110
  Burkitt's lymphoma/leukemia, 86, *86*, **87**
  Hodgkin's disease, 159
  mantle-cell lymphoma, 64
  unspecified peripheral T-cell lymphoma, 32
  see also CHOP regimen

Waldenström's macroglobulinemia, 117, 119
Waldeyer's ring, 198
WHO classification
  Burkitt-like lymphoma, 83
  follicular lymphoma, 14, 22
  peripheral T-cell lymphomas, 29, 32
Working Formulation, 1–2
  Burkitt's lymphoma, 83
  lymphoplasmacytic lymphoma, 117
  mantle-cell lymphoma, 61
  nodal marginal-zone B-cell (monocytoid) lymphoma, 124
  peripheral T-cell lymphomas, 29, 32
  primary cutaneous lymphomas, 137
  T-cell-rich B-cell lymphoma, 177